Indirect
Restorations
in Dental Practice

Second Edition

Other CBS Books by the Same Author

- **Dental Caries**
- **Textbook of Operative Dentistry,** fourth edition
- **Pre-Clinical Conservative Dentistry**, second edition
- **Fundamentals of Dental Radiology**, fourth edition
- **Community Dentistry**

Indirect Restorations
in Dental Practice

Second Edition

Vimal K Sikri

MDS, DOOP(PU), DEME(AIU), FICD

Former Professor and Head
Department of Conservative Dentistry and Endodontics
and

Principal
Punjab Government Dental College and Hospital
Amritsar, Punjab
India

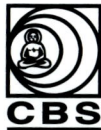

CBS

CBS Publishers & Distributors Pvt Ltd

New Delhi • Bengaluru • Chennai • Kochi • Kolkata • Mumbai
Hyderabad • Nagpur • Patna • Pune • Vijayawada

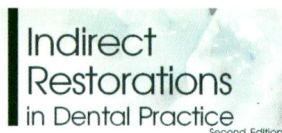

ISBN: 978-93-86217-75-2

Copyright © Author and Publisher

Second Edition 2017
First Edition 2008

Published by Satish Kumar Jain and Produced by Varun Jain for
CBS Publishers & Distributors Pvt Ltd
4819/XI Prahlad Street, 24 Ansari Road, Daryaganj, New Delhi 110 002, India.
Ph: 23289259, 23266861, 23266867   Fax: 011-23243014   Website: www.cbspd.com
e-mail: delhi@cbspd.com; cbspubs@airtelmail.in.
Corporate Office: 204 FIE, Industrial Area, Patparganj, Delhi 110 092, India
Ph: 4934 4934   Fax: 4934 4935   e-mail: publishing@cbspd.com; publicity@cbspd.com

Branches

- **Bengaluru:** Seema House 2975, 17th Cross, K.R. Road,
  Banasankari 2nd Stage, Bengaluru 560 070, Karnataka, India
  Ph: +91-80-26771678/79   Fax: +91-80-26771680   e-mail: bangalore@cbspd.com
- **Chennai:** 7, Subbaraya Street, Shenoy Nagar, Chennai 600 030, Tamil Nadu, India
  Ph: +91-44-26260666, 26208620   Fax: +91-44-42032115   e-mail: chennai@cbspd.com
- **Kochi:** Ashana House, No. 39/1904, AM Thomas Road, Valanjambalam, Ernakulam 682 018, Kochi, Kerala, India
  Ph: +91-484-4059061-65   Fax: +91-484-4059065   e-mail: kochi@cbspd.com
- **Kolkata:** No. 6/B, Ground Floor, Rameswar Shaw Road, Kolkata-700014 (West Bengal), India
  Ph: +91-33-2289-1126, 2289-1127, 2289-1128   e-mail: kolkata@cbspd.com
- **Mumbai:** 83-C, Dr E Moses Road, Worli, Mumbai-400018, Maharashtra, India
  Ph: +91-22-24902340/41   Fax: +91-22-24902342   e-mail: mumbai@cbspd.com

Representatives

- **Hyderabad** 0-9885175004   • **Nagpur** 0-9021734563   • **Patna** 0-9334159340
- **Pune**   0-9623451994   • **Vijayawada** 0-9000660880

Printed at HT Media Ltd., Sector 63, Noida, UP, India

Mother's love is the fuel
that enables a
normal human being
to do the impossible

Dedicated to

My Mother

(1930-2006)

Whose blood in my arteries made it possible

Foreword

We are in the midst of rapidly advancing technical developments in all areas of our profession. It would simply be improper to recommend anything that has not been tested satisfactorily or used in over the years. However, the vast experience of Dr Sikri coupled with his aptitude for writing, must have conceived a nice way of presenting his vision in the form of a book.

The book *Indirect Restorations in Dental Practice* comprehensively deals with clinical and theoretical needs of all types of indirect restorations. The book shows only the inherent ideas and the vision of the author. Author's emphasis on the originality and the language of the subject matter is clearly evident in the book.

I believe that the contents of the book represent a significant contribution to the original thoughts and deserve our attention where we may not comprehend all the details. Modern ideas on occlusion are excellently presented and the subject matter in other chapters is also critically analyzed. It is hoped that the dental students will find an accurate presentation of the subject and get benefited from the same.

I have great faith that in this and subsequent editions, all students, teachers and practitioners will be kept current in the field of restorative dentistry. It is advisable to consider Dr Sikri's book for application in our daily teaching and practice.

With my continued professional respect and gratitude, I wish Dr Sikri to excel in every field, especially in academics.

Ravinder Singh
Vice-Chancellor
Baba Farid University of Health Sciences
Faridkot

Preface to the Second Edition

During initial days in Academia, my professional mentor (Guru) once advised—dear, if you cannot explain the subject in simple words, that means, you have not understood the subject. Keeping his advice alive, I always put my sincere efforts to design the text in a simple and lucid language.

The second edition of this book, *Indirect Restorations in Dental Practice*, is the outcome of tremendous acceptability of the first edition. I am encouraged to revise this book based on valuable suggestions from students, teachers and practitioners. After critical examination of these suggestions and recent development in this field, new chapters and latest case history with simple design have been incorporated. Chapter on *Shade Matching* is worth mentioning, as it is pre-requisite in indirect restorations. *Principles of Tooth Preparation* is also nicely explained. The diagrams and clinical pictures have been updated along with recent advancements in the materials and techniques.

I am thankful to my colleagues, Dr Renu Sroa and Dr Baljit Sidhu for their support. I am also thankful to my students, Dr Shaveta, Dr Meghna, Dr Tejinder, Dr Komal, Dr Jasbir and Dr Neha for reading the manuscript. I am grateful to dear Dr Sumeet Rajpal for his recent photographs on componeers.

Blessings of my parents sitting near to GOD have always inspired and encouraged me for this endeavor. My elder brothers, Mr KK Sikri and Mr RK Sikri have been motivating me since childhood.

Completing this book would not have been possible without contributions from multitude of academicians and eminent teachers including my students and friends. My wife, Dr Poonam Sikri, my sons, Dr Ankit, Dr Arpit and my daughter-in-law, Dr Annupriya, cooperated whole-heartedly during completion of the book.

The book will be very useful to general practitioners and students; based on clinical aspects of indirect restorations, the practitioners and students can perform better in their clinics after reading the book.

Last but not the least, I am thankful to all those who helped me directly or indirectly in compiling the manuscript of the book.

I look forward to your suggestions, comments and criticism for future improvement of the book.

Vimal K Sikri

Preface to the First Edition

The day I conceived the idea of writing a book on 'Indirect Restorations', I had two objectives in my mind. One was to write a book 'that not only reflects the way I teach, but more importantly, conveys the fascination I used to get out of the subject matter. The second was to write a book that students, and practitioners would find useful, rather, 'not to miss' type. I don't know whether I have fully accomplished the objects, but I assure the readers of my sincere efforts in that direction.

One quotation says, 'To write a book, you are to read half the library'. Not debating the version, I would like to add that the heart and soul of the author is reflected in each chapter, every line and each word of the book. The experiences of the author and of the contributors add colour to the text. We do have plenty of books on the same subject. All are not the same. The difference lies in the vision of the author, the style of presentation and above all the language.

The book 'Indirect Restorations' is the outcome of the expanding text and syllabi of Operative Dentistry. Age old definition ' ... which don't involve the full crowns' do not sound proper. Evolution of Esthetic and Cosmetic dentistry, an offshoot of Operative Dentistry, coupled with patients' demand for better restorations, has necessitated the writing of this book.

Operative Dentistry and Prosthetic Dentistry are twins. Certain topics, subjects and chapters are not clearly defined. It is difficult to identify as to which speciality they belong to. The combined experiences of teachers of both the subjects were required; so the book in your hand has a lot of contributions from the subject experts. The originality and the lucid language of the text of the book are worth mentioning. Hopefully, this book satisfies all the requirements.

Before I thank Almighty GOD for igniting my 'thoughts', I would like to place on record, sense of gratitude to my revered teacher, Dr SS Dua for inculcating in me the urge for writing. Blessings of my parents sitting near to GOD have always inspired and encouraged me for this endeavor. My elder brothers, Mr KK Sikri and Mr RK Sikri have been motivating me since childhood.

I am sincerely grateful to all the contributors for their valuable contributions in the form of text and the photographs. I am thankful to Dr Nadig, Professor and Head, Dept of Conservative Dentistry, Oxford Dental College and Hospital, Bangalore along with his students for arranging couple of good photographs.

My thanks are due to my colleagues, Dr Renu, Dr Kusum, Dr Jaganjot, Dr Sangeeta and Dr Baljit along with my dear students, Dr Subha, Dr Ramneek, Dr Ravinder, Dr Gulwinder, Dr Namrata, Dr Payal and Dr lbadat.

Mr GB Singh and Mr Ashwani Mahajan deserve special thanks for their 'ready to help' attitude.

Certain goals are never achieved without the 'push' of your family members. My dear wife, Dr Poonam and my very dear sons Ankit and Arpit, cooperated whole-heartedly during completion of the book.

Last but not the least, I am thankful to all those who have helped me even 'indirectly' for the book 'Indirect Restorations'.

Vimal K Sikri

Contributors

Arpit Sikri
Senior Lecturer
Department of Prosthodontics
Sudha Rustagi Dental College and Hospital
Faridabad (Haryana)
Ph. 9463600555

CL Satish Babu
Former Professor and Head
Department of Prosthodontics
VS Dental College
Bengaluru (Karnataka)
Ph. 9448458424

Geetika Chawla
Research Associate
Guru Ram Das Institute of Dental Sciences
Amritsar (Punjab)
Ph. 7508165900

KH Kidiyoor
Professor and Head
Department of Conservative Dentistry and
Endodontics
PMNM Dental College and Hospital
Bagalkot (Karnataka)
Ph. 9880271017

Nandini Suresh
Professor, Department of Conservative
Dentistry and Endodontics
Meenakshi Ammal Dental College
Chennai (Tamil Nadu)
Ph. 9884292850

Sashirekha G
Professor, Department of Conservative
Dentistry and Endodontics
Shiksha 'O' Anusandhan University
Bhubaneswar (Odisha)
Ph. 9338457955

Sukhjit Kaur
Government Dental College and Hospital
Amritsar (Punjab)
Ph. 7508601789

TV Padmanabhan
Former Professor
Department of Prosthodontics
Saveetha University
Chennai (Tamil Nadu)
Ph. 9381052122

Contents

1

Indirect Restorations: An Introduction

The damaged teeth are to be restored in their form and function so as to achieve conducive stomatognathic environment. The operator may get confronted with situations where direct restorations are not feasible and advisable because of existing conditions of tooth structures and also the related factors. The treatment need is to fabricate restoration fulfilling functional and esthetic requirements keeping in mind the prevailing tooth tissue support and the patient's choice. Many a times, certain conditions warrant preparation of the restoration outside the oral cavity. Such restorations are known as 'Indirect Restorations'. 'Semi-direct' or 'semi-indirect' technique has also been tried. In case of deep proximal box, with cervical area well below the cemento-enamel junction; the cervical one-third is filled directly and the rest is restored with indirect means. Similarly, in deep occlusal cavities, the base is restored with direct restorative material and the rest is restored with indirect techniques (technique is known as semi-direct technique).

The indirect restorations can be extracoronal restorations or intracoronal restorations; both fabricated in dental laboratory by the competent person(s). A combination of intracoronal and extracoronal restoration have also been documented in literature, such as Richmond crown, Davis crown, etc.

Extracoronal restorations: These restorations cover the crown completely or partially. The retention and resistance form is gained from the external walls of the tooth and the overall surface area.

Extracoronal restorations can be fabricated using materials like all metal, metal-ceramic and all-ceramic. These restorations are of following types:

i. *Complete veneer crown:* It restores all the surfaces of the clinical crown.

ii. *Partial veneer crown:* It restores only a portion of the clinical crown. Partial veneer crowns are of following types:

- *Three-quarter crown:* This restores three out of four axial surfaces (facial surface is excluded) of the anterior teeth. In premolars, occlusal surface is also included (nomenclature can be four-fifth crown).

- *Reverse three-quarter crown:* Similar to three-quarter crown except that the lingual surfaces are excluded (preferred in lower molars with severe lingual inclination).

- *Seven-eighth crown:* As the name indicates, seven surfaces out of eight of the clinical crowns are restored (preferably, the facial axial area of the mesio-buccal cusp of the maxillary first

1

molars is excluded for esthetic reasons).

- *One-half crown:* It restores one-half of the clinical crown, may be occlusal and mesial or occlusal and distal. Such restorations are preferred in tilted molars or in mandibular second molars where third molar is erupting or abnormally erupted.
- *Laminates:* The restoration, which restores only the labial surface of the tooth, mostly fabricated with composite resin or ceramics (bonded to etched enamel surfaces).
- *Lumineers:* Thin form of laminates (cerinate porcelain is preferred); bonded to labial enamel.
- *Componeers:* Thin form of pre-fabricated composite laminates bonded to labial enamel.

Intracoronal restorations These are the restorations, which are within the confines of the coronal portion of the tooth. The retention and resistance form is gained from the intimate fit of the restoration with the opposing walls.

Intracoronal restorations can also be fabricated using materials like all metals, metal ceramics and all ceramic/composites. These restorations are of following types:

i. *Inlay:* Literally meaning 'laid inside'; the restoration is placed inside the coronal aspect of the tooth.
ii. *Onlay:* Literally meaning 'laid on'; the restoration, which along with inlay, covers one or more cusps, but not all the cusps. (In case all cusps are covered, the term 'full crown' is preferred.)
iii. *Pin-lay/Pin-ledge* is the modified form of inlay/onlay wherein one/or more pins are attached with the restoration (in one casting).

Combined intracoronal and extracoronal restorations: These restorations are of following types:

i. *Richmond crown:* Richmond crown is a single unit post retained crown. The design includes casting of post-core and crown as single unit over which ceramic is fired. Such a preparation is indicated in teeth where crown height is less and the tooth is root canal treated.

Advantages
- No stress at cervical margins
- Sufficient space for ceramic
- Eliminates cement layer between core and crown

Disadvantages
- Higher modulus of elasticity than dentin (10 times more)
- May act as wedge during occlusal functions
- In case ceramic part fractures, becomes difficult to repair

ii. *Davis crown:* Davis crown is also a single unit post-retained crown. The ceramic facing is attached to the core portion with or without making a hole (tube) in the core. Indications, advantages and disadvantages are same as for Richmond crown.

iii. *Pin retained cast crown:* Such a preparation is indicated in teeth where crown height is less and the tooth is vital. In vital teeth, the post part is prepared in dentin; the crown with attached pin is fabricated in one casting. Depending upon availability of surface, two pins can also be attached with the crown. The crown with pin can be cemented as in routine.

Decision Making in Indirect Restorations

The choice of restorative material and the technique is relatively simple. The factors which influence the choice are size of the lesion, endodontic/periodontic condition, patient's own compliance and performance, aesthetics and also the competence of the operator.

The gold standard of indirect restorative material is 'gold'. Gold, undoubtedly is an excellent material, which needs minimum tooth preparation and provides best marginal adaptation; also being biocompatible. The only drawback of color led to the use of various esthetic (tooth colored) materials.

Earlier, porcelain fused-to-metal (PFM) was the most common indirect restoration. It does provide esthetics of porcelain along with strength of the underlying metal. However, problem of adaptation of base metals underlying porcelain remained a matter of concern for the restorative dentists. Also, PFM inlays/onlays are not suited as far as requirements in cavity preparation are concerned. Indirect composite restorations demonstrated improved physical properties as good as porcelain. However, these also did not get acceptance.

The advent of all-ceramic system has revolutionized the indirect restorative protocol. The initial use of Empress (pressed ceramic) provided sufficient esthetics along with the physical properties required. It is still being used in inlays and onlays. Recently, Zirconia and allied materials have replaced the metal part of the PFM. Lithium disilicates and other related materials have provided promising results. Last but not the least, the CAD/CAM technology have given better precision and decreased costs. The paradigm has widely changed in the use of indirect restorative materials and techniques.

The decision as regard direct or indirect restoration is facilitated by considering different situations, such as:

Situation 1—where lesion is small and can easily be restored with direct restorative materials (Fig. 1.1). The decision of choosing direct restorative material (say amalgam, composite and glass-ionomer cement) depends upon operator's choice and/or patient's preference or in certain conditions needed for the tooth environment (glass-ionomer cement is considered in situations where its cariostatic effect is required).

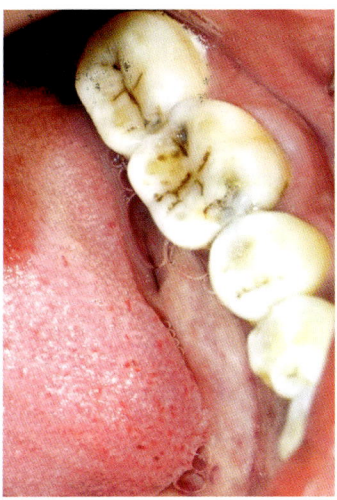

Fig. 1.1: Small carious lesion

Situation 2—where indirect restorations are mandatory; such as large cavities, failed direct restorations, teeth with large proximal area involved, teeth with missing cusps or full crowns and also where occlusal anatomy and contact/contours are to be modified (Figs 1.2 and 1.3). The choice of material (gold, base metal, porcelain fused to metal and all-ceramic) depends upon various factors listed in the beginning.

Situation 3—where decision becomes difficult at times and also certain situations create

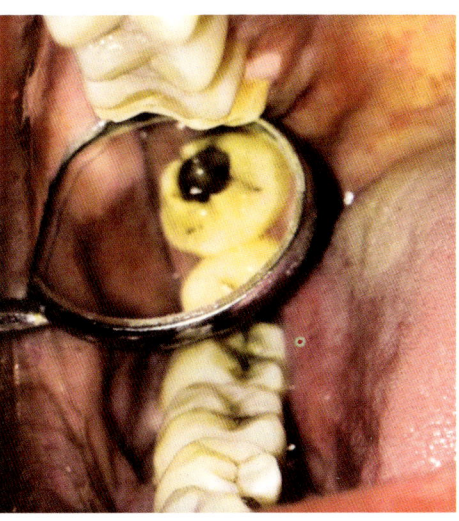

Fig. 1.2: Deep carious lesion

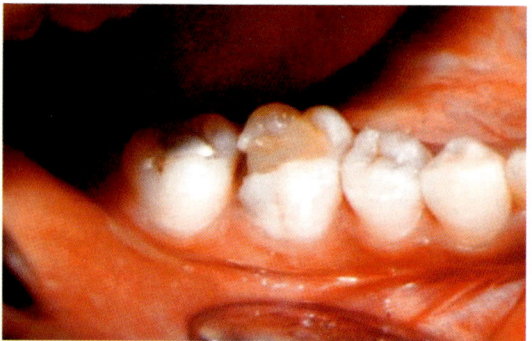

Fig. 1.3: Failed direct restoration

confusion because of lack of documentary evidence. These situations can be:

a. *Cusp replacement:* Many a times, cusp is to be replaced or there may be need to cover the cusp (one or two) of the posterior teeth. Such situation warrants decision making whether to restore directly or indirectly. Most clinicians agree that the lost cusp can be restored directly using pin retained silver or composite. The other school of thought is to fabricate the cusps indirectly so as to achieve better occlusal anatomy and also to minimize the chairside time required for direct restoration. The consensus amongst the clinician is to restore to functional cusp(s) indirectly and non-functional cusp(s) directly. A few authors also advocate replacing one cusp by direct restorations and two or more cusps by indirect restorations (Figs 1.4a and b).

b. *Wide and deep proximal lesions:* As the proximal lesions extend deeper and wider, the success of composite and/or amalgam filling is compromised (Figs 1.5a and b). Composites are considered functional and durable when the margins are situated within the confines of enamel and free from heavy loads. The subgingival area also pose problem along with difficulty in isolating the area. Such situations warrant placement of indirect restorations. A few authors recommend placing glass-ionomer or glass-cermet base at the cervical margins and inlay/onlay over it (semi-direct restorations).

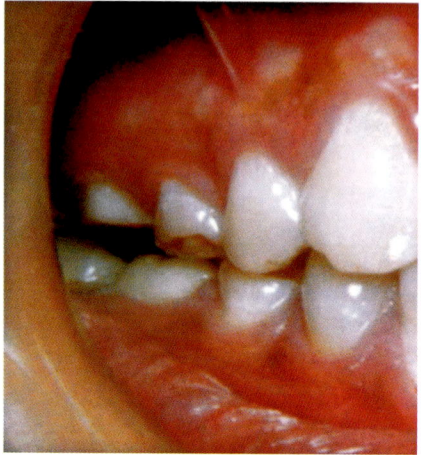

Fig. 1.4a: Fractured cusp

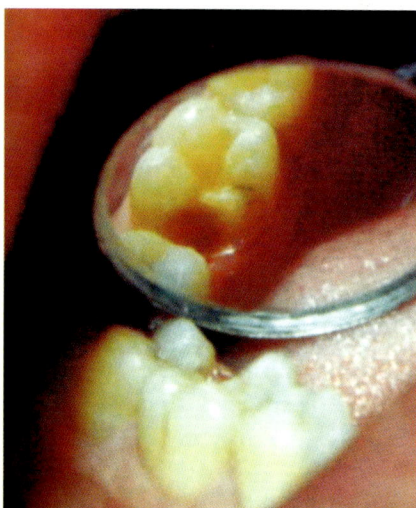

Fig. 1.4b: Fractured cusp

c. *Root canal treated teeth:* Whether root canal treated teeth be restored with full veneer crowns/onlays or with direct restorative material remained a topic of debate amongst the restorative dentists (Fig. 1.6). The root-filled teeth/pulp treated teeth are considered more prone to fracture; might be because of reduced dentin elasticity and the reduced water content. A few authors opined that loss of substantial amount of dentin, especially the dentin over the roof of pulp chamber should be the decisive criteria. The overall loss of tooth structure

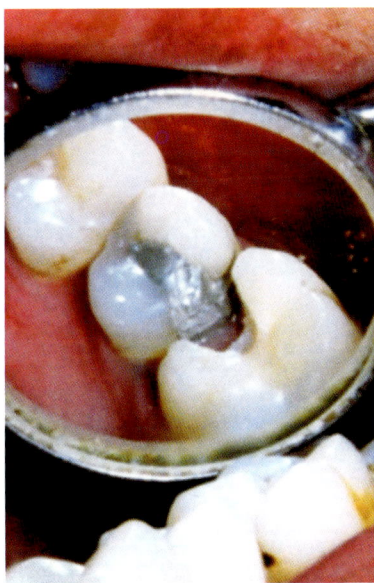

Fig. 1.5a: Wide proximal lesion

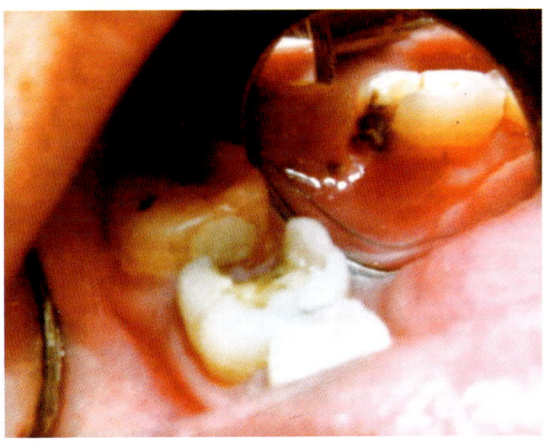

Fig. 1.5b: Wide proximal lesion

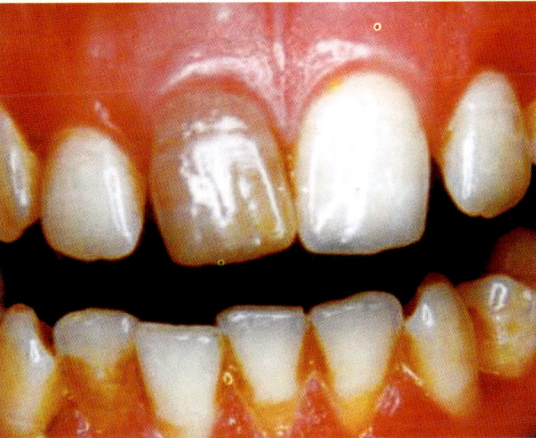

Fig. 1.6: Root canal treated tooth

fracture such teeth, especially in premolars (access cavity in premolars destroy more dentin of cusps than that of molars). Similarly in anterior teeth, the access cavity is preferably filled with direct restorative material. In case of involvement of both proximal surfaces, indirect restorations are preferred.

d. *Discolored teeth:* A variety of etiological factors lead to discoloration of teeth (Figs 1.7a and b), which can be either intrinsic, extrinsic or both. Intrinsic discolorations are more disturbing and are usually treated with bleaching (Figs 1.8a and b) or conservative laminates. Bleaching of non-vital teeth along with composite restoration is considered the preferred

should be the criteria for deciding indirect restorations, rather than change in other physical properties. For example, if there is only occlusal access preparation (other walls intact with one open wall), a direct restoration is preferred. It will preserve the remaining tooth structure and also minimizes the chances of microleakage along the margins. However, authors favouring full coverage indirect restorations opine that the presence of suspicious crack lines, coupled with occlusal load may

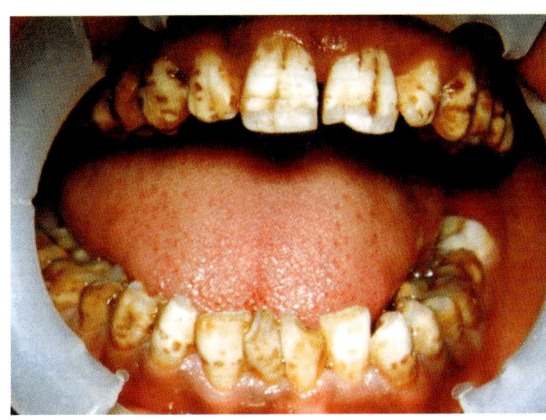

Fig. 1.7a: Discoloured teeth

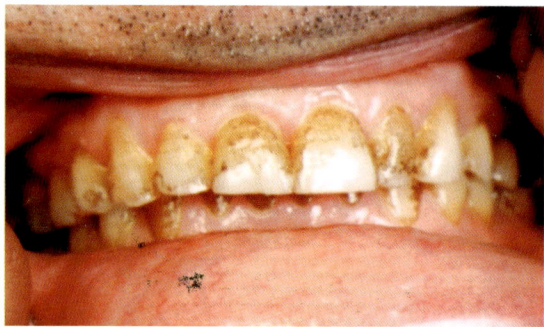

Fig. 1.7b: Discoloured teeth

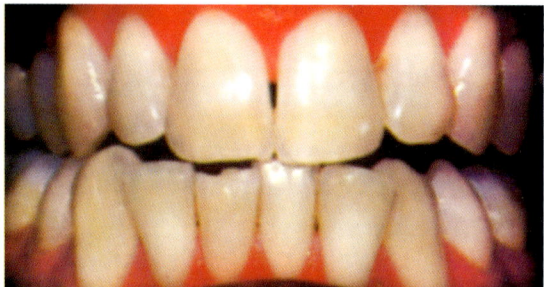

Fig. 1.8a: Preoperative before bleaching

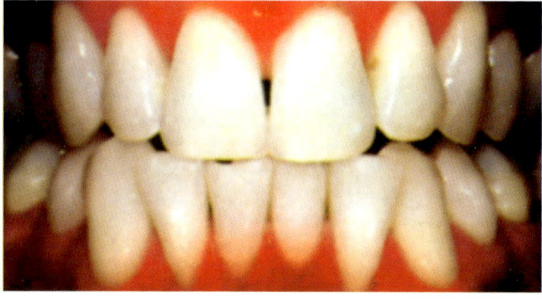

Fig. 1.8b: Postoperative after bleaching

choice of the operator. However, in tetracycline discolored teeth or fluorosed teeth, full veneers are preferred. Laminates, if extending to dentin, may fail because of retention of laminates depending upon dentin bonding rather than enamel bonding. The high elastic modules of porcelain do not match the low elastic modulus dentin; subsequently, transferring and cracking of the porcelain laminate. Long-term tooth whitening and/or direct composites with opaque base is considered effective means of restoring esthetics in

discolored teeth; however, long-term performance is better achieved with full veneer crowns (Laminates limiting to enamel may also be considered). In case the veneer depth is increased (may be because of in-depth discoloration), full veneer crowns are preferred.

Bibliography

1. Avila G, Galindo-Moreno P, Soehren S, Misch CE, Morelli T and Wang H. A novel decision-making process for tooth retention or extraction. J Periodontol: 2009;80:476–91.
2. Bardsley PF. The evolution of tooth wear indices. Clin. Oral Investig 2008; 12:15–9.
3. Becker CM and Kaldahl WB. Current theories of crown contour, margin placement and pontic design. J Prosthet. Dent.:1981;45:268–77.
4. Broadbent JM, Williams KB, Thomson WM and Williams SM. Dental restorations: a risk factor for periodontal attachment loss ? J.Clin. Preriodontol 2006;33:803–10.
5. Christensen GJ. Should resin-based composite dominate restorative dentistry today? J Am Dent. Assoc.: 2010;141:1490–3.
6. Christensen GJ. Indirect restoration use: A changing paradigm. JADA 2012;143:398–400.
7. Delgado AC, Ruiz M, Alare JA and Gonzalez E. Dentinogenesis imperfecta: the importance of early treatment. Quint. Int.: 2008;39:257–63.
8. Esteves H. Classification of extensively damaged teeth to evaluate prognosis. J Can. Dent. Assoc.: 2011;77:1–10.
9. Fills TS, Carey JP, Toogood RW and Major PW. Experimentally determined mechanical properties of, and models for, the periodontal ligament: critical review of current literature. J. Dent. Biomech.:2011; 312980.
10. Holand W, Schweiger M, Watzke R, Peschke A and Kappert H. Ceramics as biomaterials for dental restorations. Expert Rev. Med. Devices: 2008;5:729–45.
11. Kelly JR, Nishimura I and Campbell SD. Ceramics in dentistry: Historical roots and current perspectives. J. Prosthet. Dent.: 1996;75:18–32.
12. Kois JC. The restorative-periodontal interface: biological parameters. Periodontology 2000:1996; 11, 29–38.
13. Lambrechts P, Debels E, Van Landuyt K, Peumans M and Van Meerbeek B. How to

simulate wear? Overview of existing methods. Dent. Mater.: 2006;22:693–701.

14. Liebenberg W. Return to the resin-modified glass-ionomer cement sandwich technique. J. Calif. Dent. Assoc.: 2005;71:743–7.

15. Magne P. Composite resins and bonded porcelain: The postamalgam era? CDA J.: 2006;34: 135–47.

16. Magne P, Paranhos MP and Schlichting LH. Influence of material selection on the risk of inlay fracture during pre-cementation functional occlusal tapping. Dent. Mater.: 2011;27:109–13.

17. Morin D, DeLong R and Douglas WH. Cusp reinforcement by the acid-etch technique. J. Dent. Res.: 1984;63:1075–8.

18. Newsome PRH and Greenwall LH. Management of tetracycline discolored teeth. Aesthetic Dentistry Today: 2008;2:15–20.

19. Padmaja S. Biohazards associated with materials used in prosthodontics. Niger. J.Clin. Pract.: 2013; 16:139–44.

20. Poyser NJ, Briggs PFA and Chana HS. The evaluation of direct composite restorations for the worn mandibular anterior dentition–clinical

performance and patient satisfaction. J. Oral Rehab.: 2007;34:361–76.

21. Rueggeberg FA. From vulcanite to vinyl, a history of resins in restorative dentistry. J. Prosthet. Dent.: 2002;87:364–79.

22. Sherif M and Jocobi R. The ceramic reverse three-quarter crown for anterior teeth: preparation design. J. Prosthet. Dent.: 1989;61:4–6.

23. Smithson J, Newsome P, Reaney D and Owen S. Direct or indirect restorations? Int. Dent.: 2011;1: 70–80.

24. St John KR. Biocompatibility of dental materials. Dent. Clin. North Am.: 2007;51:747–60.

25. Tsitrou E, Northeast SE and Van Noort R. Brittleness index of machinable dental materials and its relation to the marginal chipping factor. J. Dent.: 2007;35:897–902.

26. Watts A and Addy M. Tooth discoloration and staining: a review of the literature. Br. Dent. J.: 2001;190:309–16.

27. Wilson NH. Curricular issues changing from amalgam to tooth-colored materials. J. Dent.: 2004;32:367–9.

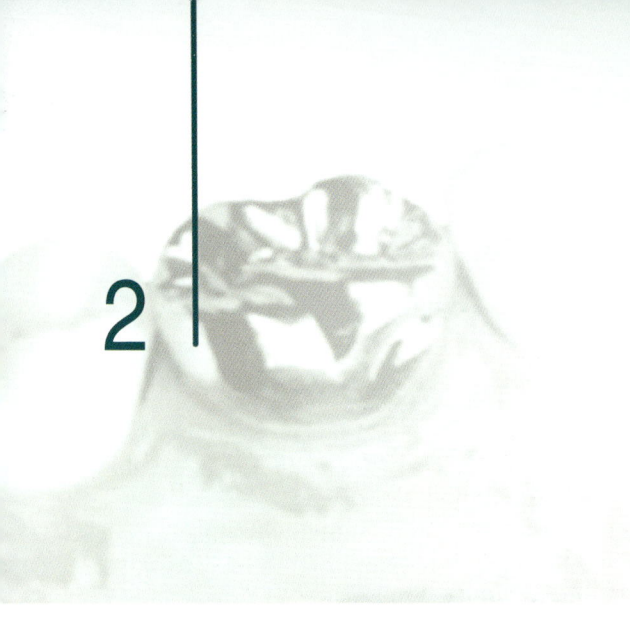

2

Treatment Planning

Sir William Ostler once wrote 'Never treat a stranger'. His statement emphasizes the need for thorough patient history. The operator must acquire complete information of the patient before planning any treatment, especially the restorative one. No set amount of historical information is required for each patient. As the patient and the doctor interact, more information comes to light facilitating the operator to be conscious regarding patient's needs and expectations. Preferably, the doctor should converse with the patient directly rather than the staff.

The relevant information about the patient can be gathered by either getting the questionnaire forms filled or direct interview of the patient. Verbal conversation is always preferred since the patient feels more confident and with the trust does not hide the facts. The operator should be a good listener (Figs 2.1a and b). Once the patient starts interacting and cooperating, the information regarding the systemic diseases, personal/psychological problems, etc. can be gathered.

The guidelines for effective conversation are:

- Start asking simple questions and make the patient feel comfortable.
- Maintain eye to eye contact with the patient; may be standing or sitting.

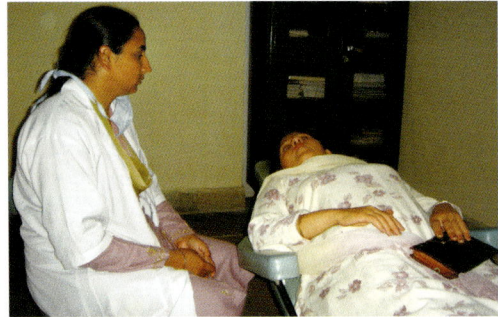

Fig. 2.1a: Eye to eye contact not proper

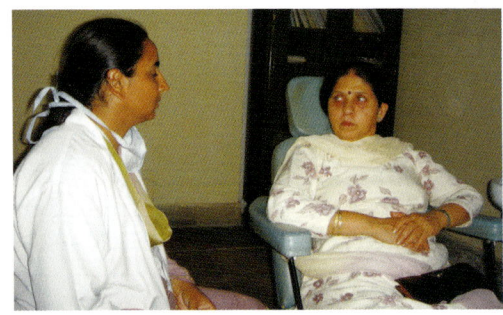

Fig. 2.1b: Eye to eye contact proper

- Be an attentive and active listener. Always listen more and talk less.
- Be objective and unbiased during interaction.
- Summarize findings and confirm the same with the patient before explaining the treatment plan.

The treatment planning precedes the features such as:

1. Recording Personal Information

The patient's name, age, sex, occupation, marital status, telephone numbers, mailing address (e-mail, etc.) and also insurance (if any), should be recorded. This information should be gathered to have fair idea of the social and professional status of the patient (at least, for the last five years).

2. Chief Complaint

Chief complaint(s) should be recorded as described by the patient. Patient's perception of his/her problems and the level of knowledge about treatment is important prior to any treatment planning.

The demand of the patient, i.e. whether he/she seeks treatment for cosmetic purposes or with regards to a functional problem must be carefully assessed as this certainly influences the treatment planning. At times of pain, the patient is to be attended quickly.

Common complaints can be pain, broken tooth, leaking restorations, etc. Control of pain by medication or supportive treatment is to be carried out first.

The acute phase is recognized during the treatment planning and is to be taken care of at the beginning. This is designated as SOAP note, commonly used in medicine and dentistry. (SOAP, acronym taken from the first initial in each of its four components.) The components are:

i. *Subjective (S):* Information regarding chief complaint and is recorded in patients own words.

ii. *Objective (O):* The operator is to generate this component by exploration, visual findings, clinical tests and interpretation of radiographs.

iii. *Assessment (A):* Practically this is tentative diagnosis. Definitive diagnosis can be arrived at gathering more information.

iv. *Plan (P):* This includes acute care plan, which is to be made clear to the patient along with other options, if any.

3. General Health Information

A comprehensive information as regard systemic problems is mandatory.

The operator should review the overall health of the patient. Significant health problems, which may affect dental treatment should be recognized. History of past illness, e.g. cardiac disorders, emotional disorders, trauma, hemorrhagic disorders and diabetes should be thoroughly assessed. Drug allergies, and/or drug reactions at any stage are to be recorded. Patients with AIDS and hepatitis B/C, etc. are potential risks to the dentist; care to be exercised prior to initiation of the treatment.

The following information should also be recorded:

- Patient's general appearance, gait and weight.
- Examine eye and skin color for any signs of anaemia or jaundice.
- Speech and ability to communicate.
- Vital signs such as respiration, pulse, temperature and blood pressure.

Special emphasis is to be given to patients with known history of cardiac problems. 'Long QT syndrome' is a cardiac abnormality encountered commonly by the dentists. These patients should be referred to a cardiologist before initiating any dental treatment. Certain drugs also affect cardiac functioning. The flowchart showing medical history especially cardiac problems is depicted in Flowchart 2.1.

The operator should also be aware of the recently confronted syndrome, known as 'Restless legs syndrome'. Restless leg syndrome is a neurological disorder leading to uncomfortable sensations in the legs especially when the patient is sitting. The visit of these patients should be scheduled for early appointments. The sitting on the dental chair should also be minimized. The patient can be referred for medical help if need be.

Flowchart 2.1: Medical history evaluating cardiac patients

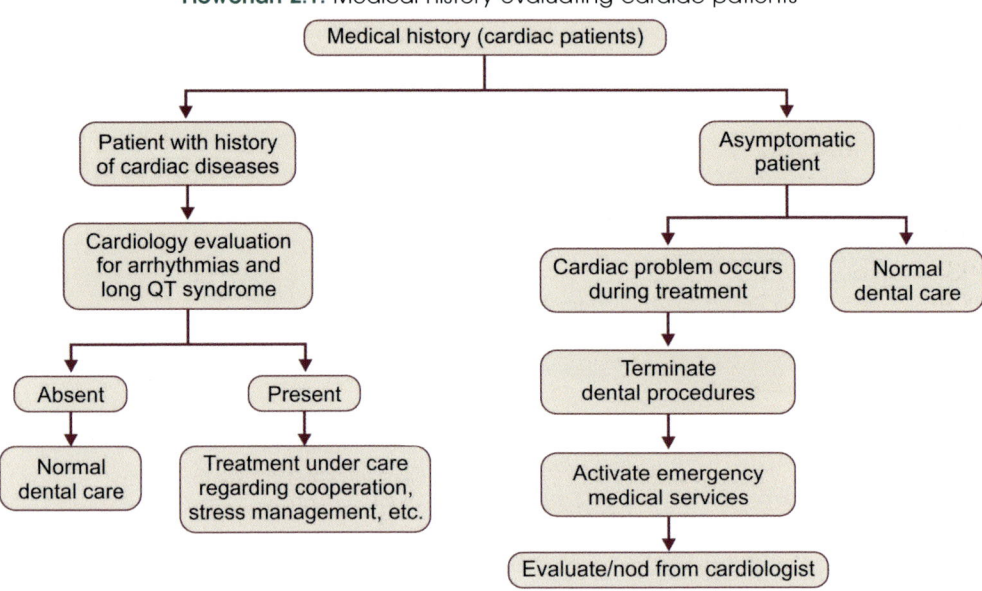

The patient's general health history is thoroughly evaluated and if the patient needs physician help, he/she should be referred for consultation. Old and debilitated patients are to be referred to physicians for advice on medication and avoidance of certain commercial products.

The common systemic diseases, which influence the oral tissues, are given in Table 2.1.

The apprehensive patients, especially the females and the geriatric ones, should be managed according to their stress level. The dentist should be able to provide the environment and also the systemic treatment so as to enable the patient cope up with the stress. Anxiety followed by stress, can lead to physical, mental or emotional events.

For managing stress, following features should be considered:
- Thorough conversation regarding individual stress level.
- Discuss in detail the treatment plan in a friendly environment.
- Appointments should be kept early and short.
- Drugs can be prescribed to have sound sleep prior to appointment.
- Plan for postoperative pain.
- Contact the patient at home, enquire about postoperative well-being.

4. Oral Health Information

The information as regards patient's past dental experiences including prior dental

Table 2.1: Oral findings relevant to common systemic diseases	
Systemic problems	**Oral findings**
Gastric reflux, bulimia, etc.	Erosion of teeth, especially the anterior teeth
AIDS, poor immunity and severely debilitated patients	Yeast and fungal infections
HIV infections	Bluish lesion on the palate
Side effect of medication, Sjögren's syndrome	Reduced salivary flow, caries, difficulty in speech
Cancer chemotherapy; cardiac medication	Gingival hyperplasia

treatment, should be recorded. Abnormal habits such as bruxism, clenching, etc. should be thoroughly evaluated.

The frequency of oral health care can be an important predictor of how effectively the patient will comply with new treatment protocol. The age and the type of previous dental treatment will provide information regarding the patient's awareness towards dentistry and also the financial conditions.

The patient's social, emotional and behavioural attitude affects the treatment planning.

5. Clinical Evaluation

A comprehensive clinical examination is mandatory prior to any treatment planning. The clinical examination includes:

a. Extra-oral evaluation

b. Intra-oral evaluation

   i. General assessment

   ii. Occlusal assessment

   iii. Examination of teeth

   iv. Examination of periodontium

c. Radiographic evaluation

a. Extra-oral Evaluation

The extra-oral evaluation implies examination of the following:

- Size, shape and symmetry of the head and neck.
- Patient profile, i.e. retrognathic, mesognathic or prognathic.
- Temporo-mandibular joint and muscles of mastication for pain or tenderness.
- Lymph node enlargements, especially in the head and neck region.

b. Intra-oral Evaluation

Any abnormality in intra-oral tissues that may influence the treatment planning should be thoroughly evaluated. The evaluation includes the following as these features affect the success of the indirect restorations.

i. General assessment

The oral cavity is assessed for:

- Oral hygiene.
- Caries activity and susceptibility.
- Quality and quantity of saliva.
- Movement of tongue.
- Any abnormal habit, which may predispose to treatment failure.

ii. Occlusal assessment

The pattern of occlusion, mandibular movements and the adjoining musculatures are assessed. The features recorded are:

- The patient's occlusion according to Angle's classification (Fig. 2.2).
- Interceptive occlusal contacts.
- The vertical and horizontal overlap of anterior teeth (Fig. 2.3).
- Any supra-erupted, rotated or mal-aligned teeth (Fig. 2.4).
- Evidence of bruxism, clenching, etc (Fig. 2.5).

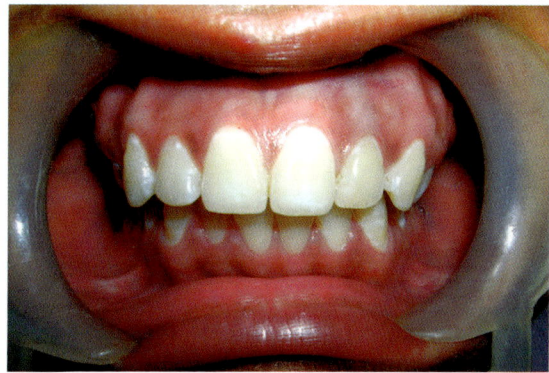

Fig. 2.2: Occlusion

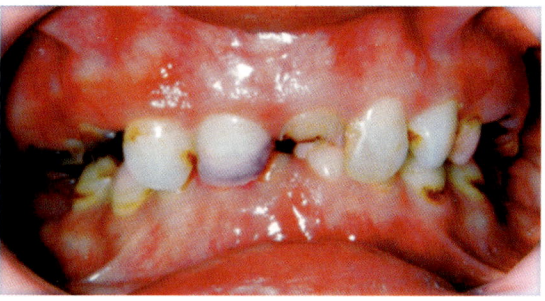

Fig. 2.3: Overlapping anterior teeth

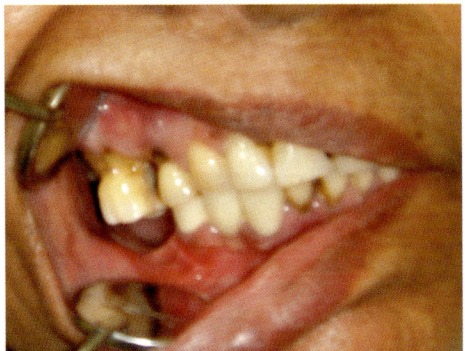

Fig. 2.4: Supra-eruption

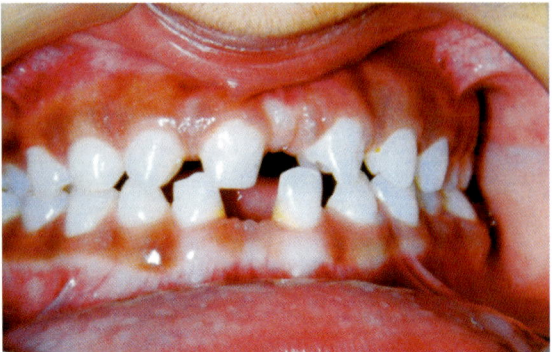

Fig. 2.6: Missing teeth

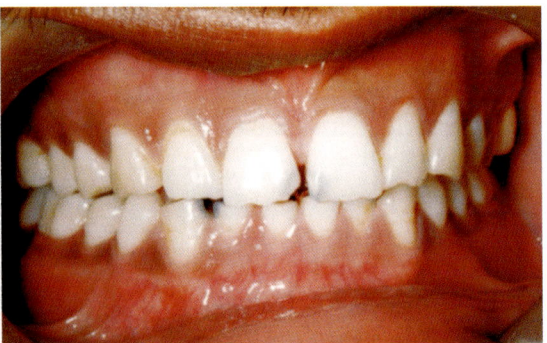

Fig. 2.5: Evidence of bruxism

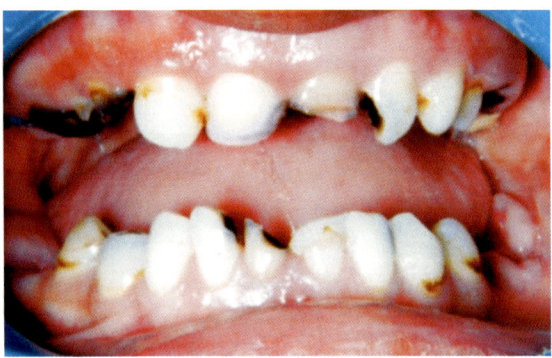

Fig. 2.7: Remaining tooth structure

The diagnostic casts are used for assessing other features such as bone contours, abnormal bony growths (tori, exostosis, etc.) and also the vestibular morphology.

The mounted diagnostic casts help in finalizing the treatment plan. A diagnostic waxing of the proposed indirect restoration on duplicate diagnostic cast provides a preview of the anticipated occlusal scheme.

iii. *Examination of teeth*
The teeth should be thoroughly examined for:
- Missing teeth and the number of remaining teeth (Figs 2.6 and 2.7).
- Presence of caries, decalcifications, erosion, abrasion, attrition and fractures (Figs 2.8 to 2.11).
- Defects including the non-carious defects or recurrent caries in restored teeth.
- Abnormalities in crown configuration, contours and overall alignments (Fig. 2.12).

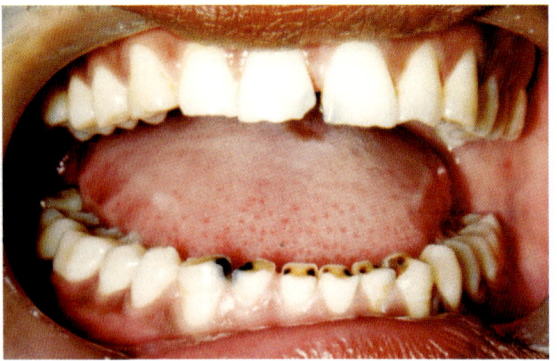

Fig. 2.8: Presence of caries

iv. *Examination of periodontium*
The periodontium is examined for:
- Mobility of teeth/tooth
- Inflammation, may be local or general
- Pocket depths
- Recession
- Anatomy of the margins

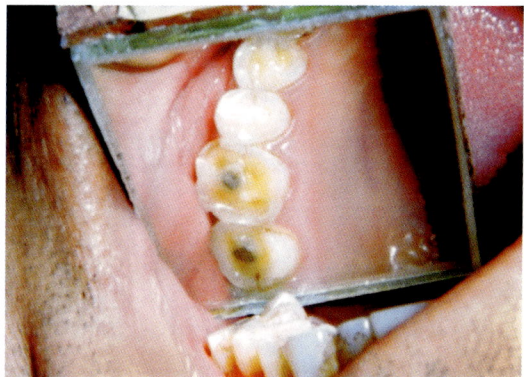

Fig. 2.9: Attrition

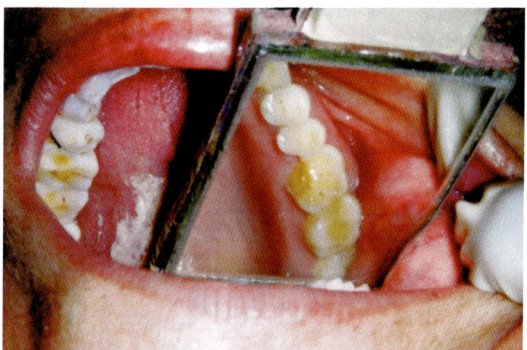

Fig. 2.10: Cusp fracture

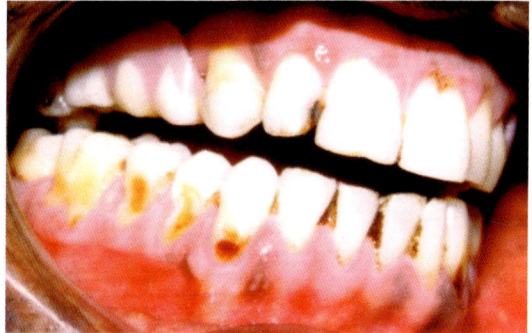

Fig. 2.11: Erosion

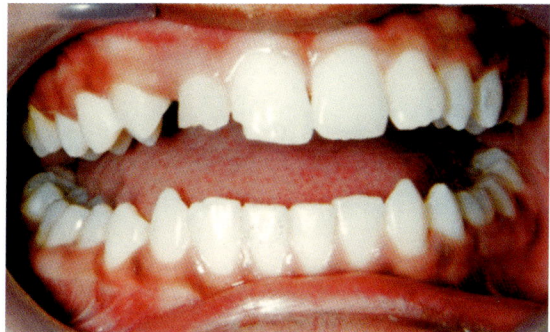

Fig. 2.12: Abnormal crown configuration

are observed at six sites around each tooth. A numerical score between 0 and 4 is recorded for each sextant of the mouth, based on the deepest recorded probing in the sextant.

R	2	1*	2	L	Day	Month	Year
	1	1	2				

Periodontal screening and recording (PSR) system (*added to the score denotes furcation involvement, mobility, muco-gingival problems or recession greater than 3.5 mm)

Periodontal screening and recording serves as a screening tool, assisting the clinicians in deciding whether the patient is to be referred to periodontist for treatment prior to restoration or not.

c. Radiographic Evaluation

Although radiographs are an adjunct and not the sole source of diagnostic information, these are widely used to assess the conditions of oral tissues. Intra-oral periapical and bite wing radiographs are preferred in analyzing conditions such as:

- Presence of periapical pathology (Fig. 2.13)
- Morphology of roots
- Integrity of lamina dura
- Quality and quantity of supporting bone (Fig. 2.14)
- Width of periodontal ligament (Fig. 2.15)
- Areas of furcation involvement
- Root resorption, fractures, etc.
- Evidence of trauma from occlusion

- Previous restorations, if any, impinging upon the periodontium

The periodontal screening and recording (PSR) system is usually used for evaluating the extent of periodontal problem for an individual patient. To perform PSR examination, a special periodontal probe is inserted through the gingival crevice and measurements

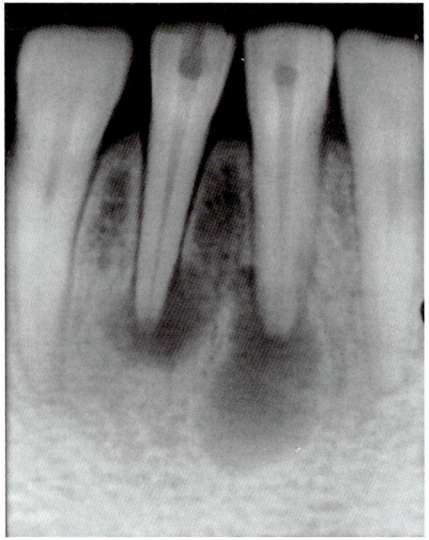

Fig. 2.13: Periapical pathology

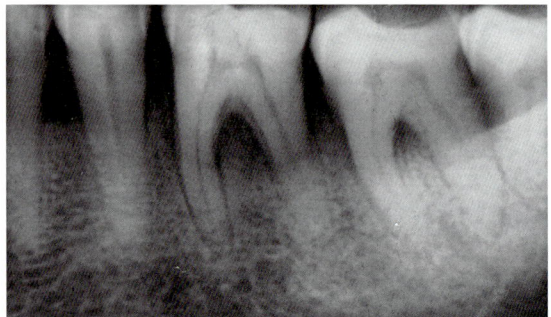

Fig. 2.14: Remaining bone support

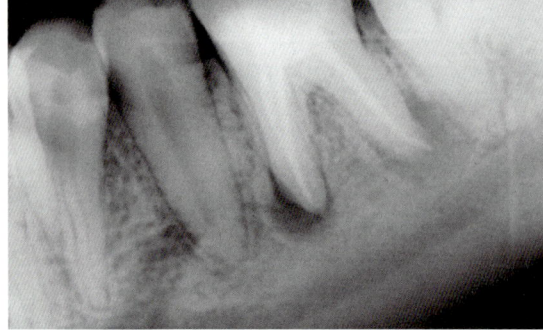

Fig. 2.15: Widened periodontal ligament

- Condition of existing restorations
- Presence of clinically undetectable (hidden) caries (Fig. 2.16)

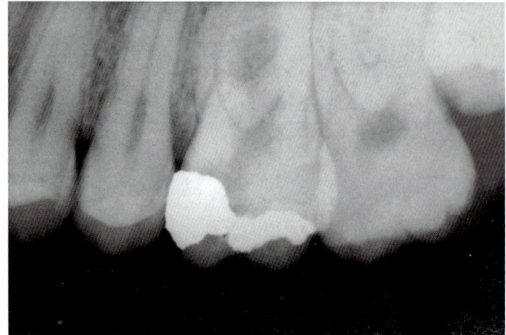

Fig. 2.16: Hidden caries

- Area of bone resorption (Fig. 2.17)
- Retained roots, impacted teeth (Fig. 2.18)

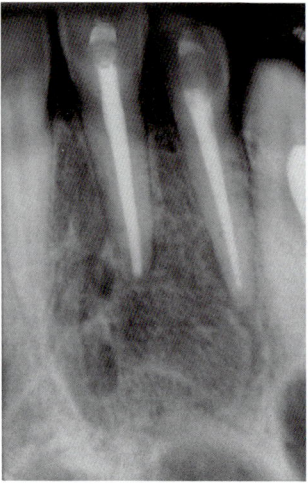

Fig. 2.17: Periapical bone resorption

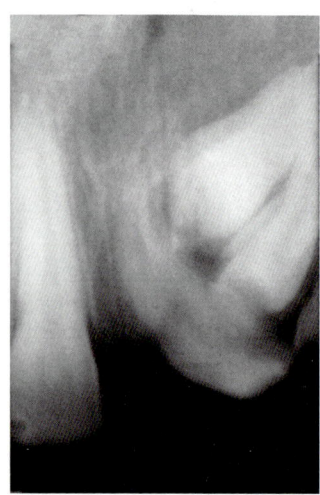

Fig. 2.18: Impacted tooth

After thoroughly reviewing all the recorded information and examining the patient clinically, coupled with findings of laboratory tests and radiographs, etc. a definitive diagnosis is arrived at and subsequently treatment modalities can be logically planned.

TREATMENT PLANNING

Treatment planning involves formulating a logical sequence of treatment to restore the patient's dentition to optimum function and appearance. Earlier, the patients used to comply with the operator for all treatment decisions; however, currently, the treatment planning is becoming a discussion platform where patient is fully involved. The decision pathways, a common planning protocol provide directions in identifying the range of treatment options, indicating some of the key decisions taken earlier; subsequently, leading to an appropriate treatment decision. Decision pathways have been developed to cover a wide range of dental situations and procedures. The limitation of adopting this approach is that they tend to be somewhat cumbersome for routine use, especially for the experienced and busy practitioners. Another approach is 'decision trees', which not only specify key decisions and treatment options, but also include research based success rates for each of these options.

Decision analysis is being applied to several areas including radiographic interpretations. The operator should not show autonomy in assessing, diagnosing and planning for the needs of the individual patient. The consent also includes the current and future risk and the expected outcomes of the whole process.

The process of treatment planning in general is summarized in Flowchart 2.2.

In planning for indirect restorations, the features to be assessed are:

a. Identification of patient needs
b. Periodontal factors
   i. Inflammation
   ii. Crown contour

Flowchart 2.2: Process of treatment planning in general

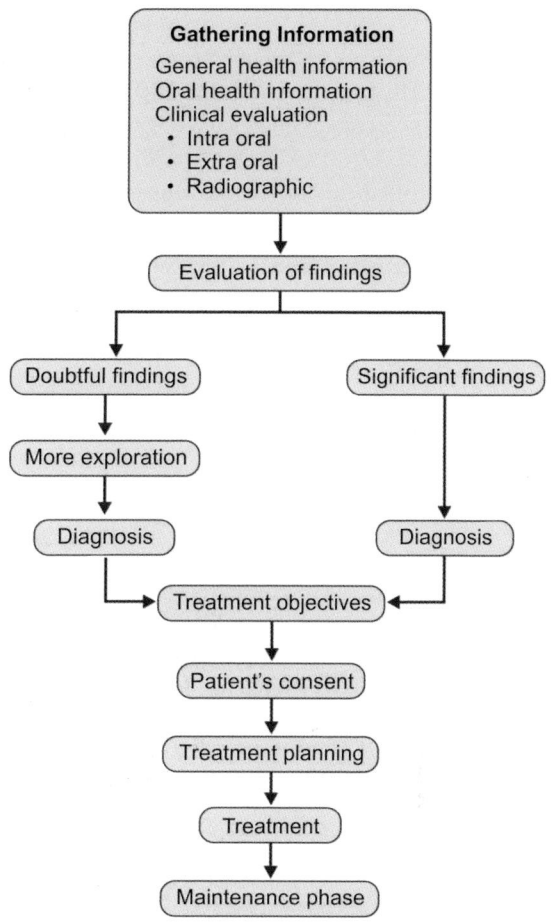

iii. Placement of margins
   iv. Biological width
   v. The pontic design
c. Abutment teeth selection
   i. Bone support and root surface area
   ii. Root shape
   iii. Root angulation
   iv. Periodontal disease
   v. Endodontically treated abutments
   vi. Span length
   vii. Path of insertion
   viii. Pier abutments
   ix. Design of the fixed prosthesis
d. Amount of remaining tooth structure
e. Esthetics

a. Identification of Patient Needs

Successful treatment planning is based on proper identification of the patient's needs, expectations and desires. The treatment option is to be discussed as regard 'need based dentistry', i.e. what is academically required to be carried out on the particular patient and 'want based dentistry', i.e. what is the preference of the patient. The balance is to be maintained between these two modalities. The patient's preferences are to be ignored, especially if they lead to future problems and also many a times, academic treatment options are also compromised. *Time* and *Cost* are two major factors, which govern the balance between need dentistry and want dentistry. In no case, unethical treatment option be adopted to please the patients. Treatment protocol should be finalized keeping in mind the long-term prognosis of the restoration along with the esthetics. The restoration, in no way, should disturb the stomatognathic system.

b. Periodontal Factors

The physiological periodontal climate is to be maintained at all times. The preparation of the tooth surface, placement of margins, anatomical contours and contacts and even the luting cements used, affect the periodontal health. The most important among all is the crown contours and the margins.

i. Inflammation

The inflammation of periodontium must be resolved before commencing the tooth preparations. If surgical intervention is required to restore periodontal health, 6–8 weeks of healing should be allowed before the start of restorative procedures. In case tooth preparation is initiated while the periodontium is inflamed, the final impression must be delayed till the inflammation subsides. The margins vis-à-vis the gingival contours should be evaluated before final impression.

ii. Crown Contour

The crowns are contoured simulating the original tooth anatomy in the oral cavity. Abnormal contouring may lead to gingival/periodontal problems, leading to discomfort and subsequently failure of the restoration. The proper contouring provides:
- Gingival protection
- Oral hygiene accessibility
- Muscle action

Gingival protection: It has been established that the crown contours protect the gingiva from mechanical irritants. Other than protection, the gingival stimulation and the self-cleansing of the area is also to be taken care of. The over-contoured crowns may overprotect the gingival margins but the stimulation aspect will be lacking. Similarly under-contoured crowns may lead to over-stimulation, but the self-cleansing aspect will not be proper. The lack of protection coupled with the over-stimulation pushes the gingivaa apically. Many authors are of the view that cervical constriction of the crown hypothetically protects the gingiva, minimizing the accumulation of microbial plaque. However, gingival stimulation is more important. As and when food is masticated and passes over the gingiva, that leads to increased keratinization and the keratinized epithelium is more resistant to periodontal breakdown. A few authors are of the view that the masticatory mechanism has a little effect on the gingival stimulation. It is believed to be because of the functional movement of the cheeks and tongue. The word 'self-cleansing' is also debatable as crown contours may not exactly provide self-cleansing of the gingival margins.

Oral hygiene accessibility: The over-contoured crowns minimize the access for the oral hygiene measures. The buccal and lingual surfaces are kept flat or under-contoured, which help in proper oral hygiene procedures. Normally, the bucco-cervical bulge should not be more than 0.5 mm than the cemento-enamel junction. The inter-proximal areas or the embrasures should be planned in such a manner so as to facilitate the cleaning process. An over-contoured embrasure reduces the space intended for gingival papilla. This affects oral hygiene. A few authors are of the view that embrasures may lead to lateral food impaction; however, others are of the view that even with open embrasures lateral food impaction does not occur. The effective way is to keep the embrasures open and instruct the patient to use inter-proximal brushes so as to avoid any periodontal problem at the inter-proximal areas. The contact areas should be placed as far occlusally as possible and preferably buccally. These provide easy cleaning of gingival areas beneath the contact area. In case of furcation, the crowns are extended up to the periodontally exposed roots leaving the furcation triangle so as to overcome the problem of cleaning in such areas. This type of 'fluting' is indicated in mandibular/maxillary molars with furcation involvements.

Muscle action: It is desirable that the crown contours should allow both gingival protection and muscular action. Action of the muscles during various functional movements should be assessed.

iii. *Placement of Margins*

The margins of the crowns are placed supragingival, subgingival or equi-gingival (touching at the crest) depending upon the clinical requirement. In no circumstances, the margins should impinge upon the biological width area. The supragingival margins are definitely preferred than the subgingival margins as far as periodontal health is concerned. Placement of margins (1.0–1.5 mm) away from the gingival crest is preferred for healthy periodontium. Plaque accumulation, inflammation and other related problems are associated with subgingival crown margins.

The subgingival margins are, however, indicated in following conditions:
- Esthetic needs
- To gain crown length (surface area)
- To cover subgingival restoration
- To achieve favourable crown contour

In case, the margins are to be extended subgingivally, care should be taken to keep the margins supragingivally first and slowly extend the same subgingivally, using end-cutting burs. This will minimize gingival damage during preparation of the crowns. The cement excess should also be removed with care in case the margins are placed subgingivally.

iv. *Biological Width*

The area of dento-gingival attachment is referred to as 'biological width' and has significant implications in treatment planning. When even an intra-crevicular margin is indicated, it should terminate at least 2.0 mm above the alveolar crest. Severing off the 'biological width' area produces chronic inflammation, pocket formation and osseous defects. The impinging of biological width area is to be avoided by all means.

v. *The Pontic Design*

The pontic (free area in a bridge) should be designed in such a way that it should not interfere with the cleansing mechanism. The embrasure between pontic and abutment is designed in such a manner so as to facilitate the cleansing. The embrasure space between two adjacent pontics usually is closed to provide added strength, reduce plaque retention and facilitate oral hygiene procedures. The pontic should be designed in such a way so as not to cause any adverse effect on the underlying mucosa. For example, increased inflammation of mucosa may occur with ridge lap pontic design as compared to a modified ridge lap or sanitary pontic. However, sanitary pontics are not preferred for replacing missing anterior teeth.

c. Abutment Teeth Selection

The selection of abutments for fixed prosthesis (bridge) is influenced by the following factors:

i. Bone Support and Root Surface Area

This is assessed according to 'Ante's law', which states that the abutment teeth should have a combined pericemental area equal to or greater than the tooth/teeth to be replaced. A ratio of 1:1 or greater will satisfy 'Ante's law'. However, the divergent oral conditions may influence abutment tooth selection, requiring modification of Ante's law (Table 2.2).

ii. Root Shape

Single rooted teeth with elliptical cross-section offer better support than a tooth with circular cross-section. A molar with divergent roots will provide better support as compared to conical roots.

iii. Root Angulation

The teeth with aligned roots will provide better support than the tilted one. The tilted roots would be subjected to abnormal occlusal forces; subsequently, early periodontal breakdown.

iv. Periodontal Disease

Healthy periodontium is a prerequisite for all indirect restorations. The root surface area is exposed as a sequelae of periodontal disease. When one-third of the root length is exposed, half the supporting area is lost. In addition, the forces applied are magnified because of the greater leverage due to longer clinical crowns.

v. Endodontically Treated Abutment

The endodontically treated teeth serve as an excellent abutment. If apicoectomy is indicated, care should be taken not to shorten the root excessively as this reduces the bone support. In case of excessive shortening of root, additional abutment involvement should be planned so as to distribute the forces equally.

vi. Span Length

Excessive flexing under occlusal loads may cause failure of long span fixed prosthesis. The deflexion is proportional to the cube of span length, i.e. when the span length is doubled, deflexion is eight times greater. When a long span fixed prosthesis is mandatory, connectors and retainers should be made bulky to ensure optimum rigidity. The excessive span can be managed by placing implants, if need be. Generally replacing more than three molars, especially in mandibular area prevents poor prognosis.

Table 2.2: Abutment teeth selection	
Existing condition	**Preferred number of abutments**
• Bone loss (periodontally affected teeth)	• Increase the number of abutments
• Mesial/distal tipping of teeth	• Increase the number of abutments
• Bodily movement (migration) of teeth decreasing mesio-distal length of edentulous area	• Decrease the number of abutments
• Unfavourable relation of opposing teeth causing increased load	• Increase the number of abutments
• Endodontically restored teeth especially with root resection	• Increase the number of abutments
• Arch form causing increased leverage	• Increase the number of abutments
• Tooth mobility even after surgery	• Increase the number of abutments

vii. *Path of Insertion*

Abutment teeth must have a common path of insertion. If the long axes of teeth diverge or converge from the line of parallelism by more than 25°, preparations on teeth become more cumbersome. Such a situation may be encountered in case of mesio-lingually tilted mandibular second molar. This would require a tooth preparation for proximal half crown rather than the customary full coverage metal preparation.

viii. *Pier Abutment*

A pier (intermediate) abutment is one with edentulous areas on both mesial and distal sides. It has the potential to produce unfavourable leverage and unseating effect on the terminal retainers. A non-rigid connector with the female portion being placed on the distal side of the intermediate abutment is preferred.

ix. *Design of the Fixed Prosthesis*

- *Replacement of single tooth:* The replacement of a single tooth can usually be carried out with a three unit fixed prosthesis with one mesial and one distal abutment. However, in case of replacing the canine, both lateral and central incisors of the side are used as abutments to prevent lateral drift of the prosthesis.
- *Cantilever prosthesis:* The pontic when attached to a single retainer on an abutment is referred as being cantilevered, e.g. lateral incisor may be cantilevered to the canine. The cantilever designs should be avoided as they introduce lateral stresses; subsequently leading to drifting or tipping of the abutment teeth.
- *Replacement of several missing teeth:* Replacing multiple missing teeth with fixed prosthesis is generally difficult.

When four mandibular incisors are missing, they can be replaced by a fixed prosthesis with retainers on each canine. One remaining incisor is preferably removed since it may complicate the fabrication of the fixed prosthesis. Mandibular incisors, because of their small size, generally make poor abutments.

When the four maxillary incisors are missing, the canines and first premolars are used as abutments. This is because unlike their mandibular counterparts, the maxillary incisors are not positioned in a straight line but in a curve, and forces directed on the pontics will tend to tip the abutment teeth.

If three or more posterior teeth (maxillary or mandibular) are missing, the removable partial denture is preferred.

d. Amount of Remaining Tooth Structure

The amount of remaining tooth structure before and after tooth preparation is important for the long-term success/failure of the restoration (Fig. 2.19). The remaining tooth structure also help in decision making as regard type of indirect restoration, preferred material and the probable technique to be employed. The methods commonly used are:

  i. *Laser profilometer:* The remaining dentin volume can be calculated either by scanning the cast using a laser profilometer or weighing the remaining die stone and calculating the equivalent dentin volume.

 ii. *Tooth restorability index:* A tooth restorability index (TRI) was developed to

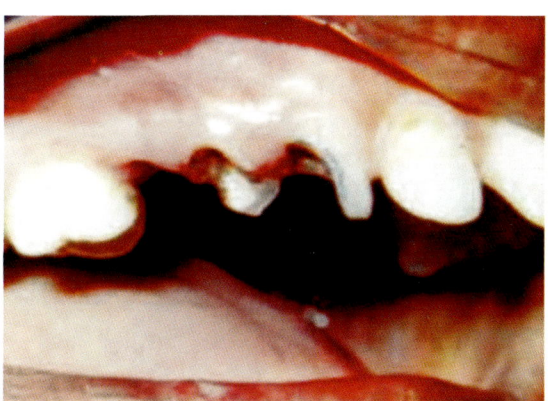

Fig. 2.19: Amount of remaining tooth structure

provide a structured assessment using defined parameters to evaluate remaining coronal tissue (Fig. 2.20).

- Two or even more operators should evaluate the remaining dentin (may be directly or on casts).
- The tooth is divided into six equal sextants: 2 proximal, 2 buccal and 2 lingual areas.
- The scores of 0-3 is assigned to each tooth sextant (maximum score being 18 per tooth).

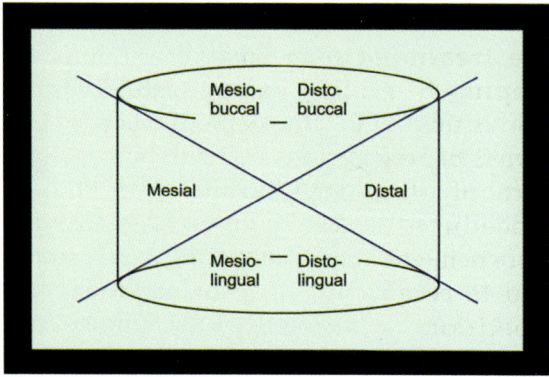

Fig. 2.20: Diagrammatic representation of TRI

Score 0–3 is assigned as follows:

'0'—None: Throughout two-thirds or more of the tooth sextant under consideration, there is no axial wall of dentin (i.e. a box or missing cusp) or any dentin present above the finishing line is so lacking in height that it may not be able to contribute to retention and resistance form. The score is appropriate where a margin is visible just apical to the limit of a missing wall but there is only a small bevel or chamfer comprising the preparation dentin.

'1'—Inadequate: Although coronal dentin is present in the tooth sextant but in terms of thickness, height or configuration (for example, an undercut) that is insufficient to make any predictable contribution to retention and resistance form as opined by the operator. Dentin walls are less than 1.5 mm thick or more than twice as high as their thinnest part would be included in this category.

'2'—Questionable: More dentin is present than in '1', but clinically it will not make predictable contribution to retention and resistance. This score should only be assigned where the operator finds it difficult to determine whether a score of '1' or '3' is more appropriate.

'3'—Adequate: There is sufficient coronal dentin in terms of height and thickness and the operator is confident that the distribution for the forces would provide resistance and retention form to the final restoration.

The possible TRI score and the clinical decisions thereof are depicted in Table 2.3.

e. Esthetics

The esthetics in indirect restorations, especially crowns and also the bridges is compromised in certain conditions such as:

- Drifting of teeth into available pontic space
- Diastemas resulting in excessive mesio-distal width for pontic
- The high lip line that defines finish lines, especially in maxillary anterior crowns
- Longer clinical crowns resulting from surgical periodontics and/or recession pose difficulty in achieving esthetics

Bonded laminates can be a conservative alternative to full crowns and restore tooth esthetics without excessively compromising the tooth structure. The indications and the clinical limitations are discussed in Chapter 9.

Table 2.3: Tooth restorability index (TRI)	
Tooth structure remaining	**Clinical decision**
TRI score >12	Acceptable
TRI score 9–12	Questionable (In 3 or less sextants score three, can be acceptable)
TRI score <9	Unacceptable (consider crown lengthening and post and core)

Sequencing of Treatment Plan

The treatment plan must be sequenced keeping in mind the ongoing treatment modalities. The treatment sequence must always be well planned, since it is an integral part of the comprehensive treatment procedure for each patient. Improper sequencing can be most unfortunate and may lead to compromised efforts, unnecessary repetitions and finally poor restoration. Therefore, a rational sequence of treatment is indicated for symptomatic relief, stabilization, definitive therapy and finally follow-up care. The sequence may need to be modified during the course of treatment keeping in view the altered objectives for the betterment of the patient. In case, the planning is required for complex needs, the treatment plan is divided into phases. The guidelines for sequencing dental treatment are elaborated in Table 2.4.

The keys to decision-making as regard the single tooth restoration is elaborated in Table 2.4.

Once the treatment plan is complete and organized in consultation with patient, the same is conveyed to the patient and the relatives around. Usually, the patient has gained confidence by the time treatment is planned and it becomes comparative easier for the operator to explain. The guidelines are:

- Maintain eye to eye contact with the patient, whether in upright or sitting position.
- Use simple terminology; avoid anxiety-producing terms.
- Straight talk to the patients and do not preach; maintain positive body language.
- Do not discuss minute details and the minor possibilities
- Models, wax up casts should be used to make the patient understand the plan.
- Finally, confirm the patient has understood the treatment plan.

Table 2.4: Keys to decision making in single tooth restoration		
Condition	*Treatment options*	*Recommendations*
Deep caries in posterior teeth	• Amalgam/composite/sandwich • Indirect restoration (inlay/onlay)	• Recommended for small lesions depending upon tooth condition and choice of the patient • Indicated where the remaining tooth structure is not sufficient to retain direct restoration.
Caries in anterior teeth involving one proximal surface	• Composite/glass-ionomer restoration	• Preferred because of esthetics/anticaries effect
Caries in anterior teeth involving both the proximal surfaces	• Composite • Full crowns	• Can be preferred in case the lesion is small • Recommended, provides better esthetics
Cusp(s) fracture or undermining cusp(s)	• Pin retained amalgam • Pin retained composite • Full crowns	• Provides functional protection (esthetic if not priority) • Recommended, if esthetic is priority. • Provides durable and fracture resistant restoration.
Cervical lesions	• Composite/glass-ionomer • Amalgam restoration	• Recommended, when esthetics is important and margins are not subgingival (GIC for anticaries effect) • Preferred in inaccessible areas/areas where deep subgingival margins create difficulty in isolation.

Bibliography

1. Ahmed MF and Elseed AI. The medical management and dental implications of long QT syndrome. Dent. Update: 2005;32:472–4.

2. Al-Quran EA, Al-Ghalayini RE and Al-Zubi BN. Single tooth replacement: factors affecting different prosthetic treatment modalities. BMC Oral Health: 2011;21:34.

3. Anusavice KJ. Decision analysis in restorative dentistry. J. Dent. Educ.: 1992;56:812–22.

4. Bandlish RB, McDonald AV and Setchell DJ. Assessment of the amount of remaining coronal dentine in root-treated teeth. Journal of Dentistry: 2006;34:699–708.

5. Bateman G and Tomson P. Trends in indirect dentistry: Case Selection. Dent. Update: 2005;32: 190–2.

6. Borghi N. To silanate or not to silanate: Making a clinical decision. Compend. Contin. Educ. Dent.: 2000;21:659–62.

7. Cortellini D, Valenti M and Canale A. The metal-free approach to restorative treatment planning. Clin. Appl.: 2006;1:128–45.

8. Fernandes AS and Dessai GS. Factors affecting the fracture resistance of post-core reconstructed teeth: a review. Int. J. of Prosth.: 2001;14:355–63.

9. Grossman Y and Sadan A. The prosthetic concept of crown-to-root ratio: A review of the literature. JPD 2005;93:559–62.

10. Heintze SD, Cavalleri A, Forjanic M, Zellweger G and Rousson V. Wear of ceramic and antagonist— a systematic evaluation of influencing factors in vitro. Dent. Mater.: 2008;24:433–49.

11. McDonald AV and Setchell DJ. Developing a tooth restorability index. Dent. Update: 2005;32: 343–4.

12. Raigrodski AJ. Contemporary all-ceramic fixed partial dentures: A review. Dent. Clin. North Am.:2004;48:531–44.

13. Sairon I, Saucier CL, Rues S and Sadan A. The pier abutment: A review of the literature and a suggested mathematical model. Quint. Int.: 2006;37:345–52.

14. Seow LL, Toh CG and Wilson NHF. Remaining tooth structure associated with various preparation designs for the endodontically treated maxillary second premolar. Eur. J. Prosth. Rest. Dent.: 2005;13:57–64.

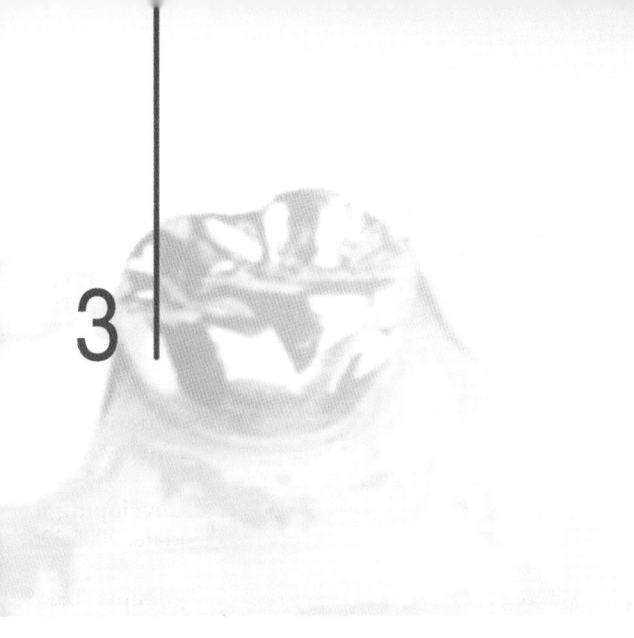

3

Functional Occlusion

The basic need in restorative dentistry is to restore the form and function of the tooth and the arch. The form and functions are restored so as to provide conducive environment to the stomatognathic system. Contact between the opposing teeth is one of the functions of the masticatory system, which stabilizes mandible and maxilla during mastication and swallowing. The term 'occlusion' in simple words means the contact between upper and lower teeth. The static contact is the occlusion and the dynamic contact during function is referred to as 'articulation'.

An ideal occlusion is defined as 'the most dynamic position, arrangement and relationship of one tooth with another tooth, one arch with another arch and both the arches with base of the skull so as to optimally perform the functions of mastication, swallowing and contribution for phonetics, esthetics and help in maintaining the integrity and longevity of the individual teeth and the stomatognathic system'.

The restorative dentists should follow, physiologic/functional occlusion. Physiologic occlusion is the one whereby teeth when in contact are in harmony with each other and create no damaging effect to the underlying periodontium. The occluded teeth function normally and efficiently without causing any pain or discomfort to the individual and also helps in maintaining the periodontium in a healthy state. The characteristics of functional occlusion are:

- In centric relation, the condyles articulate with the thinnest avascular portion of their respective discs with the complex in the antero-superior portion against the slopes of the articular eminences.
- The maxillo-mandibular relations should have correct vertical dimensions. There should be an acceptable intra-occlusal clearance between the vertical dimensions at rest and vertical dimension during occlusion.
- The contact between the opposing cusps should be such that there should be even and axial distribution of occlusal forces.
- The initial contact in centric relation should be bilateral. When there is an anterior slide between CR and CO, it should be within the limits, preferably less than 1.0 mm.
- No premature contact should be present in any of the mandibular movements.
- During lateral excursion, on the working side, there should be either canine guidance or group function with no contacts on non-working side.
- During protrusion, posterior teeth should be in disclusion (no posterior contacts).

- During maximal intercuspal position (MIP) there should be axial loading of occlusal forces.
- Forces of occlusal contact should be distributed over as many teeth as possible in maximal intercuspal position.
- Bilateral contacts should be present between posterior teeth in maximal intercuspal position.

Let us have a clear concept of basics in occlusion and its terminology.

Centric Occlusion

The occlusion of opposing teeth when the mandible is in centric relation (Fig. 3.1).

Maximal Intercuspal Position

It is the complete intercuspation of the opposing teeth independent of condylar position, sometimes referred to as the best fit of the teeth regardless of the condylar position, also called maximal intercuspation (Fig. 3.2). This may or may not coincide with the maximal intercuspal position (MIP).

Normally in MIP, the palatal cusps of maxillary molars contact the central fossae or the marginal ridges of mandibular molars. These cusps are known as 'supporting cusps'. The cusps that do not contact the opposing fossae and ridges in MIP are called 'non- supporting cusps' or shearing cusps. In centric occlusion, the maxillary teeth overlap mandibular teeth.

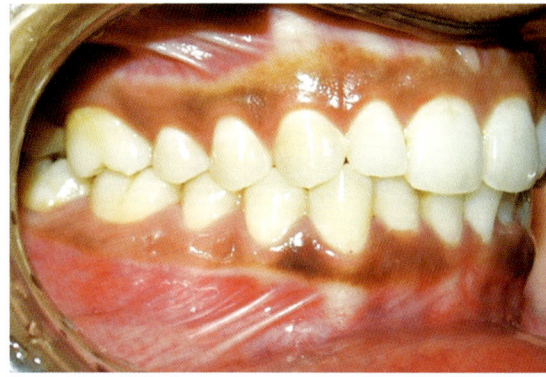
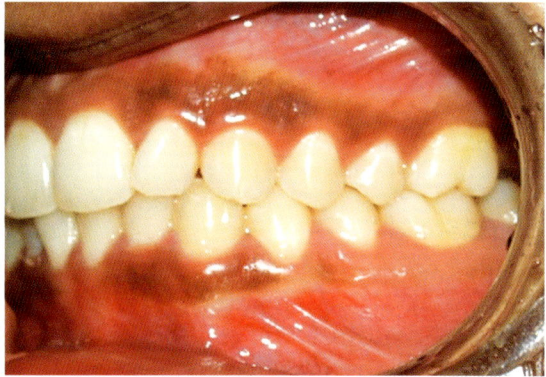

Fig. 3.2: Maximal intercuspal position

The horizontal overlap of maxillary incisors to mandibular incisors is called 'overjet' and the vertical overlap of maxillary incisors is known as 'overbite'.

Centric Relation

The maxillomandibular relationship in which the condyles articulate with the thinnest avascular portion of their respective disks with the complex in the anterior-superior position against the shapes of the articular eminences. This position is independent of tooth contact (Fig. 3.3).

The mandibular condyles rotate around a horizontal axis termed 'hinge axis'. When the hinge axis is in the terminal position, it coincides with centric relation. In centric relation, the condyles rotate around a terminal hinge axis and the lower incisors rotate around an arc, which ranges between 20 and 25 mm.

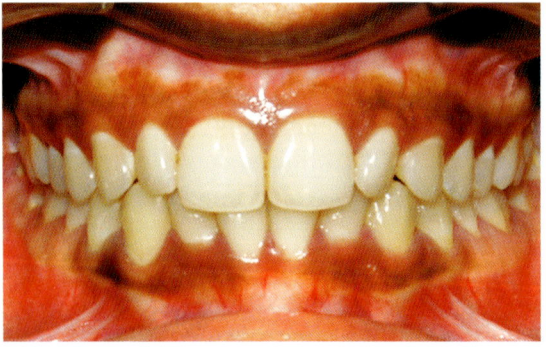

Fig. 3.1: Centric occlusion

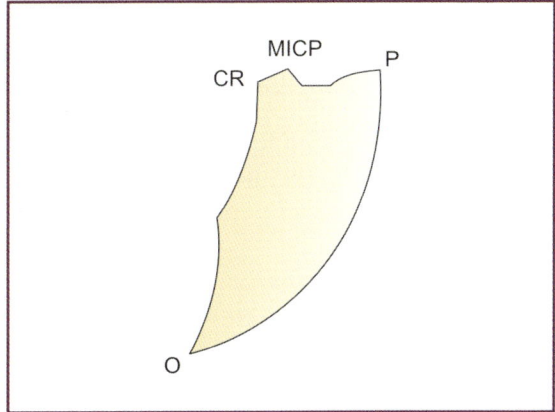

Fig. 3.3: Centric relation and maximum intercuspal position as viewed from lateral border movements. MICP: Maximum intercuspal position; CR: Centric relation; P: Protrusive; O: Opening of mandible

Long Centric Occlusion

It is the range of tooth contact in MIP. This movement occurs without any occlusal interferences. This slide, varies from individual to individual, is rarely more than 1.0 mm. In case, where centric relation coincides with the centric occlusion, there is no slide of the mandible.

In 90% of the population, CO and CR are not coincident as CO is, on an average, 1.0 mm anterior to CR. In 10% of the cases, ICP and RCP are coincident, especially in patients who have undergone therapeutic reorganization of their dentition. This is termed 'point centric' and involve restoration of teeth to inter-digitate in CR. The term 'long centric' relates to the ability to close the mandible into CR or slightly anterior to it.

Factors of Occlusion

The factors which control the movement of mandible are:
- Incisal guidance
- Condylar guidance
- Curve of Spee
- Curve of Wilson and Curve of Monson
- Bennett movement or Bennett shift
- Intercondylar distance

Incisal Guidance

The path followed by the incisal edges of mandibular teeth as it glides over the palatal surfaces of maxillary teeth is called incisal guidance (Fig. 3.4). When the incisors are in class I position, protrusive movement is guided by the tips of the lower mandibular incisors gliding down the palatal surfaces of the maxillary incisors. The incisal guidance depends on the overjet and overbite. The protrusive incisal guidance varies with different incisor relations. When the incisors are in class I relation, protrusion from centric occlusion is guided by the movement of the incisal edges of mandibular incisors against the palatal surface of the maxillary incisors and the posterior teeth become disoccluded. When the incisors are in class II division II relations, the angulations of teeth create very steep incisal guidance. Disclusion of the posterior teeth is quick. When the incisors are in class III relation, and there is anterior crossbite, there is no incisal guidance and the protrusive movement is guided by the contacting inclines of posterior teeth.

Condylar Guidance

Mandibular guidance generated by the condyle and articular disc traversing the contour of the glenoid fossae. Condylar guidance (Fig. 3.5) also refers to the mechanical

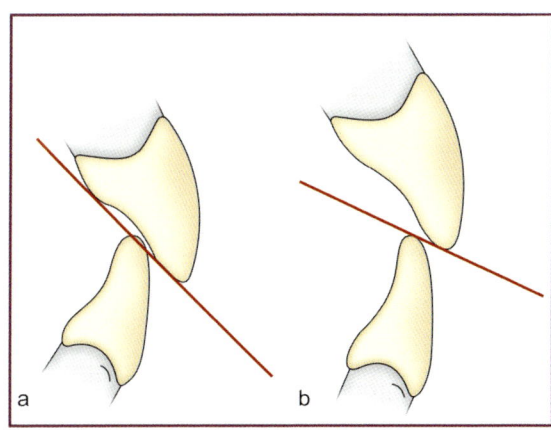

Fig. 3.4: Incisal guidance. a. Steep; b. shallow

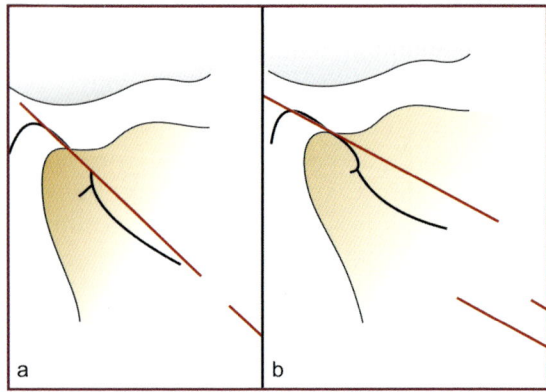

Fig. 3.5: Condylar guidance. a. Steep; b. Shallow

form located in the upper posterior region of an articulator that controls movement of its mobile member.

During protrusive movements, the separation of maxillary and mandibular teeth is controlled by the two end factors, i.e. incisal guidance and condylar guidance.

The angle formed by the condyles as it moves from its terminal position in the glenoid fossa forwards is called condylar guidance. The condylar guidance is dictated by the slopes of the articular eminence and the incisal guidance.

Curve of Spee

Curve of Spee or anteroposterior curve (Fig. 3.6): The anatomic curve established by the occlusal alignment of the teeth, as projected onto the median plane, beginning with the cusp tip of the mandibular canine and following the buccal cusp tips of the premolar and molar teeth, continuing through the anterior border of the mandibular ramus, ending with the anterior most portion of the mandibular condyle.

The distal and superior curvature of the occlusal plane is known as curve of Spee. If we look at teeth from a point opposite the first molar buccally, a curve following the occlusal and incisal surfaces is observed. This is the curve of Spee. Curve of Spee influences the anteroposterior movement of the teeth.

Curve of Wilson

It is also known as mediolateral curve (Fig. 3.7).

The curve in the lower arch being concave and consequently the one in the upper arch being convex. The curvature in the lower arch is affected by an equal lingual inclination of the right and left molars so that the tip points of the corresponding cross-aligned cusps can be placed into the circumferences of a circle. The transverse cuspal curvature of the upper teeth is affected by the equal buccal inclinations of their long axes.

The curvature of the plane of occlusion viewed in the frontal plane is known as curve of Wilson. The curvature of mandibular teeth is concave and that of maxillary teeth is convex. Curve of Wilson influences the lateral movement of the teeth.

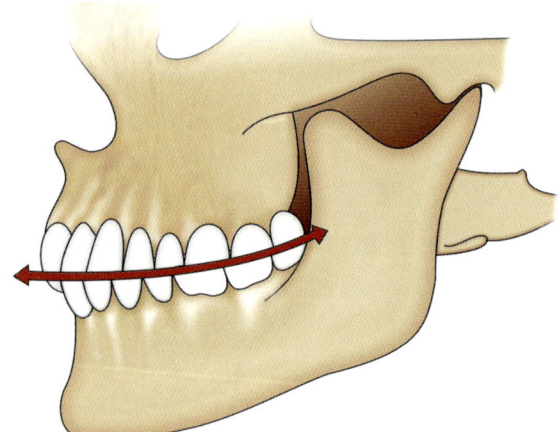

Fig. 3.6: Curve of Spee

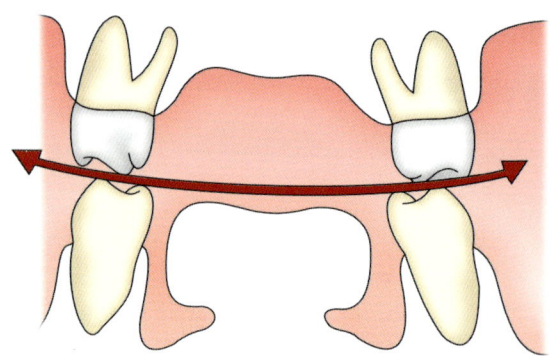

Fig. 3.7: Curve of Wilson

Bennett Movement or Bennett Shift

Bennett movement laterotrusion (Fig. 3.8): Lateral and downward movement of the condyle on the working side.

Bennett shift/mandibular translation: It is the bodily side shift of the mandible towards the working side during the lateral excursions. Also described as the translatory (mediolateral) movements of the mandible, when viewed in the frontal plane. It could theoretically occur in an essentially pure translatory form in the early part of the motion or in combination with rotation in the latter part of the motion or both.

The Bennett movement influences the width of the fossae on the working side—the Bennett angle which forms on the non-working side between protrusion and lateral movements influences the slopes of the cusps on the non-working side.

Intercondylar Distance

Intercondylar distance (Fig. 3.9) is the distance between the rotational centers of two condyles or their analogues.

The distance between the two condyles and the distance of each tooth from the working condyle influences cuspal inclines. Wider the intercondylar distance shallower will be the cuspal inclines. Narrower the intercondylar distance steeper will be the cuspal inclines. The cuspal inclines are also influenced by the

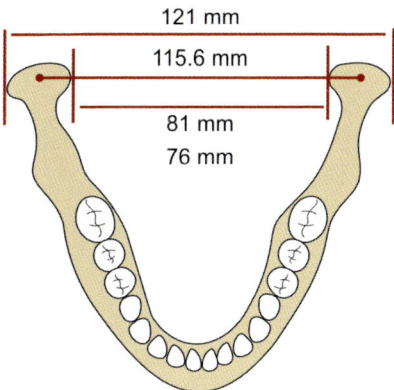

Fig. 3.9: Intercondylar distance

incisal guidance. Shallower the incisal guidance, shallower will be the cuspal inclines. Steeper the incisal guidance, steeper will be the cuspal inclines.

Mutually Protected Occlusion

Mutually protected occlusion (Figs 3.10 and 3.11) is an occlusal scheme in which the

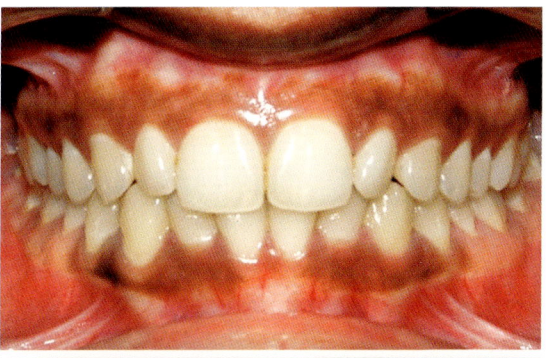

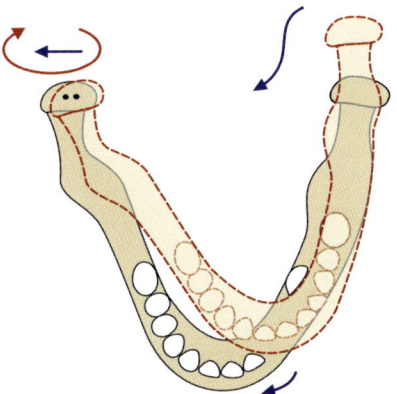

Fig. 3.8: Bennett movement and Bennett angle

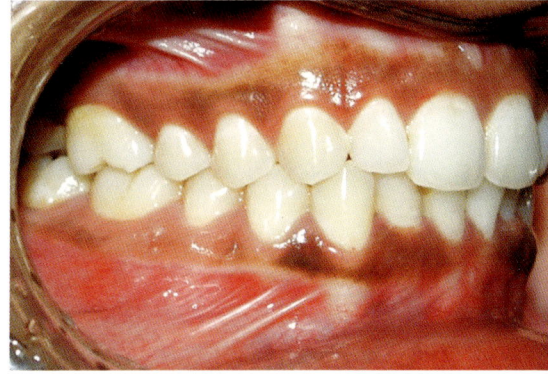

Fig. 3.10: Mutually protected occlusion—posterior teeth protect the anterior teeth

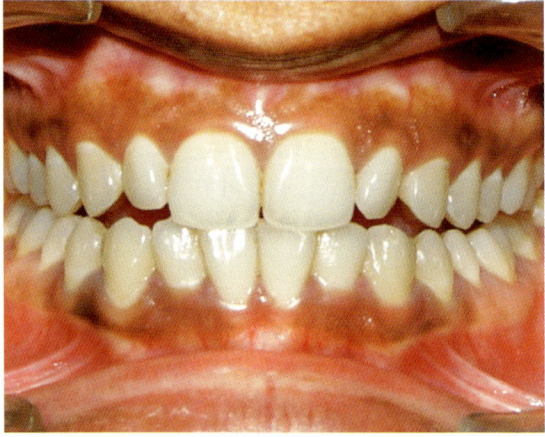

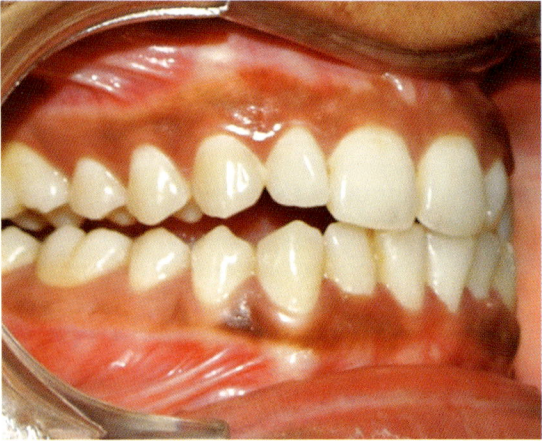

Fig. 3.11: Mutually protected occlusion. In protrusion and lateral excursion the anterior teeth protect the posterior teeth

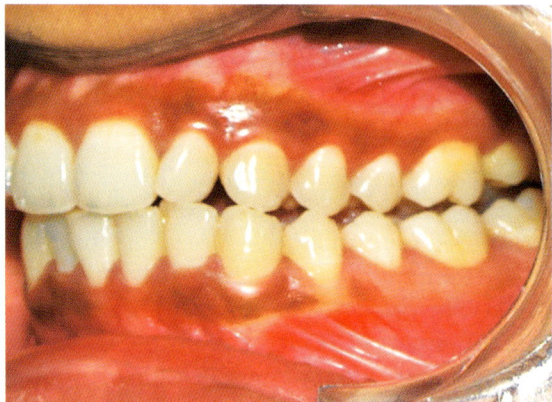

Fig. 3.12: Canine guided occlusion

that the posterior teeth are disoccluded in lateral excursions (Fig. 3.12). During this type of occlusion, the posterior teeth during working movements become free as the mandible moves away from the centric occlusion. The teeth on the non-working side also get separated. The canines being strong and reinforced by sufficient radicular support can absorb the lateral forces.

Group Function Occlusion

During lateral excursions on the working side the canines along with a few posterior teeth simultaneously glide over the buccal cuspal inclines of the mandibular teeth. The working guidance in group-function occurs on all or most of the teeth on working side. The buccal inclines of buccal cusps of mandibular posterior teeth glide against the palatal inclines of buccal cusps of maxillary posterior teeth. Similarly, during protrusive movements, incisal edges of the mandibular anterior teeth glide over the palatal surfaces of the maxillary anterior teeth (Fig. 3.13).

Analysis of Occlusion Prior to Restoration

Before any restoration is planned, it is mandatory for the restorative dentist to examine and analyze the pre-existing occlusion keeping in mind not only the desirability of satisfactorily restoring the dentition, but also the patient's adaptability

posterior teeth prevent excessive contact of the anterior teeth in maximum intercuspation, and the anterior teeth disengage the posterior teeth in all mandibular excursive movements. Alternatively, an occlusal scheme in which the anterior teeth disengage the posterior teeth in all mandibular excursive movements, and the posterior teeth prevent excessive contact of the anterior teeth in maximum intercuspation.

During lateral excursions, the teeth can be either in canine protected occlusion or in group function.

Canine Protected Occlusion

In this design of occlusion, the maxillary canines guide the mandibular movement so

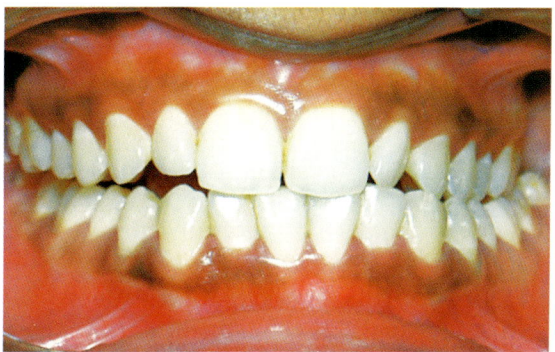

Fig. 3.13: Group function occlusion

to it. The occlusion can best be examined by consultation, physical examination and analysis of occlusal functions. Further analysis can be carried out using articulators, etc. A preliminary diagnosis of the disturbances in occlusion should be made prior to restoration.

The initial conversation with the patient in a congenial environment is important. The objective is to receive accurate information from the patient regarding occlusal disharmony. Certain questions, which can lead to initial diagnosis, are:

• Any difficulty in eating or prefer eating on one side only
• Clicking of teeth or joints during eating
• Grinding or occasional sliding of teeth
• Any difficulty in opening of mouth
• Any para-functional habits such as opening hair pin, biting nails, etc.
• Bleeding of gums during eating
• Discomfort with the previous restorations, if any.

These questions/answers will provide evidence in diagnosing mandibular and maxillary masticatory dysfunction. A dental and medical history suggests the possibilities of pathological states leading to altered occlusal functions.

Clinical Examination

During clinical examination, noting of routine missing, carious and filled teeth is important. The gingiva and associated oral hygiene is also

to be looked into. Other particular features which should be taken care of are:

• The pattern of occlusal wear on both mandibular and maxillary teeth
• Inclination of teeth
• Cusp-fossa and cusp-ridge relationships showing any type of interferences
• Individual contacts of teeth. Any open contact and plunger cusp
• Supra-eruption of one or more teeth
• Periodontal conditions of the teeth

All the information gathered in routine clinical examination should be further evaluated in the light of radiographs and the casts.

Panoramic radiographs (Fig. 3.14) will give us a bird's-eye view of the changes in the alveolar bone structure, teeth, periodontal condition and any other gross pathology.

Intraoral periapical radiographs (Fig. 3.15) are more focused and gives us a clear picture of

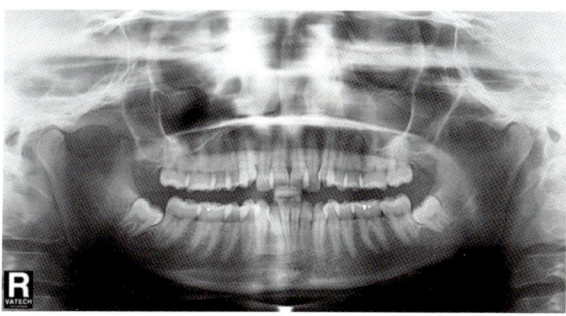

Fig. 3.14: Orthopantomograph

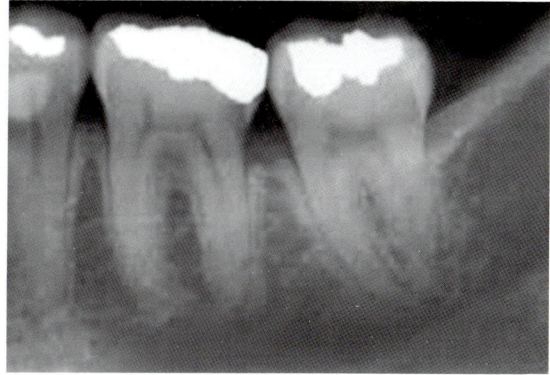

Fig. 3.15: Intraoral periapical radiograph

the coronal and the radicular portions of the teeth.

Bitewing radiographs (Fig. 3.16) give an excellent view of proximal caries.

The study of upper and lower casts in occluded form will provide the information regarding tipping of teeth, supra-occlusion in teeth, migration, and the presence of plunger cusps. The localized attrition of one or more cups or of marginal ridge can also be examined. The horizontal and vertical overlap and the crowding of teeth should be noted which will help planning the restorative regime. The ideal dynamic relationships are not present in a significant proportion of the population and yet they do not have signs and symptoms of disorder. Adaptation within the stomatognathic system is important. The adaptive capacity may be reduced with age, illness and/or stress. Thus, in some individuals, a minor occlusal disturbance (tilted teeth), which previously was within the physiologic limits of tolerance may become pathological. Generally, in the absence of any sign and symptom, prophylactic removal of non-ideal contacts is not advisable. These non-ideal contacts do have potential to become interferences, which may require occlusal adjustments at that time.

Restoration of one or a few teeth can be done in maximal intercuspal position only when full mouth rehabilitation has to be undertaken, the occlusion can be developed to coincide with the centric relation position of the patient.

Articular Analysis

The occlusal movements, both functional and non-functional, are difficult to examine in the mouth, since even after opening the lips, one can see only the buccal/labial aspects. The occlusal contacts between the mandibular and the maxillary teeth on the lingual side are not visible. To examine these contacts from both buccal and lingual side, along with the contacts during movements, the casts are examined over articulators, which simulate movements of the jaws.

Let us first study the types of articulators, process of articulation and its significance in restorative dentistry.

ARTICULATORS AND ARTICULATION OF CASTS

Many a times, the ignorance or poor knowledge of occlusion lead to flat restorations or cuspless restorations. Such restoration affects the underlying periodontium as well as the overall health of the stomatognathic system. The cuspal occlusion maintains the forces of mastication along the long axis of the tooth. Such an occlusion also helps in proprioception, controlling the mandibular movements.

Articulator is a mechanical instrument that represents the temporomandibular joints and jaws, to which maxillary and mandibular casts may be attached to simulate some or all mandibular movements.

Articulation is the process by which the casts are mounted on an articulator simulating the patient's mandibular movement and occlusion. There are four classes of articulators.

* *Class I articulator:* A simple holding instrument capable of accepting a single static registration; vertical motion is possible, e.g. Hinge articulator.

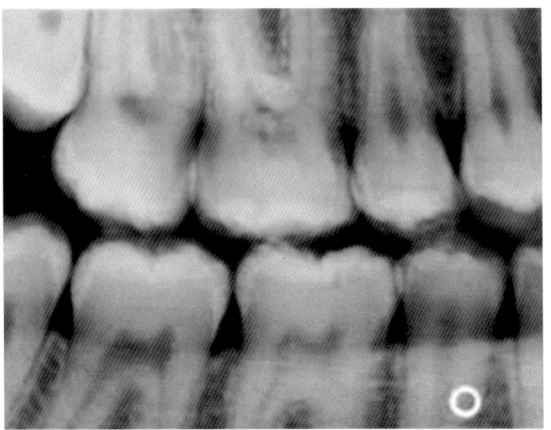

Fig. 3.16: Bitewing radiograph

- *Class II articulator:* An instrument that permits horizontal as well as vertical motion but does not orient the motion to the temporomandibular joints, e.g. Plane line or average value articulator.
- *Class III articulator:* An instrument that simulates condylar pathways by using averages or mechanical equivalents for all or part of the motion; these instruments allow for orientation of the casts relative to the joints and may be Arcon or non-Arcon instruments, e.g. Arcon articulator—Whipmix 3040 , Denar Mark II; non-Arcon articulator—Dentatus, Hanau H2 articulator.
- *Class IV articulator:* An instrument that will accept three-dimensional dynamic registrations; these instruments allow for orientation of the casts to the temporomandibular joints and simulation of mandibular movements, e.g. Denar DSA and Stuart articulators.

Hinge articulator (Fig. 3.17): The hinge articulator basically is a cast holder. Only opening and closing movement is possible. There is no possibility of simulating lateral or protrusive movements. Its application is limited to restoration of a single tooth in an otherwise dentate arch. Such an articulator cannot be used for diagnostic purposes.

Plane line or average value articulator (Fig. 3.18): Apart from opening and closing, these articulators permit lateral and protrusive movements based on average values. Usually 30° for condylar guidance and 15° for incisal guidance. These are best suited for small bridges, say three units or a couple of posterior crowns. Some intraoral adjustments, if necessary, can be carried out later especially with lateral excursion movements.

Semi-adjustable articulator (Figs 3.19 and 3.20): These semi-adjustable articulators are routinely used in restorative dentistry. The horizontal and lateral condylar guidances of

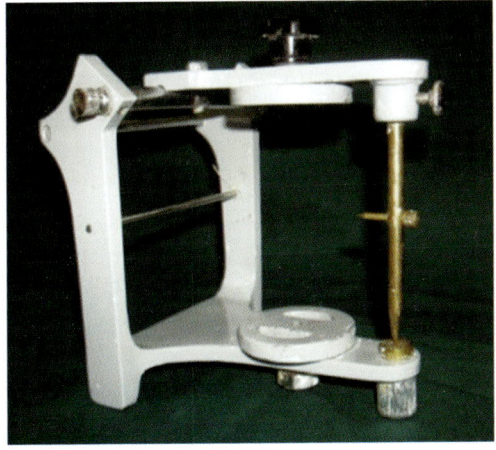

Fig. 3.18: Mean value articulator

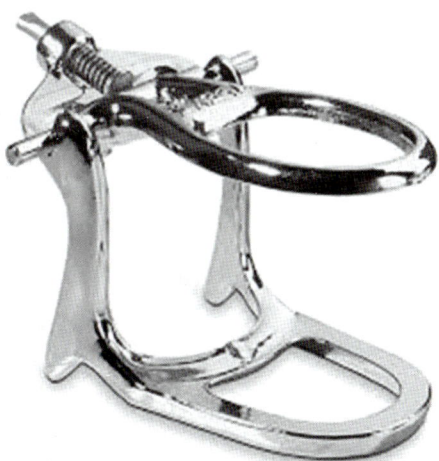

Fig. 3.17: Hinge articulator

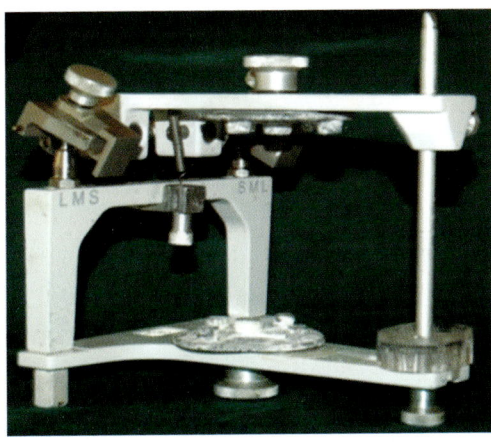

Fig. 3.19: Semi-adjustable articulator-Whipmix-Arcon

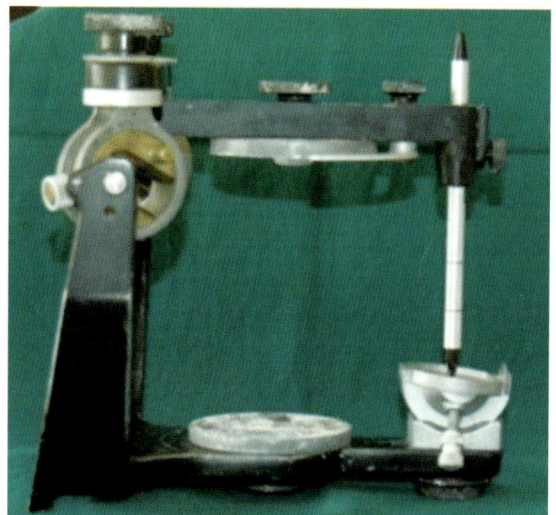

Fig. 3.20: Semi-adjustable articulator-Hanau-H2-non-Arcon

these articulators can be customized using interocclusal records from the patient to simulate the patient's mandibular movements.

Based on whether the condyles are attached to the upper or the lower member of the articulator, they can be classified as Arcon or non-Arcon articulators. The term Arcon derived from two words, articulators and condyles. The first two letters of articulators and the first three letters of condyle forms the term "Arcon". In Arcon articulators, the condylar elements are attached to the lower member of the articulator as it is in the mandible. In non-Arcon articulators, the condylar elements of the articulator is attached to the upper member of the articulator. Though, both of them simulate the mandibular movements, the Arcon articulators have the advantage as they simulate the mandibular movements more closely.

After transferring the orientation relation from the patient to the articulator, these articulators can be customized using protrusive and lateral interocclusal records to simulate the patient's mandibular movements.

However, there are certain shortcomings using these semi-adjustable articulators, which are:

- The path between the positional records are straight line approximation of the actual condyle movements.
- The arbitrary face bow is an approximation of the actual retruded axis.

To overcome these shortcomings, fully adjustable articulators are also available and are being used.

Fully Adjustable Articulators

These articulators provide more adjustments and greater accuracy as far as dimensions and movements are concerned. Examples are: 'Denar D5A' and 'Stuart' (Fig. 3.21).

These articulators require pantographic tracings to set the adjustments. The pantograph tracing has also been utilized for diagnostic purposes in TMJ dysfunction. The Pantographic Reproducible Index (PRI) was developed to confirm dysfunction and also to monitor progress of the treatment.

These instruments, besides being expensive, are also technique sensitive, therefore they are rarely used in restorative dentistry. Recently electronic jaw tracking devices have also been developed by which the mandibular movements are digitized and displayed onto the projector, thereby reducing chair side time.

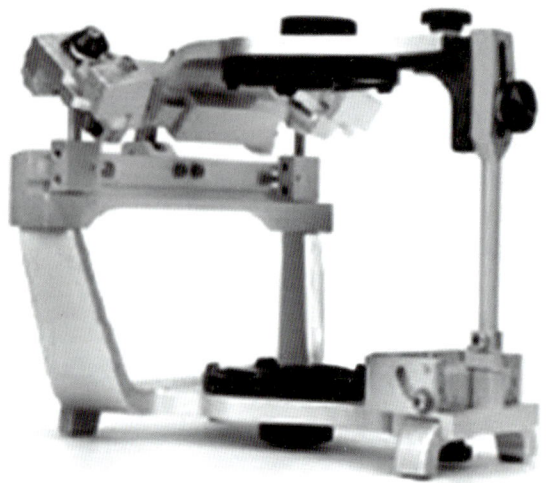

Fig. 3.21: Fully-adjustable articulator-Denar

Face-bow and Face-bow Records

Face-bow is a caliper-like instrument used to record the spatial relationship of the maxillary arch to some anatomic reference point or points and then transfer this relationship to an articulator. It orients the dental cast in the same relationship to the opening axis of the articulator as it is in the patient.

There are two commonly used face-bows with the articulators; arbitrary face-bow and kinematic face-bow.

In arbitrary face-bow, the condylar elements of the bow relates to the arbitrary marks located thirteen millimeters anterior to the tragus on a line drawn from tragus to the outer canthus of the eye to transfer the orientation relation.

In one of the arbitrary face-bows (ear piece type) (Fig. 3.22), the ear rods of the face-bow can be placed in the external auditory meatus. The design of the face-bow compensates for

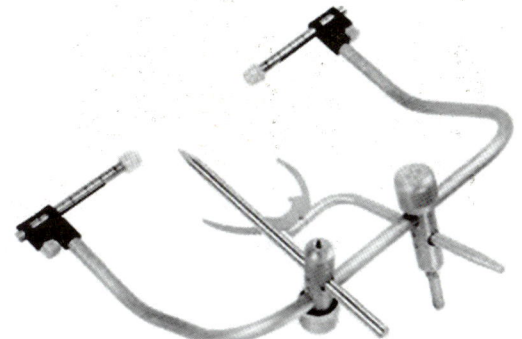

Fig. 3.23: Orbital face-bow—Hanau

the distance between the arbitrary location of the hinge axis and the external auditory meatus. These type of face-bows are user friendly.

The third reference point relates the maxillary cast to the Frankfort plane. Some face-bows use the infraorbital notch (Fig. 3.23) and others have a plastic 'nose piece' that rests on the bridge of nose during recording to orient the maxillary cast three dimensionally.

Interocclusal Records

Interocclusal record (Fig. 3.24) is the registration of the positional relationship of the opposing teeth or arches; a record of the positional relationship of the teeth or jaws to each other. The types of interocclusal records, articulators and potential interferences with various types of restorations are depicted in Table 3.1.

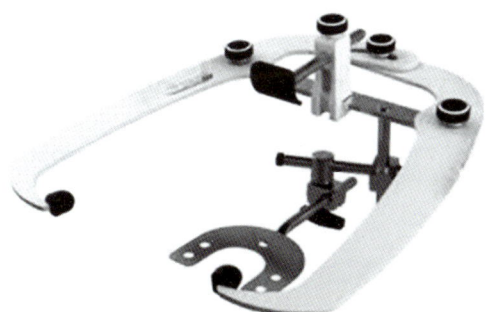

Fig. 3.22: Ear piece face-bow—Whipmix

Table 3.1: Types of interocclusal records, articulators and potential interferences with various types of restorations

Type of restoration	Interocclusal records	Articulators	Potential interferences
Single anterior unit	MICP	Simple hinge or mean value	Protrusive/lateral
Single posterior unit	MICP	Simple hinge or mean value	Protrusive/lateral
Last molars	MICP	Simple hinge or mean value	Protrusive/lateral
Multiple anteriors	MICP Lateral and protrusive	Semi-adjustable with face bow transfer	Nil or marginal
Multiple posteriors in one arch	MICP Lateral and protrusive	Semi-adjustable with face-bow transfer	Nil or marginal
Multiple posteriors in both arches	MICP Lateral and protrusive	Semi-adjustable with face-bow transfer or fully adjustable	Nil or marginal

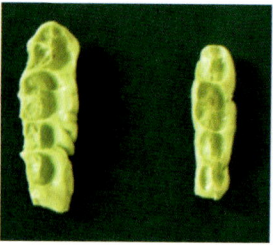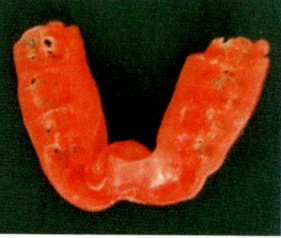

Fig. 3.24: Interocclusal records

The ideal recording material should have following requisites:
- It should be soft and mouldable
- It should not displace the soft tissues or teeth
- It should not interfere with mandibular movements
- It should be stable and accurate once it sets.

The routinely used materials include impression plaster, elastomers and hard base plate wax. Two thickness of base plate wax, which do not distort during removal, is usually used.

Interocclusal records are made in centric relation or centric occlusion to articulate the casts. Interocclusal records made in protrusive or lateral excursions are used to program the articulator to simulate the horizontal or lateral condylar guidances.

Occlusal records for one, a few or all the posterior teeth in a quadrant has to be restored

When one, a few or all the teeth in a quadrant needs to be restored on one side of the mouth, the following technique is employed. The record is made covering only the prepared teeth with the unprepared teeth in occlusion. The stepwise procedure is:
- The base plate wax is softened in warm water.
- Two thickness of wax is shaped according to the preparation and placed over the prepared tooth/teeth. The mandible is guided according to the intercuspal position (ICP).

- Keep the occluded wax in position till cool and then removed.
- If need be, it can be further improved by using zinc oxide eugenol paste or temporary cements.

It is important to maintain the horizontal and the vertical relationship of the jaws. After articulation, an anterior jig can be prepared to relate the maxillary and the mandibular teeth on the articulated casts or in the patient's mouth and can be used while making interocclusal records.

Occlusal records for all posterior teeth is to be prepared in one arch

After all the posterior teeth are prepared, the base plate wax is softened, shaped and placed over the teeth using an anterior jig. The wax interocclusal record can then be made and relined with zinc oxide eugenol, if necessary.

When there are insufficient number of teeth available to support a stable interocclusal record in wax, occlusal rims on a stable acrylic base can be used to make the interocclusal records.

PRINCIPLES OF EDEC

A few authors opine following EDEC (examine, design, execute and check the occlusion) principle for producing the desired restoration. The principle is useful in both direct and indirect restoration.

EDEC Principle for Indirect Restorations

In case of indirect restoration, the laboratory technician is also involved in decision making. The operator records the occlusion and the same is transferred accurately to the technician. During the time gap of fabrication of the restoration, the operator has the responsibility of maintaining the occlusion with provisional restorations.

Examine

The occlusion is examined prior to the start of preparation. Both static and dynamic occlusion is to be analyzed, using appropriate articulating papers and/or foils. The cast models with marked occlusal problems are sent to technician for analysis. The anatomical information can be transferred by using photographs, bite records or by occlusal sketching. Both static and dynamic records are taken and transferred to the technician.

Design

The designing of tooth preparation depends upon the material to be used for fabrication of the restoration. Minor adjustments in the model can be carried out by the technician after due discussion with the operator. Such adjustments in the model is named 'model grooming'. Many authors, however, do not favor this type of adjustments. They are of the view that any adjustment in the model will lead to defective restoration; preferably the preparation is to be modified accordingly and the impression is repeated.

Execute

The preservation of patient's occlusion is mandatory, till the time the permanent restoration is placed. Interim restorations provide the necessary relief, duplicating the occlusion and maintaining till the procedure lasts.

Check

The occlusion is to be checked thoroughly during the preparation and also after placing the restoration. The occlusal interferences, if any, are to be noted and cleared. The final, finished and polished restoration should simulate the functional occlusion of the patient.

RESTORING INDIVIDUAL TEETH

The occlusion is to be examined prior to restoring the teeth. The restorations should be in harmony with the functions of the supporting structures and the stomatognathic system. These restorations should not introduce any premature contacts and the cuspal interferences. The contours, contacts and embrasures of these restorations should be optimally placed so as to prevent caries and periodontal problems.

Occlusal Adjustments Prior to Restoration

The occlusal adjustments, being irreversible, should be judiciously made by using slow speed, small diamond wheel. Before eliminating the prematurities, they should be examined on the articulated casts and confirmed clinically by marking them. After each adjustment, see that the interference is eliminated by using an articulating paper. Generally, cusp tips are not ground down, only cuspal inclines are adjusted. The cusp tips are not ground to maintain the vertical dimension. Only the cusp slopes need to be modified to eliminate the occlusal prematurities.

The occlusal examination involves the following steps:

a. History

A complete history elicited during a conversation with a patient in a congenial atmosphere will help us in gathering important information regarding occlusal disharmony.

b. Clinical Examination

Judicious clinical examination will help us in observing the signs and symptoms of non-physiologic occlusion.

c. Radiographic Examination

The intraoral radiographs and/or panoramic radiograph will help us in observing the changes around the tooth structure and the alveolar bone (Figs 3.14 to 3.16).

d. Articulated Casts

The occlusal movements, both functional and nonfunctional are difficult to be observed and examined intraorally. The occlusal contacts between the mandibular and the maxillary teeth, on the lingual side are not visible (Fig. 3.25).

Study casts articulated on a semi adjustable articulator with face-bow transfer helps us in examining the occlusal contacts not only from buccal and lingual aspects but also during occlusion and excursive movements.

e. Evaluation of Traumatic Tooth Contacts

The traumatic tooth contacts can be primary or secondary.

  i. Primary occlusal trauma (mobility due to excessive occlusal load despite the presence of intact periodontium).
  ii. Secondary occlusal trauma (mobility due to periodontal breakdown in the presence of normal occlusal load).

Procedure for Occlusal Examination

1. Patient's cooperation and feedback is of great help in examining the occlusal contacts that need adjustment.
2. Wipe the articulating surfaces dry using gauze wipes, as the markings will be clearly visible when teeth are dry.
3. Occlusal contacts or interferences during grinding can be identified by
   • Visual inspection
   • Use of articulating paper
   • Shim stock

Detecting Occlusal Contacts

The occlusal contact areas in an occlusal set up, both static and dynamic, are to be analyzed

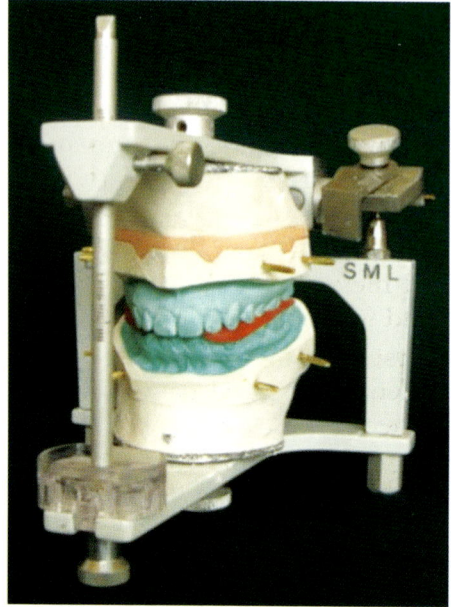

Fig. 3.25: Articulated casts

thoroughly by the operator and the technician. Various types of papers, silk, foil and waxes are used to precisely analyze tooth contact relations in static and dynamic occlusion.

Articulating papers are most commonly used to mark and indicate the position of occlusal contacts. The articulating paper is available in different thickness (8 to 200 μm) and in different colors (red, blue, white). The thinner ones are preferred in natural dentition (non-resiliency of teeth), whereas thicker ones are preferred in denture teeth (resiliency of acrylics). In ceramics and metals, middle thickness is preferred.

The sponge-like nature of the articulating paper store the color, which is released under

Table 3.2: Difference between paper and foil	
Paper	**Foil**
Size 40 to 200 μm	Size 8 to 12 μm
Mark under pressure	Mark on stroke
Contact marks are larger	Contact marks are pinpoint
Shows different pressure areas	Visualize high spots precisely
To check static occlusion	To check static and dynamic occlusion
Marks well on wet surfaces	Equally good in wet conditions

pressure. At the area of greater masticatory stresses (heavy contacts), more color is squeezed and produces dark marks, whereas in light masticatory stresses (light contacts), less color is squeezed producing less marks. Translucase bonding agent is added to articulating papers and foils to mark on wet surfaces, glazed porcelain or the highly polished metal surfaces. The differences in paper and foil is depicted in Table 3.2.

The first step is to carry out marking with blue articulating paper (preferably 100 µm thick). The contacts are immediately evident. The second step is to take a thin film (Art foil 8–12 µm) preferably red, to visualize clearly the light spots. (Thin areas of the articulating foil marks will clearly differentiate the high spots.)

The smooth fiber reinforced papers (100 µm thick paper impregnated with hydrophilic waxes and pharmaceutical oils) are useful in locating high spots in highly polished metals and ceramics.

Articulating silk, made from high quality silk (silk is tear resistant and flexible) adapts perfectly to the anatomy of tooth. Articulating silk is specially suitable for use on laboratory model because one strip can be used for more than once.

The micro-thin articulating papers (40 µm thick) are suited for two way recording of occlusion, static and dynamic. The first step is to inspect the concentric contact (static occlusion) in blue color followed by second step to inspect the eccentric contact (dynamic occlusion) in red. The color sequence can be changed as per operator's choice.

The unique combination of metal foil (Shimstock 8–12) with two-sided color coating enables clear marking on the occlusal surfaces. The centric and eccentric contacts can be shown consecutively with one foil because of the two colors. (Single color coating and without color foils are also available for conventional use.) A white film specially designed for colored modeling waxes is available (white contact points appear nicely on dark background). This film also marks effectively on polished metal surfaces.

The horseshoe shaped articulating papers are especially useful for patients who tend to bite unilaterally during the occlusion test due to diminished resilience.

Various types of articulation forceps are available for the convenience of the operator. The forceps are also designed for the analysis of proximal contact areas. High spot indicators are also available for testing the accurate fit of crowns, inlays and also the denture clasps (Arti-spot). Arti-spot is a contact color, which can be applied with a small paint brush. The solvent evaporates leaving a thin film on the surface. The heavy contact destroys the color at that area, visualizing the shining spot (high spot area). After use, the Arti-spot dye can easily be removed with mechanical cleaning and/or in alcohol.

A color spray (air-spray) is available, which is sprayed over the occlusal surfaces of the restoration. A thin film left over the surface, if grinded during occlusal contacts, shows the areas of high contacts. The same can be used for crowns and inlays to note the high-spot areas. The layer left over the restorations can easily be washed off.

Signs and Symptoms of Traumatic Tooth Contacts

A tooth in traumatic contact may exhibit one or more of the following clinical features:
- Cracked/fractured teeth
- Root resorption
- Pulpal hyperemia
- Pulpitis
- Degenerative pulpal changes
- Tooth mobility
- Fremitus
- Fractured restoration
- Alveolar/ periodontal pain
- Large wear facet
- Loose teeth
- Flaring of anterior teeth

Objectives of Selective Grinding

1. To achieve a stable non-traumatic occlusal contact relationship between the maxillary and mandibular teeth in maximum inter-cuspation/centric occlusion and in all functional excursive positions.
2. To provide stability of the temporomandibular joint in maximum inter-cuspation/centric occlusion.
3. To improve structural and functional relation of the dentition.
4. Bringing occlusal forces within the limits of tolerance of the periodontium.
5. To achieve occlusal stability.
6. To permit condyle disc complex to move and function normally or within the tolerable limits.
7. To permit neuromuscular system to function within adaptive potential of the patient.
8. To reduce the effects of parafunctional activities of the patient.
9. To improve esthetic needs of the patient.

Occlusal Adjustment Procedures

The simplest treatment that accomplishes the treatment goals is generally the best and the treatment should never begin until the end result is visualized.

Armamentarium (Fig. 3.26)

1. Hand piece (slow speed, high speed)
2. Green stones
3. White stones
4. Rubber wheel
5. Articulating paper
6. Paper holding forceps
7. Gauge wipes
8. Green wax sheets

Preparation of Patient

- Explain the purpose of the adjustment and what to expect during and after the procedure.

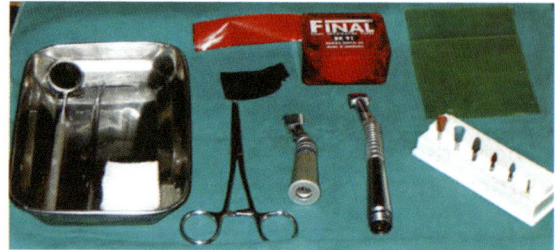
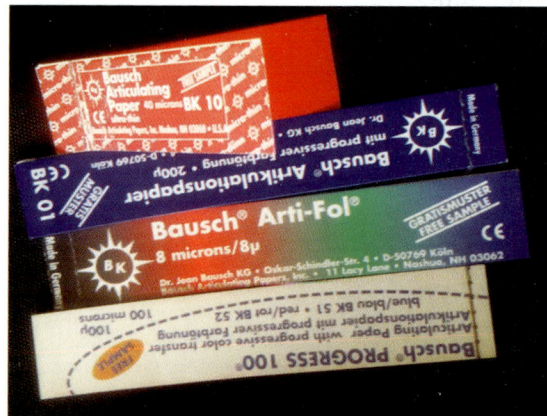
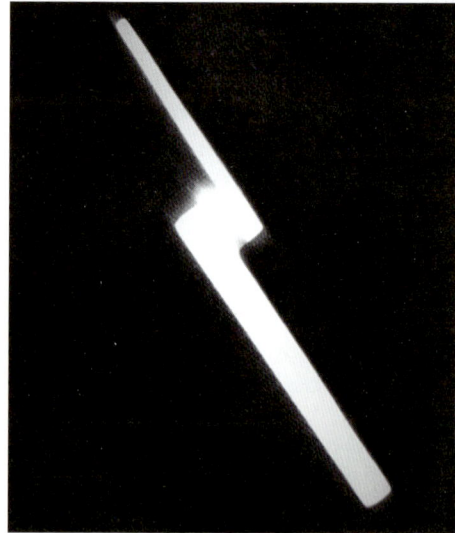

Fig. 3.26: Armamentarium for occlusal adjustments

- After the initial adjustment, the occlusion will feel more comfortable and stable. The occlusion will be re-evaluated after two weeks; during this period loose teeth may become firm and muscles may relax. The occlusion may change slightly after the correction, hence the need for re-evaluation and refinement.

Diagnostic Cast Adjustment Procedures

- Mount the casts accurately on an articulator with face-bow transfer in the same relation in which coronoplasty has to be done.
- Mark the casts for adjustment using the articulating paper.
- Make the necessary changes on the casts following the guidelines of correcting the natural dentition.

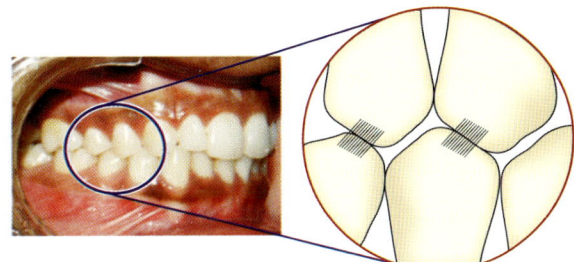

Fig. 3.27: Elimination of protrusive interferences

Sequence of Occlusal Adjustments

Occlusal correlations should always begin with identification and elimination of the interferences in maximal intercuspal position by the following procedures:

- Shorten extruded teeth
- Reduce plunger cusp
- Correct marginal ridge relationship
- Correct rotated, mal-positioned or tilted teeth
- Round sharp cusps
- Create ability to voluntary tap into a constant centric occlusion with patient's head in erect posture.

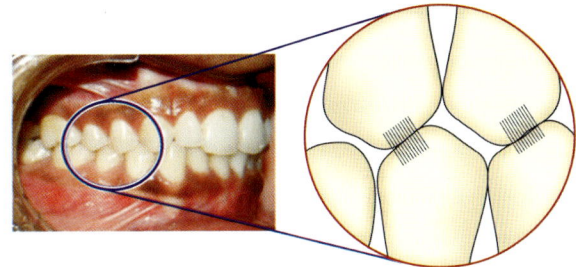

Fig. 3.28: Elimination of retrusive interferences

Elimination of the slide between centric relation and maximal intercuspal position

Identify the anterior components to the slide and eliminate the interference by correcting the forward facing incline of maxillary teeth and backward facing incline of mandibular teeth.

As a general rule, widen the fossae or embrasure areas at the occluding cusps.

Elimination of protrusive interferences (Fig. 3.27)

Interferences during protrusive movements can be eliminated by correcting the distal inclines of maxillary teeth and the mesial inclines of mandibular teeth.

Elimination of retrusive interferences (Fig. 3.28)

Interferences during retrusive movements can be eliminated by correcting the mesial inclines of the maxillary teeth and the distal inclines of mandibular teeth.

Elimination of working side prematurity (Fig. 3.29)

The working side prematurity is commonly seen in extruded teeth rather than in normal

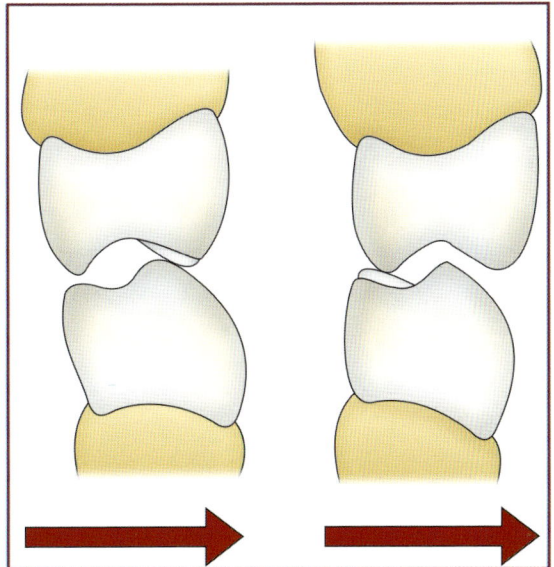

Fig. 3.29: Elimination of working side interferences—BULL's law

dentition. For such type of interferences, BULL (buccal upper and lingual lower) rule is applied to correct the occlusal prematurities on the working side since these are non-supporting cusps. The palatal upper and the buccal lower cusps should not be adjusted.

Elimination of non-working side prematurity (Fig. 3.30)

The premature contacts pose special problem in the non-working side as they occur on supporting cusps. Their removal, however, is indicated, as they are associated with an increased risk of bone loss, TMJ dysfunctions and mobility. The palatal slopes of the maxillary buccal cusps and the lingual slopes of the mandibular buccal cusps are modified to eliminate the interferences.

Occlusal Consideration during Tooth Preparation

Preferably, the restoration is so planned that the natural crown is not completely covered. The intact buccal and lingual surfaces of the crown guide the accurate contouring of the restoration (Fig. 3.31) and help preserve the gingival environment. Full coverage restorations and the onlays are indicated where the

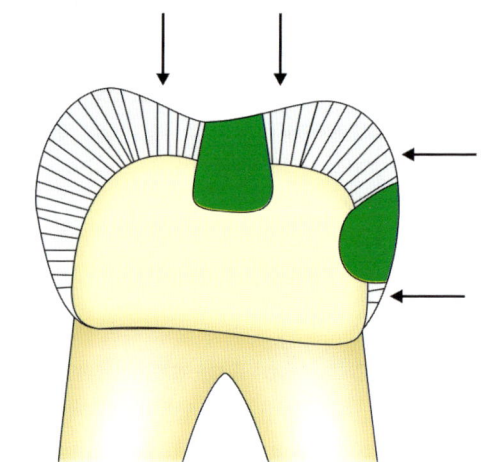

Fig. 3.31: Natural contours guide the contours of the restorations

cusps are severely damaged or fractured and also where the occlusion is to be modified.

During tooth preparation, the gingival health is to be taken care of, since the impinging of biological width area and the gingival margins can lead to periodontal problems. Adequate tooth preparation is to be carried out depending upon the choice of the material. A shoulder and chamfer (Fig. 3.32) preparation provides sufficient bulk for the material. The cervical areas should not be

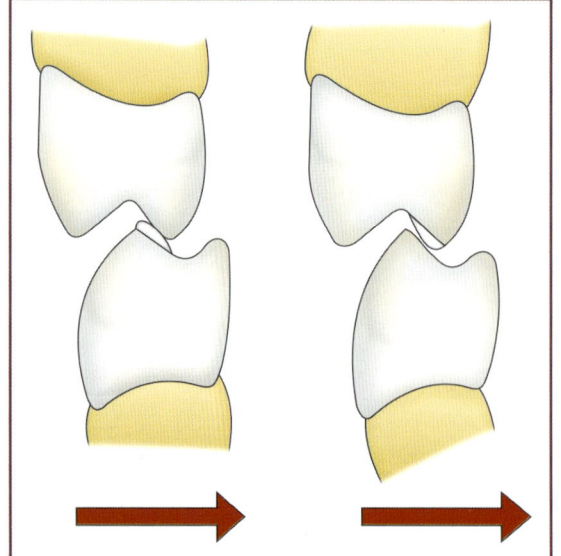

Fig. 3.30: Elimination of non-working side interferences

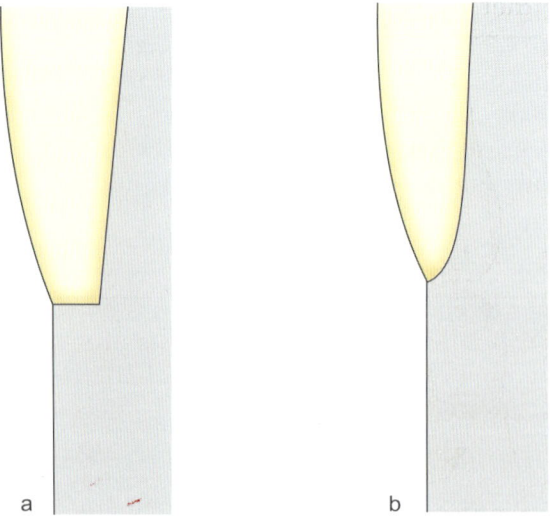

Fig. 3.32: Adequate tooth preparation. a. Shoulder; b. Chamfer

over-contoured. Inadequate tooth preparation at the margins of the shoulder or chamfer leads to overcontouring of the restoration which is not conducive to the health of the periodontium. The shape of the embrasures and contact points should be reproduced to prevent food impaction.

During the preparation of the teeth for inlays and onlays, the margins should not be placed at the occluso-buccal line angle of the mandibular teeth and the occluso-palatal line angles of the maxillary teeth. Such cases are indicated for cusp covering. The depth of occlusal preparation will vary depending upon the choice of the restoration, however, usually the working cusps are reduced by 1.0–1.5 mm and the non-working cusps by 0.5–1.0 mm for metal onlays and crowns. In case of full crowns, the height of the clinical crown should be examined and evaluated thoroughly. At least 3 to 4 mm of occlusal height is required for proper retention. The crowns with lesser heights need extra retentive features like grooves. The occlusal table is kept narrower during preparation and restoration to minimize the interferences during lateral excursions and to reduce the occlusal forces on the tooth (Fig. 3.33).

The tooth preparation needs to be checked either by wax interocclusal records perio-dically during the tooth preparation to avoid under or overpreparation of the occlusal surfaces. The temporary restoration, prior to cementation, should be examined for occlusal interference, and if any, should be corrected. The occlusal thickness of the temporary restorations act as guide to evaluate the adequacy of the preparation. The appearance of thin acrylic at certain areas indicates the need for further tooth preparation in those areas.

Need for Restoring the Anatomic Form of the Teeth

- The physiologic relationship with the adjacent teeth will enable the dentition bear the masticatory stresses in a better way. Such relationships promote deflection of food through embrasures and prevent food impaction.
- The correct relationship with opposing teeth during mastication will prevent deflective occlusal contacts, which otherwise can lead to pain and periodontal problems and even fracture of the teeth.
- The proper bucco-lingual contour will allow deflection of food over the gingiva protecting the periodontal tissue.
- For maintaining oral hygiene
- Esthetically pleasing

Anterior Restorations

The dynamic balance of anterior teeth is maintained by tongue, lips, occlusal relationships and also the alveolar bone support. The teeth should be restored in this balanced envelope to achieve stability and longevity of the restoration. Changes, if any, will lead to unwanted movements leading to migration, rotation or over-eruption.

The anterior teeth should be examined thoroughly regarding incisal guidance, protrusive movement and also the horizontal and vertical overlap. The incisal guidance varies with different individuals depending

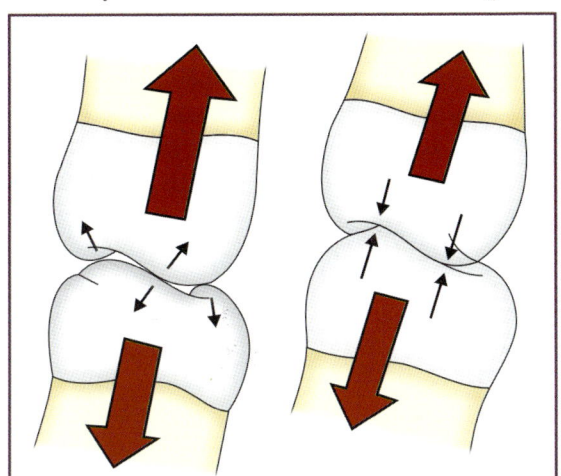

Fig. 3.33: Occlusal forces directed along the long axis of the tooth

upon the type of occlusion and the jaw relations.

During lateral excursions, both in canine protected occlusion and in group function, canines play a very important role. Therefore, particular care should be exercised in restoring canine in both group function and canine guided occlusion.

Anterior guidance where mandibular incisors glide over palatal surfaces of the maxillary incisors should provide smooth even contact on as many anterior teeth as possible from MICP through the protrusion leading to the disocclusion of the posterior teeth. If single tooth is to be restored, it can be done using the existing guidance (Fig. 3.34). When all the anterior teeth need to be restored, some changes to incisal guidance and position of teeth can be made only if necessary.

The relationship of mandibular anterior teeth to maxillary anterior teeth, especially in class II division 1, where the incisal edges touches the dento-gingival junction is not favorable. It becomes necessary to shorten the mandibular incisors. The edges are reduced horizontally to produce flat rather than beveled incisal edge to improve the prognosis.

The canine has a favorable crown/root ratio for absorbing occlusal forces. The root length and configuration provides greater surface area and more proprioception than the adjacent teeth. This tooth is best suited to guide lateral excursive movements. The canine guidance allows easy access in front of the mouth for adjustments.

Posterior Restoration

Most of the teeth requiring indirect restorations are the posterior teeth. The occlusion of the tooth to be prepared for cast restoration should be thoroughly examined before the tooth preparation. Examination of the occlusion both by using articulated study casts and clinically using an articulating paper will help us in identifying any premature contacts. Such contacts should be eliminated before beginning the tooth preparations.

The occlusion of the complete veneer restorations can be satisfactorily restored using articulators. However, when inlays, onlays and partial veneer crowns are to be used to restore the teeth, then the occlusion should be examined and the occlusal contact points should be marked. During tooth preparation, the occlusal contact points should either be included or excluded from the outline form of the restoration (Fig. 3.35). Avoid placing the occlusal contacts on the margins of the tooth preparation.

Restoring Posterior Teeth-Occlusal Scheme

When restoring one or a few posterior teeth, the occlusion should be examined, interferences if any on the teeth to be prepared, should be corrected. The restorations can then be placed to be in harmony with the existing occlusion.

When a large number of posterior teeth needs to be restored, then the existing

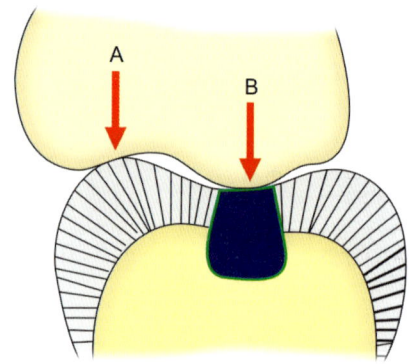

Fig. 3.35: Outline form. A. Contact area excluded in the outline form; B. Contact area included in the outline form

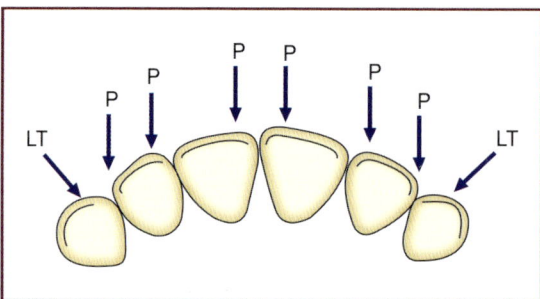

Fig. 3.34: Anterior guidance

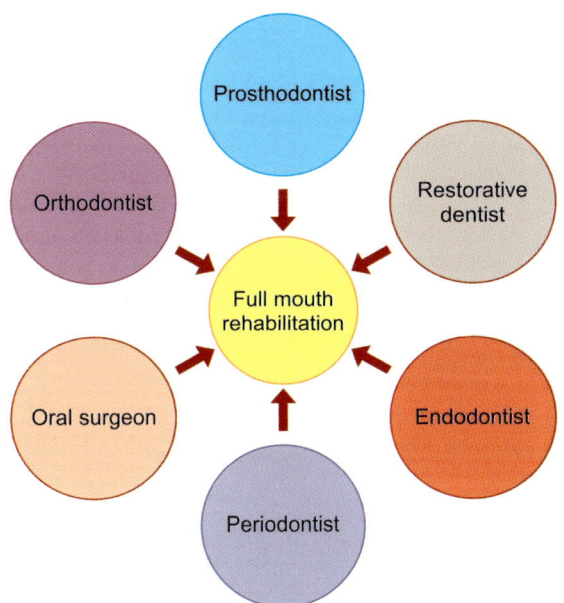

Fig. 3.36: Full mouth rehabilitation. A multidisciplinary approach

occlusion should be examined and in the absence of any signs and symptoms of pathological occlusion, the teeth can be restored in the existing occlusion.

When full mouth rehabilitation is planned, the centric occlusion should be developed to coincide with the centric relation of the patient. Full mouth rehabilitation is a multidisciplinary approach where one or more specialists may be required to complete the case (Fig. 3.36).

Bibliography

1. Adams SH and Zander HA. Functional tooth contacts in lateral and centric occlusion. JADA: 1967;69:437–65.
2. Beyron HL. Optimal occlusion. Dent. Clin. North Am. : 1969;13:537–54.
3. Brizuela-Velasco A, Alvarez-Arenal A, Ellakuria-Echevarria J, Rio-Highsmith J, Santamaria-Arrieta G and Martin-Blanco N. Influence of articulating paper thickness on occlusal contacts registration: A preliminary report. Int. J. Prosthodont.: 2015;28: 360–2.
4. Carey JP, Craig M, Kerstein RB and Radke J. Determining a relationship between applied occlusal load and articulating paper mark area. Oper. Dent. J.: 2007;1:1–7.
5. Clayton JA. Centric: Factors to consider in their use. Aust. Dent. J.: 1986;16:41–9.
6. Cotter S and Oshea D. Traumatic overbite: A restorative solution. Dent. Update: 2002;29:136–40.
7. Darveniza M. Full occlusal protection : Theory and practice of occlusal therapy. Aust. Dent. J.: 2001;46:70–9.
8. Davies SJ and Gray RMJ. The examination and recording of the occlusion: why and how. Br. Dent. J.: 2001;191:291–302.
9. Davies SJ, Gray RMJ and Smith PW. Good occlusal practice in simple restorative dentistry. Br. Dent. J.: 2001;191:365–81.
10. Fattore LD, Malone WFP, Sandrik JL, Mazur B and Hart J. Clinical evaluation of the accuracy of inter-occlusal recording materials. JPD: 1984;51: 152–7.
11. Frederick CSC, Adam SC, Philip RH, Tak WC and Smales RJ. Restorative management of the worn dentition : 2. Localized anterior tooth wear. Dent. Update: 2002;29:214–22.
12. Frederick CSC, Adam SC, Philip RH, Tak WC and Smales RJ. Restorative management of the worn dentition : 3 Localized posterior tooth wear. Dent. Update: 2002;29:267–72.
13. Frederick CSC, Adam SC, Philip RH, Tak WC and Smales RJ. Restorative management of the worn dentition: 4 Generalized tooth wear. Dent. Update: 2002;29:318–24.
14. Freilich MA, Altieri JV and Wahle JJ. Principles for selecting inter-occlusal records for articulation of dentate and partially dentate casts. JPD: 1992; 68:361–7.
15. Haruaki H, Atsuyoshi O, Yoko I, Youichi Y and Minoru N. Occlusal Contact Area of Mandibular Teeth During Lateral Excursion. J. Int. Prosthodont.: 2004;17:72–6.
16. Ishigaki S. Classification of maximal opening and closing movements. Int. J. Prosthod.: 1989;2:148–54.
17. Jenat T, Lundquist S and Hedegard B. Group function or canine protection. J.P.D.: 1982;91:719–24.
18. Keshvad A and Winstanley RB. An appraisal of the literature on centric relation. Part III. J. Oral Rehab.: 2001;28:55–63.
19. Loos LG. Clinical criteria used to select an articulator. Compend. Contin. Educ. Dent.: 1993; 14:80–8.

20. Lundeen HC. Occlusal morphology considerations for fixed restorations. Dent. Clin. North Am. 1971;15:649–61.

21. McCullock AJ. Making occlusion work: 1. Terminology, occlusal adjustments and recording. Dent. Update: 2003;30:150–7.

22. McCullock AJ. Making occlusion work: 2 Practical consideration. Dent. Update: 2003;30:211–6, 218–9.

23. Melntyre FM and Jureyda O. Occlusal function: Beyond centric occlusion. DCNA: 2001;173–80.

24. Milosevic A. Occlusion 1: Terms, mandibular movements and factors of occlusion. Dent. Update : 2003;30:359–61.

25. Milosevic A. Occlusion 2: Occlusal splints: Analysis and adjustments. Dent. Update: 2003;30:416–22.

26. Milosevic A. Occlusion 3: Articulators and related instruments. Dent. Update: 2003;30:511–5.

27. Mullick SC, Stackhoyse JA and Vincent GRV. A study of interocclusal record materials. J. Prosthet. Dent.: 1981;25:304–7.

28. Murray MC, Smith PW, Watts DC and Wilson NFH. Occlusal registration: science or art ? Int. Dent. J.: 1999;49:41–6.

29. Reynolds JM. Occlusal wear facets. J. Prosthet. Dent.: 1970;24:367–72.

30. Saad MN, Weiner G, Ehrenberg D and Weiner S. Effects of load and indicator type upon occlusal contact markings. J. Biomed. Mater. Res. B. Appl. Biomater.: 2008;85:18–22.

31. Schuyler CH. An evaluation of incisal guidance and its influence in restorative dentistry. JPD: 1959; 9:374–85.

32. Schuyler CH. The function and importance of incisal guidance in oral rehabilitation. J. Prosthet. Dent.: 1963;13;1011–29.

33. Starcke EN. The history of articulators: early attempt to reproduce mandibular movements. J. Prosthodont.: 2000;9:161–5.

34. Starcke EN. The history of articulators: Scribing Articulators: Those with Functionally Generated Custom Guide Controls, Part I. J. Prosthodont.: 2004;13:118–28.

35. Starcke EN. The history of articulators: Scribing Articulators: Those with Functionally Generated Custom Guide Controls, Part II. J. Prosthodont. 2005;14:198–207.

36. Starcke EN and Engelmeier RL. The history of articulators: the wonderful world of 'Grinders'. Part IJ Prosthodont: 2006;15:129–40.

37. Steele JG, Nohl FSA and Wassell RW. Crowns and other extracoronal restorations: occlusal considerations and articulator selection. Br. Dent. J.: 2002;192:377–87.

38. Stuart CE. Why dental restoration should have cusps? J. South Calif. Dent. Assoc.: 1959;27:198.

39. Trushkowsky RD and Burgess JO. Complex single tooth restorations. Dent. Clinic North Am.: 2002; 46:341–65.

40. Warren K and Capp N. A review of principles and techniques for making inter-occlusal records for mounting working casts. Int. J. Prosthodont.: 1990; 3:341–8.

41. Wilson PHR and Banerjee A. Recording the retruded contact position: a review of clinical techniques. Br. Dent. J.: 2004;196:395–402.

42. Woda A, Vigneron DC and Douglas Kay DC. Non-functional and functional occlusal contacts: A review of the literature. JPD: 1979;42:335–41.

4

Principles of Tooth Preparation

The main goal of the operator is to restore the tooth to its form and function in a restorative phase of the treatment. The tooth is to be prepared to receive the restoration, may it be direct or indirect.

Tooth preparation is defined as the process of removal of diseased and/or healthy tooth tissue so as to shape a tooth to receive the restoration. The amount of tooth structure removed and also preserved, while providing final form to the tooth preparation contribute to the success of the restoration. The decision of the choice of indirect restoration also depends upon the remaining tooth structure. The preservation of remaining tooth structure warrants choice of indirect restoration over direct restoration. Further, the type of indirect restoration should be selected keeping in mind preservation of the remaining tooth structure.

Teeth require appropriate preparation to receive the pre-selected restoration. The principles of tooth preparation governing indirect restorations are described here. As tooth has no regenerative ability, the preparation principles are to be followed in precision. Careful attention to every guideline is imperative during tooth preparation. The accepted guidelines are:

a. Permissible occlusal convergence
b. Height of axial walls (incisal/occlusal-cervical length)

c. Geometric form of the prepared tooth (surface area)
d. Depth of reduction
e. Location and form of finish lines
f. Auxiliary retentive features
g. Assessing final form of the preparation
h. Confirm uniformity of preparation before impression making

a. Permissible Occlusal Convergence

The occlusal convergence (the angle of convergence between two opposing axial walls) is considered as one of the important aspect in the success of both intracoronal and extracoronal restorations. Former authors recommended 2–6° (average 5°) occlusal convergence, focusing mainly on the forces parallel to the long axis of the tooth (Figs 4.1a and b). Later, it was established that lateral/oblique forces are the determining factors in the restoration's resistance to dislodgement.

It is established that the operator prefers 6–10° convergence angle in anterior teeth and 10–20° in posterior teeth. Various studies have confirmed that occlusal convergence is kept more in posterior teeth as compared to anterior teeth. Mandibular teeth are prepared with more occlusal convergence than maxillary teeth.

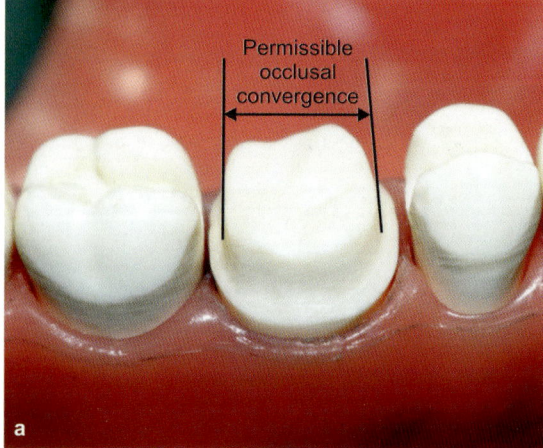

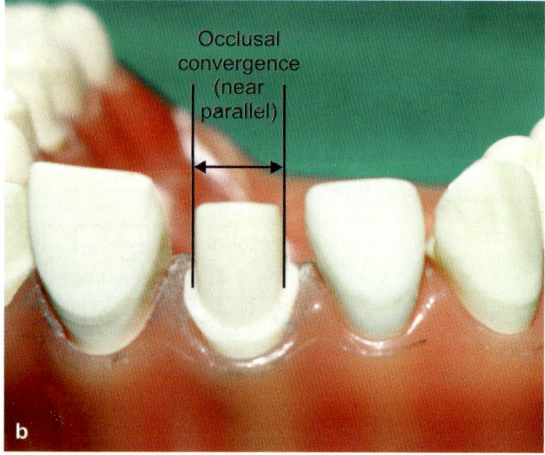

Figs 4.1a and b: Permissible occlusal convergence: Should be kept near parallel

It is confirmed that the occlusal convergence is inversely proportional to retention (more the taper; less the retention); however, taper is increased (10–15°) in case of ceramic/composite indirect restorations (providing easy path of insertion, since the material is brittle).

With the advent of resin luting agents coupled with advanced bonding agents, the occlusal convergence of 10° is considered appropriate for indirect restorations.

b. Height of Axial Walls (incisal/occlusal-cervical length)

The height of two opposing axial walls and their corresponding taper contribute to the retention of the extracoronal indirect restorations (onlays and crowns). Similarly, height of two opposing cavity walls contribute to the retention of intracoronal restorations (inlays). A minimum of 3.0 mm of incisal/occlusal-cervical height with appropriate taper (up to 10°) is recommended for extracoronal restorations; however, 3.0 mm height may provide inadequate resistance and retention at 20° taper. With increase of taper, the height is to be increased correspondingly (for example, in molars, 4.0 mm height is recommended, since the usual taper is kept above 10°) (Fig. 4.2). The teeth that do not possess the requisite height of the axial walls, should be modified with auxiliary retentive features.

c. Geometric Form of the Prepared Tooth (surface area)

The surface area of the prepared tooth (dimensions of occluso-cervical and facio-lingual) contributes mainly in achieving the resistance and retention form of the teeth. The ratio of occluso-cervical to facio-lingual surface is also considered important (ratio of 0.4 or higher is appropriate for all teeth). Prepared molars have more facio-lingual dimension than pre-molars and incisors, producing lower ratio and subsequently poor resistance. More so, the occlusal divergence

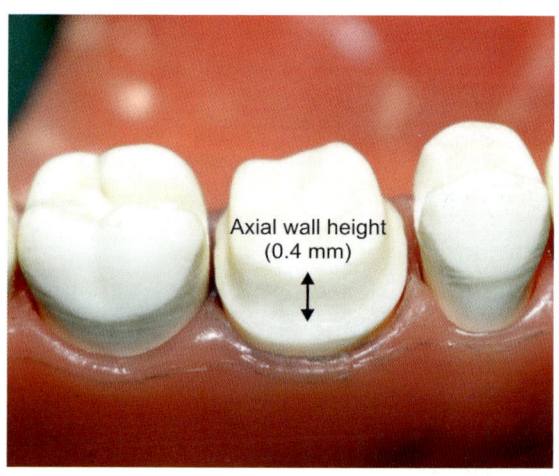

Fig. 4.2: Height of opposing axial walls

is also more on molars, which accentuates the unfavourable ratio (Figs 4.3a and b).

It is established that adequate resistance/retention can be achieved even if the ratio is 0.1 provided the taper is less than 6°. As the taper increases, the ratio is to be increased. A ratio of 0.4 is considered adequate for all type of preparations.

d. Depth of Reduction

The facial, lingual and occlusal reduction in extracoronal restorations and the depth of cavity in intracoronal preparations is important aspect for the success of these restorations. The mal-aligned teeth may require greater reduction of the protruding

surfaces to permit restoration alignment and also the resistance and retention form. The depth of reduction varies with the type of material to be used for the fabrication of the restoration. The depth of reduction should allow development of normal contours, esthetics and adequate strength; however, over-reduction may jeopardize the health of the underlying pulp (Figs 4.4a–c). The increase in depth or over-reduction can be compro-

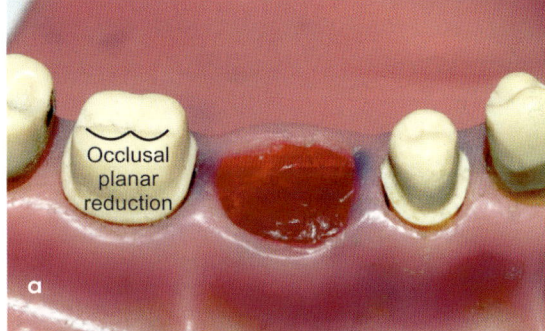

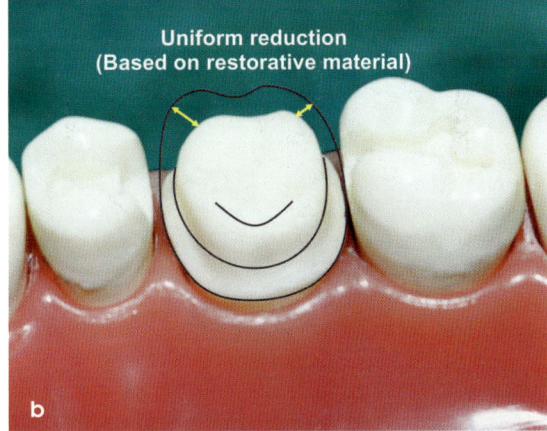

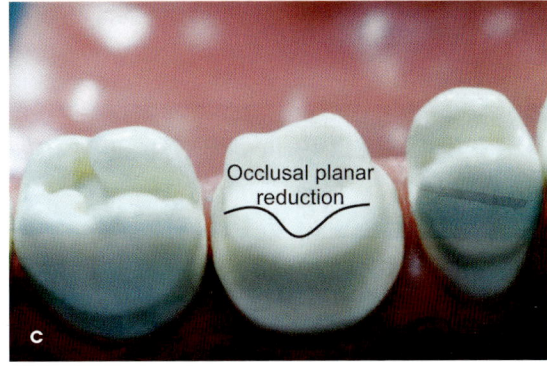

Figs 4.4a–c: Depth of reduction in occlusal plane

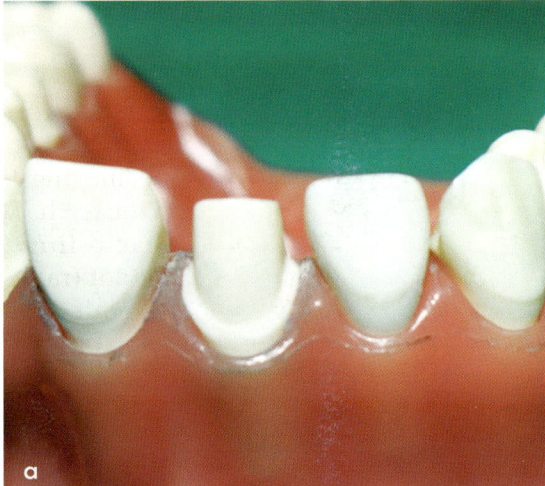

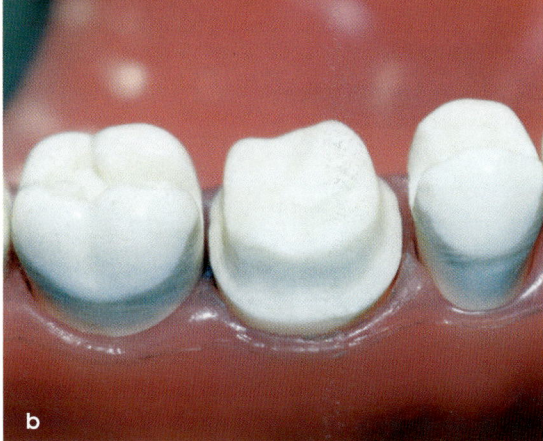

Figs 4.3a and b: Geometric form of prepared tooth

mised in non-vital teeth. The less reduction will lead to over-contouring of restoration, subsequently resulting in periodontal problems.

The depth of grooves and other retentive features should also be considered (depth should be more than width for grooves and for slots, the width should be more than depth). Overprepared teeth should be modified with creation of grooves and/or slots, depending upon the need. The reduction should definitely be uniform to achieve better results. Sometimes, the depth of reduction is increased, especially in all-ceramic restorations, to achieve the desired color and translucency of the ceramic (1.0–1.5 mm is ideal depth in all-ceramic restorations).

e. Location and Form of Finish Lines

The margins of the restoration should be uniform and follow the gingival contour (Figs 4.5a–c). It is established that supra-gingival finish lines enhance periodontal health; however, subgingival finish lines are preferred in case of undermining caries or to achieve sufficient surface area for the restoration. When subgingival finish line is required, extension up to epithelial attachment is to be avoided. The restoration must be properly contoured and exhibit good marginal fit. The soft tissues should be protected carefully during tooth preparation.

The form of finish lines depend upon the material to be used for fabrication of indirect restorations. For all-metal crowns, 1.0 mm shoulder or heavy chamfer is considered adequate, whereas for porcelain fused to metal crowns, the depth is increased to 1.75–2.0 mm. In case of all-ceramics, 1.0 mm uniform shoulder is preferred.

f. Auxiliary Retentive Features

The auxiliary retentive features are created to achieve better resistance and retention form (Figs 4.6a–e). Grooves, when indicated, are placed extracoronally on buccal and lingual

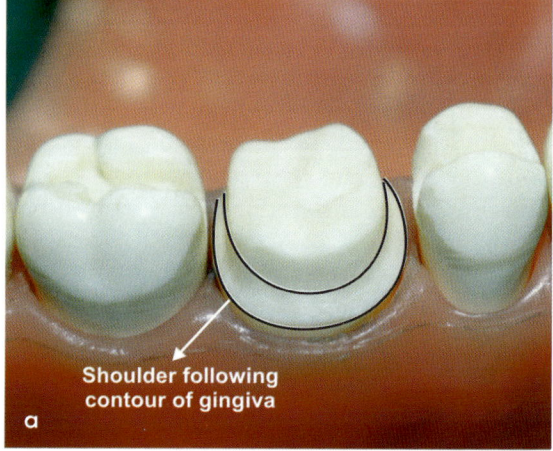

Shoulder following contour of gingiva

a

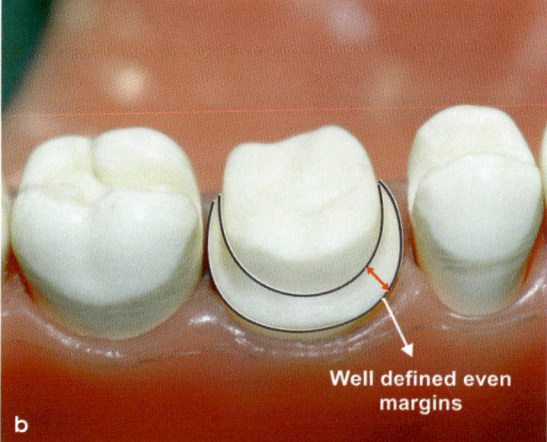

Well defined even margins

b

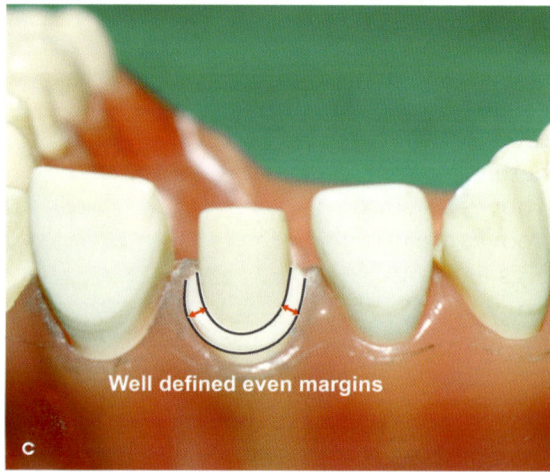

Well defined even margins

c

Figs 4.5a–c: Location of finish lines: even margins following gingival contours

surfaces of the teeth (preferably molars) (Fig. 4.6c). The tooth structure where groove

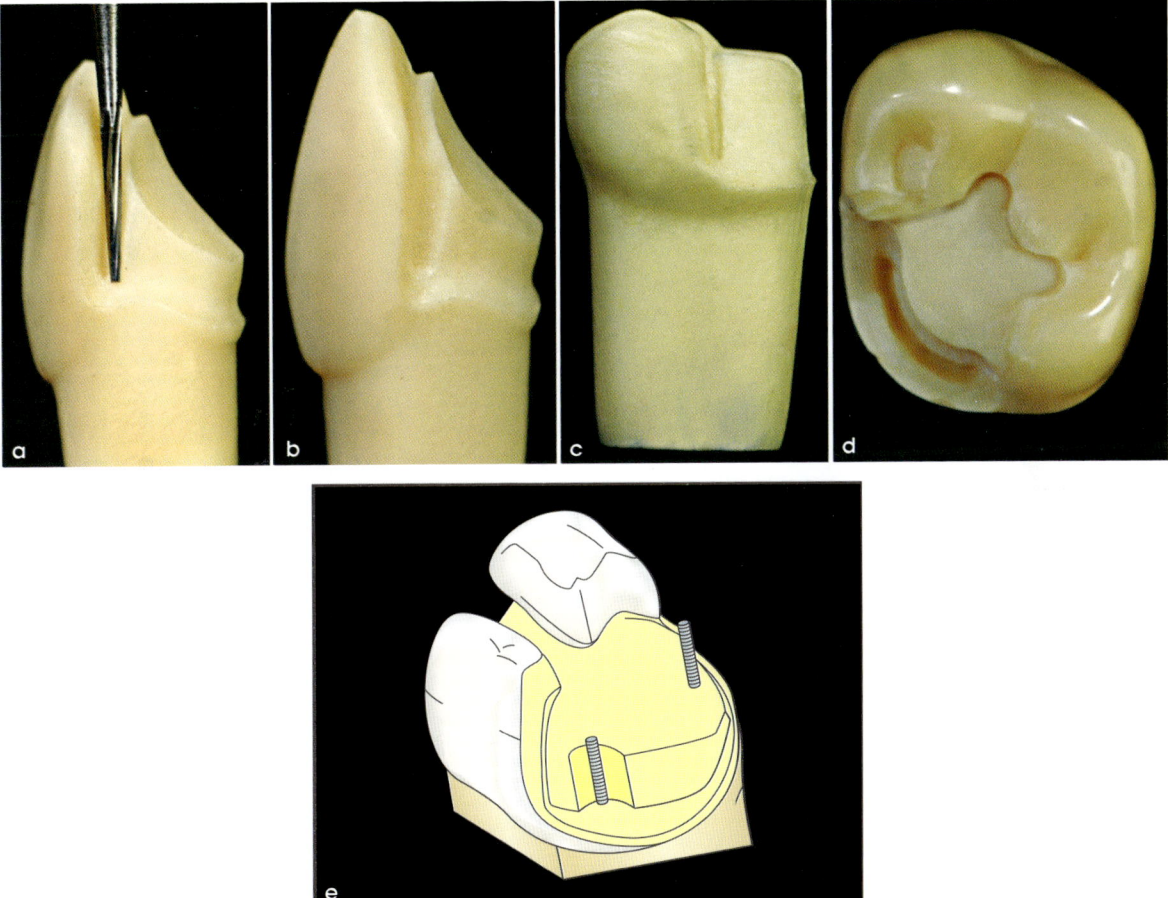

Figs 4.6a–e: Auxiliary retentive features. a, b. proximal groove in anterior tooth, c. proximal groove in posterior tooth, d. slot preparation, e. pin placement

is to be placed will withstand the torquing forces to prevent rotation of the restoration; therefore, it should be sound (always create grooves in sound tooth structure). Proximal grooves are usually preferred in anterior teeth (Figs 4.6a and b). In intracoronal restoration, grooves are placed at axial-proximal box wall line angles at the expense of dentin. Slots, if required, are placed at the occlusal wall or sometimes at the cervical wall (Fig. 4.6d). Other retentive features, such as pins, are placed inside the dentino-enamel junction (minimum 1.0 mm within dentin) (Fig. 4.6e). In case, more than one pin is required, each pin should be surrounded by minimum of 1.0 mm of dentin.

g. Assessing Final Form of the Preparation

All line angles should be rounded, since sharp angles create stress concentration (Figs 4.7a–d). The rounded line angles also provide the requisite structural durability to the restoration. The round line angle facilitates laboratory fabrication of all indirect restorations, apart from facilitating impression pouring.

It is established that smooth tooth surfaces in the preparation enhance marginal fit of the restoration. The surface roughness may improve binding to some extent, but smooth surface is considered beneficial for the long-term success of the restoration.

The bevels are placed according to the need of the material (inverted bevel is preferred on

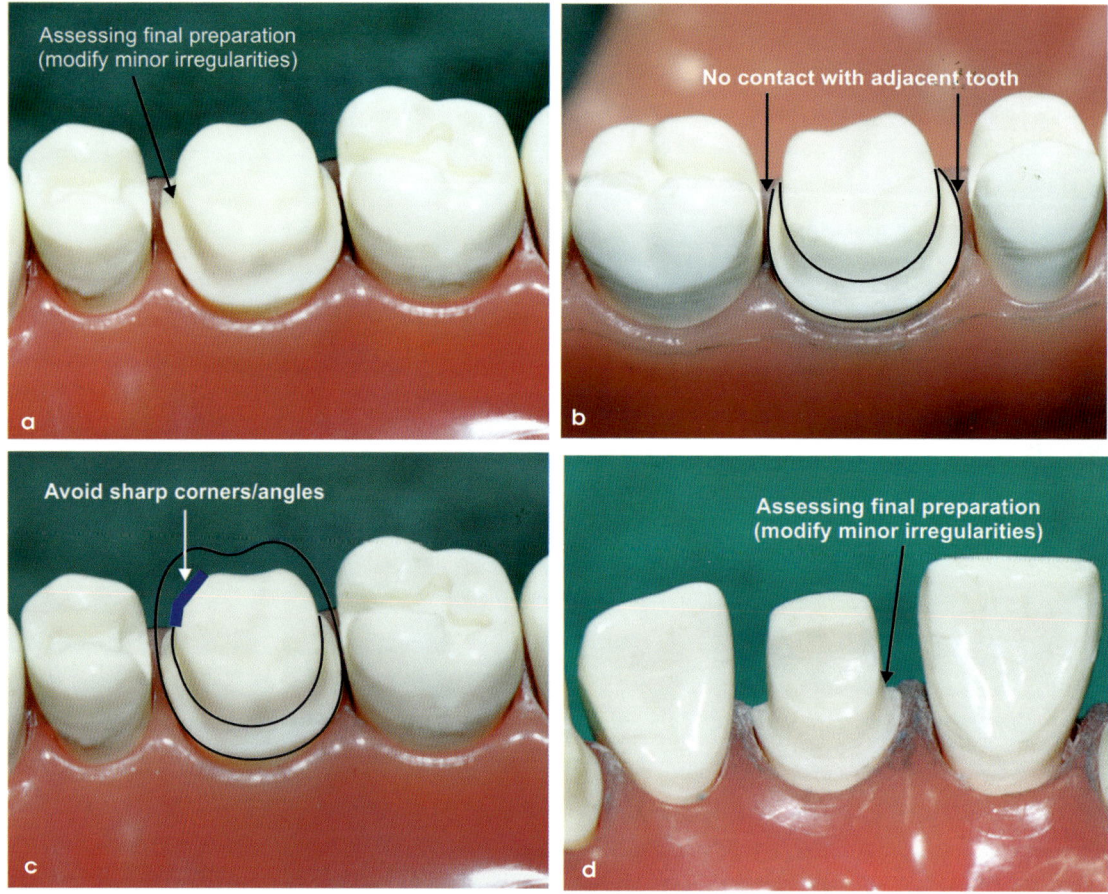

Figs 4.7a–d: Assessing final form of preparation

the labial shoulder in porcelain fused to metal crowns).

h. Confirm Uniformity of Preparation before Impression Making

The prepared tooth is analyzed, either directly or after making a cast, as regard uniform depth of reduction, uniform finish line all around and also the requisite convergence on the axial walls (Figs 4.8a–d). Usually, visual inspection with mirror is sufficient; however, inspection of cast from occlusal direction, with one eye closed (monocular vision) is considered more effective. Visual inspection is recommended from a distance of 30 cm and with one eye. For indirect vision, the mouth mirror should be held at an angle and half a inch above the preparation. Undercutting or overcutting and also the deficient finish line, if any, is to be analyzed and modified accordingly before impression making.

The tooth preparation is carried out keeping in mind three main factors. The factors are:

A. Biological factors (affect the health of oral tissues)
B. Mechanical factors (affect the integrity and durability of the restoration)
C. Esthetic factors (affect the appearance of the patient)

A. Biological Factors

Once the tooth is planned for any type of preparation, care should be taken to preserve gingival, periodontal and pulpal tissues along

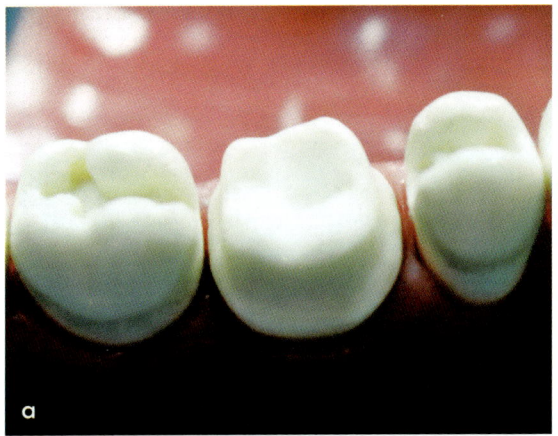

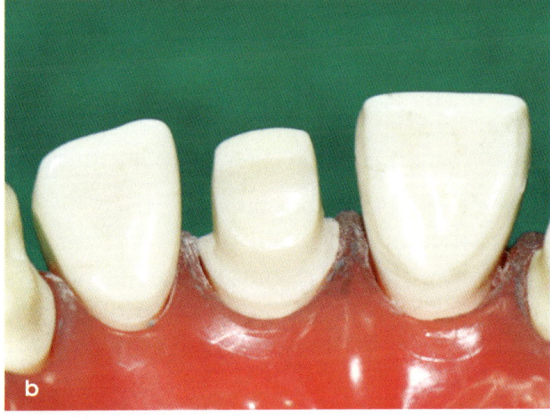

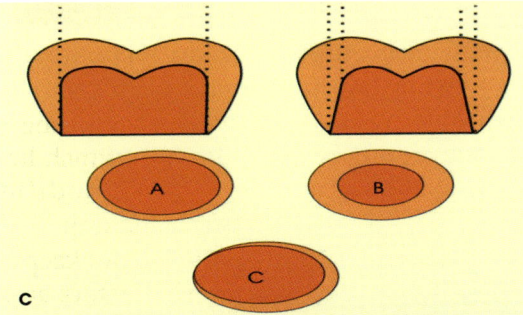

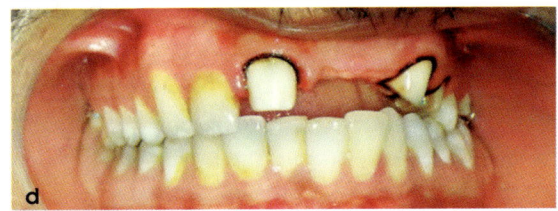

Figs 4.8a–d: a,b,c. Confirm uniformity of preparation before impression making, d. gingival retraction

Guidelines summarized as:
- The permissible occlusal convergence for indirect restorations is 10°. In case of ceramic/composite restorations, the taper is increased to 16–20° (accepted rule is less taper, more retention).
- The height of axial walls, parallel with the opposing walls, should be minimum 3.0 mm. In case of molars, because of increased taper, the recommended height is 4.0 mm.
- The accepted ratio of incisor/occlusal/cervical dimension of the prepared tooth with facio-lingual dimension should be at least 0.4 or higher for all teeth.
- The facio-proximal and linguo-proximal corners are rounded for better resistance form.
- Short teeth after preparation or teeth without circumferential morphology should be modified with auxiliary retentive features, such as grooves, slots, etc.
- Grooves should preferably be placed on buccal and lingual surfaces of posterior teeth and proximal surface of anterior teeth (depth of groove should be more than width).
- Supragingival finish line is preferred; however, sub-gingival finish lines are indicated for increasing the surface area of the preparation or when caries extending up to the sub-gingival area (In no case, the epithelial attachment area should be disturbed).
- 1.0 mm shoulder is preferred for all-ceramic and for all-metal preparations (Heavy chamfer can be given in metals having some malleability). 1.7–2.0 mm shoulder is must for porcelain fused to metal (PFM) crowns (Depending upon the physical properties of underlying metal, chamfer can be given on the lingual side).
- The depth of occlusal, proximal and buccal/lingual reduction depend upon the material used (1.0 mm is adequate for metals, whereas 1.5–2.0 mm is for porcelain fused to metal and 1.0–1.25 mm for all ceramic restorations).
- All sharp angles are rounded to avoid stress concentration.
- Bevels are created depending upon the need.
- The surface of the teeth should be smooth for better marginal fit.
- Any undercut, amount of taper and uniformity of reduction is evaluated, both clinically and also on cast, before impression making.

with other soft tissues, which are liable to be injured during preparation. These features are called biological factors.

The biological factors are:

1. Prevention of Damage to Adjacent Teeth

The proximal reduction should be carried out in a way that the adjacent tooth should not be damaged. During preparation of proximal surfaces, a thin lip or fin of enamel should be kept intact at the contact area with the adjacent tooth. This thin fin should be removed gently with hand instruments later. A thin metal strip can also be placed inter-proximally so as the bur/diamond points should not touch the adjacent proximal surface.

2. Prevention of Damage to Oral Tissues (cheeks, lips and tongue)

The damage to oral tissues (cheeks, lips and the tongue) can be prevented by using appropriate isolation methods, viz. rubber dam, suction devices, mouth mirror, etc.

3. Pulp Protection

The underlying pulp is to be protected from external stimuli and its vitality must be preserved during and after the tooth preparation. The irritants, which can affect the pulp, are:

- Mechanical irritants due to grinding procedures
- Heat produced during cutting and grinding
- Chemical irritants like saliva, drugs or any other ingredient of food
- Bacterial irritants which may affect pulp through exposed dentinal tubules

   i. *Painless tooth preparation:* Utmost care is mandatory to avoid any type of irritation to pulp (irritant/stimulus is responded as pain). The pulp protection features involved during tooth preparation are:
  - The patient should be mentally prepared and psychologically motivated to undergo minor implications associated with tooth preparation. The psychological motivation depends upon the age and sex of the patient.

The patients can be shown tooth preparation on the casts so as to minimize the fear factor. Preoperative and postoperative photographs can also be useful.

- New and sharp instruments should be used along with intermittent cutting so as to minimize heat generation.
- The cutting field should be kept wet; coolant, water spray should be used.
- Undue pressure during cutting procedure should be avoided.
- Frictional heat produced during finishing and polishing should be kept minimum.
- The cutting instruments should be sterilized thoroughly so that bacteria should not enter the open tubules.
- Local anesthesia can be used, if need be.

A few authors prefer administering local anesthesia before tooth preparation as it enhances patient's comfort during tooth preparation and also gingival retraction. Local anesthesia also leads to reduced salivation and minimizes anxiety. However, authors who do not prefer local anesthesia, opine that anesthesia may block vital responses from pulp, compromising the depth of preparation.

   ii. *Maintaining pulp vitality after tooth preparation:*
  - The prepared tooth should be washed with 3.0% hydrogen peroxide followed by saline solution.
  - After gently drying, the prepared tooth should be coated with copal varnish, which will seal the dentinal tubules against ingress of bacteria and saliva.
  - Intracoronal preparations can be sealed with zinc oxide eugenol and in extracoronal, temporary crowns are given (Refer to Chapter 11). In case, temporary crowns cannot be given

because of certain reasons, the area should be covered with periodontal packs.

- All restorations, may be interim, should be adjusted in occlusion. The functional occlusion should be checked thoroughly to minimize the mechanical trauma due to incorrect occlusion.

4. Gingival and Periodontal Protection

The maintenance of gingival and periodontal health is important for longevity of the restoration. Healthy periodontium along the restoration also provides better esthetics. The over-contoured and under-contoured restorations should be avoided, since both these features are injurious to gingival health.

i. *Protection of gingiva during tooth preparation*

- Retraction of gingival tissue with any means (mechanical, chemical and/or surgical) should avoid injury to the gingiva during tooth preparation. During preparation of gingival finish lines, especially below the gingiva, end-cutting burs are preferred for extending the finish lines subgingivally. In case, the surface area permits, the finish lines in extracoronal preparations should preferably be kept above the gingiva.

- The supragingival margins are best suited for the marginal adaptation of the restoration especially inlays and onlays; however, subgingival margins are preferred in certain clinical conditions, viz. esthetic needs (especially in anterior teeth), caries extending subgingivally and teeth having insufficient surface area (the axial extension needs to be extended subgingivally to achieve the required surface area).

- The subgingival finish line should be in between the epithelial attachment and the crest of gingiva. The biological width area (defined as the dimension of soft tissues which is attached to the portion of tooth coronal to the crest of the alveolar bone: Sum total of epithelial attachment and the connective tissue attachment. The average of dimension of biological width area is 2.04 mm; 0.97 mm epithelial attachment and 1.07 mm connective tissue attachment) should not be disturbed. The margins of the preparation should not be kept at the gingival crest area, since most of the plaque activity is initiated there, which may lead to secondary caries. Such margins are also a continuous source of mechanical irritation of the gingiva. The over-contoured restorations, especially at the cervical third area and line angles, should be avoided.

- The inter-dental col area should also be taken care of during and after the preparation of extracoronal restorations. The proximal finish line should approximate the gingival papillary outline rather than keeping it in a straight line. The anatomical contour of gingival papilla must be followed during proximal preparation to avoid injury to the epithelial attachments.

- In case of metal-ceramic crowns, the depth/width of the shoulder should be extended uniformly till its planned position along the proximal areas, without injuring the inter-proximal gingiva. The over-contouring of the restoration, especially at the line angles will interfere with the physiological gingival stimulation. Such restorations are not esthetically pleasing either.

ii. *Protection of gingiva after tooth preparation*
   The gingival tissue should be protected till the placement of final restoration. The following features should be considered:

- The margins of the restoration should be smooth and even; the uneven margins will keep impinging the gingiva and may hinder with the adaptation of restoration. The restoration if not properly adapted at the margins will result in secondary caries, tooth sensitivity and other associated complications.
- During impression making, the gingival tissues should not be impinged upon (especially with copper band impressions, the band should be shaped according to the contour of gingiva so as not to injure the adjoining tissues).
- The occlusion must be in harmony even with temporary/interim restorations. The cuspal inclines should be maintained properly so as to enable the periodontal fibers to withstand the forces in a better way.

5. Conservative Tooth Preparation

The tooth preparation in indirect restorations may require ample amount of cutting of tooth structure. The thickness of remaining dentin after tooth preparation is inversely proportional to the pulpal response. Overcutting leading to less remaining dentin, in any form and any area, is harmful to the health of pulp (utmost care should be exercised while preparing the vital teeth). The tooth structure is to be conserved by all means.

Selecting partial veneer crown instead of full veneer crown, uniform and planar reduction of teeth, supragingival margins (avoid unnecessary gingival extension), appropriate finish lines and less taper of axial walls are the features which help maintaining the future health of the prepared tooth.

6. Margin Adaptation of Restoration

The margins of an extracoronal indirect restoration play important role in the longevity of the restoration, as well as longevity of the prepared tooth. The tooth-restoration interface in a cemented restoration is always a potential site for recurrent caries because of dissolution of cement at the site. The dissolution of cement exposes dentinal tubules leading to hot and cold sensations, which are clinically disturbing to the patient. Poor margin adaptability is considered as the main cause of failure, not only in restoration, but also of the prepared tooth. Since, the process of leakage is slow, subsequently the damage of the underlying tooth, the margin adaptability is to be thoroughly analyzed at the time of placement of the restoration and also periodically.

It has been established that a gap of 50–100 μm is left at the interface even after precisely fabricating the restoration. The luting cement exposure is minimized at the junction by selecting appropriate restorative materials, judicious margin designs and also the less soluble luting agents. The process of seating of the restoration clinically also affects the margin adaptability.

7. Occlusal Considerations

In case of tilted or supra-erupted teeth, the occlusal plane should be given more importance than conservation of tooth structure. Incorrect occlusal plane can lead to traumatic occlusal forces, which are not conducive to the success of the restoration. Sometimes, it may necessitate endodontic treatment of the involved tooth to bring the occlusal plane at the desired level.

8. Preventing Tooth Fracture

The large intracoronal restorations (inlay) may create wedging action leading to fracture of teeth. The proper isthmus width of the inlay is to be maintained to avoid such fractures. Alternatively, the weaker cusps are covered, making extracoronal (onlay) preparation. Full veneer crown restorations are considered as an effective way of preventing tooth fracture, since full crowns hold the cusps together.

B. Mechanical Factors

The features responsible for resistance and retention form, structural durability and marginal integrity of the restoration are called mechanical factors.

The mechanical factors are described under the following heads:
1. Resistance and retention form
2. Structural durability
3. Margin integrity

1. Resistance and Retention Form

Lateral forces tend to displace the restoration by causing rotation around gingival margin. Resistance form involves the features of a tooth preparation that enhance the stability of restoration and resist dislodgement along an axis other than the path of placement. It prevents dislodgement of a restoration by forces directed in an apical, oblique or horizontal direction, e.g. mastication and para-functional activity cause substantial horizontal or oblique forces.

The following factors affect resistance and retention form of all the indirect restorations (inlays, onlays and crowns).

a. Magnitude of dislodging forces

The functional forces (vertical and oblique) coupled with sticky food tend to dislodge the restoration. The magnitude of the dislodging forces depends on the stickiness of food, working and lateral movement of the jaws and surface area of the restoration being pulled.

- More tapered a preparation, less is the resistance.
- If there is no taper, the resisting area covers half the axial wall.
- In ideal taper, the resistance area covers less than half the axial wall.
- In over-tapered preparations, small resisting area is present near the occlusal surface.
- Permissible taper of a preparation is directly proportional to height: width ratio.
  Taper that permits an effective resisting area for a preparation in which height equals width is double than in a preparation where height is only half of the width.

The resistance and retention form is better achieved in normal occlusion (axially directed forces). The resistance decreases in case of habits such as, pipe smoking and bruxism (oblique forces) followed by eccentric interferences and anterior guidance.

b. Geometry of the tooth preparation

The retention of indirect restoration depends mainly on geometric form of the preparation. The geometrical form of the tooth is prepared according to the need of the selected material for indirect restoration.

The geometrical forms generally responsible for retention are:

i. *Taper:* A basic requirement of tooth preparations for the intracoronal and extracoronal cast restoration is that the cavity walls must diverge occlusally. This concept of taper facilitates the removal of wax pattern and subsequent insertion of casting. As long as the taper is small, the movement of the cemented restoration will be effectively restrained by limited path of withdrawal. As the taper increases, there will be free movement of the restoration along the path of withdrawal and consequently retention will decrease.

Each intracoronal and extracoronal preparation has a line of draw that describes the path of insertion and removal of the casting, which determines the axis of taper. The lines of draw for class I and II preparations parallel the long axis of the tooth and for class V preparations the lines are perpendicular to the long axis of the tooth.

Line of draw intersects the angle formed by convergence of the tapered cavity walls to a point of their intersection. The angle of intersection is the convergence angle and describes the amount of taper upon opposing cavity walls. A range of 2–6° taper is used since it provides adequate retention and convenience of seating of the casting.

The axial length of the preparation influences the amount of taper. For longer preparation, higher angle of taper can be given. For shorter preparation, a very steep taper angle is required.

The taper should not be so great as to lose the frictional grip between tooth and restoration. At the same time, it should be sufficient to allow complete seating of restoration in/on the prepared tooth.

ii. *Surface area and ratio of tooth height: Base of preparation:* The retention is dependent on the length of the path of withdrawal collectively on the surface area in contact. Therefore, restorations with long axial walls are more retentive than those with short axial walls; for example, anterior restorations are more retentive than posterior restorations. The retention of a complete crown is double than that of partial coverage crowns. Grooves do aid in retention, since they limit the path of withdrawal.

Resistance form is easily obtained on anterior teeth, although it is more difficult to obtain with posterior teeth because they are shorter and wider, making the height-to-base ratio less. A wider preparation has a greater retention but a narrow tooth can have greater resistance to tipping. Because of smaller diameter, a tangent line falls low on the wall opposite to axis of rotation resulting in a large resisting area.

Weak resistance can be enhanced by placing vertical grooves/ boxes/ pinholes because these features shorten the arc of rotation and hence increase the resistance area (Fig. 4.9).

iii. *Stress concentration:* It is established that a retentive failure occurs due to cohesive failure in the cement layer, because the strength of the cement is less than the induced stresses. These stresses are concentrated around junction of the axial and occlusal surfaces, which may not be uniform throughout the cement layer.

The geometric configuration of tooth structure must place the cement in compression to provide the necessary resistance.

Leverage occurs when the line of action of a force passes outside the supporting tooth structure. If the force passes within the margin of a crown, no tipping of the restoration occurs when compared to the line of action passing outside the margins of the restoration.

For example, wide occlusal table of restoration, crowns on tipped teeth, retainers for cantilever bridge and functional/ para-functional force at an oblique angle (Fig. 4.10).

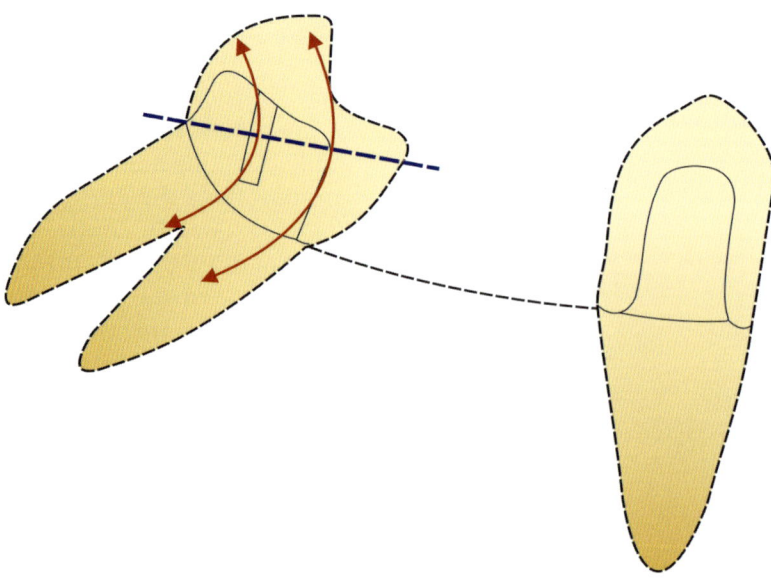

Fig. 4.9: Placement of a groove shortens the arc of rotation and increases the resistance area

c. *Type of preparation:* Partial coverage restoration may have less resistance than a complete crown because it has no buccal resistance area.

A partial veneer crown which has no grooves offers a little resistance to rotation. The axial symmetry of a complete veneer crown preparation may allow rotation of the restoration.

d. *Roughness of the surfaces being cemented:* A smooth internal surface of a restoration decreases retention since the cement does not adhere properly. Air abrasion of the internal surface with 50 µm alumina particle increases retention. Since traditional cements are non-adhesive, the grains of the cement help increasing the frictional resistance between cavity wall and the restoration. This is analogous to the effect of dust particles within the machinery. They do not have specific adhesion to metal, but do increase friction between the sliding metal parts. Acid etching of the tooth surface and that of the inner surface of the restoration do aid in retention with certain luting agents.

e. *Restorative materials being cemented:* The adhesion of cement with the metal depends upon the reactivity of the metal. The more reactive the alloy is, the more will be adhesion with the luting cement. Therefore, base metal alloys are better retained than less reactive noble and high noble metals.

f. *Physical properties of luting agent:* The luting agents because of their low tensile strength do not offer much retention to the restoration. However, adhesive resin cements do aid in retention to some extent. The cement is effective only if the restoration has a single path of withdrawal, i.e. the tooth is prepared in a manner so as to restrain the free movement of the restoration.

Resistance to deformation is affected by physical properties of the luting agent, such as compressive strength and modulus of elasticity. The order of luting agents in terms of resistance to displacement is

Adhesive resin > Glass ionomer cement > Zinc phosphate cement > Polycarboxylate > Zinc oxide eugenol

The effect of film thickness of luting agents on retention form is not confirmed.

Methods to Analyze Resistance Form

If a line is drawn from the center of rotation perpendicular to the cement film on the opposite wall of the preparation, the point where the line intersects the cement film is known as tangent point.

If the tangent points of all the arcs of rotation around a given axis are connected, they form the tangent line. The area above the tangent line is resisting area. Rotation is prevented by any areas of the tooth preparation that are placed in compression and are called resistance area. To have effective resistance, the tangent line should extend at least halfway down the preparation.

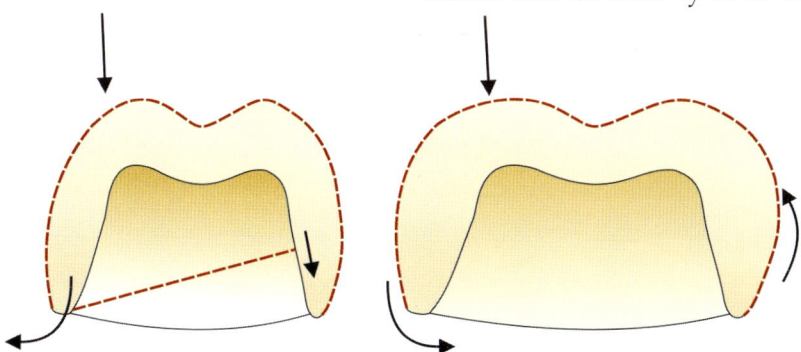

Fig. 4.10: Wide occlusal table of restoration increases leverage and decreases resistance

The techniques employed for analyzing the resistance form are:

i. *Lewis method* employs a perpendicular drawn from one margin as centre to the opposite wall. The area above the point where the perpendicular intersects this opposite wall, is resistance area (Fig. 4.11).

ii. *Zuckerman circle* is drawn with centre of the base of tooth preparation as origin. The points outside the circle are resistance areas, whereas points inside this circle do not resist dislodgement (Fig. 4.11).

iii. *Weed circle* considers width of base as radius of a circle drawn on one margin of tooth preparation. If all the points are kept inside the circle, less or no resistance area results in posterior teeth (Fig. 4.11).

2. Structural Durability

A restoration must have sufficient strength to prevent permanent deformation during function. The ability of a restoration to withstand destruction due to external forces is known as structural durability.

Factors affecting structural durability are:
a. Adequate tooth reduction
    i. Occlusal reduction
    ii. Axial reduction
    iii. Functional cusp bevel
b. Selection of the alloy
c. Metal-ceramic framework design
d. Margin design

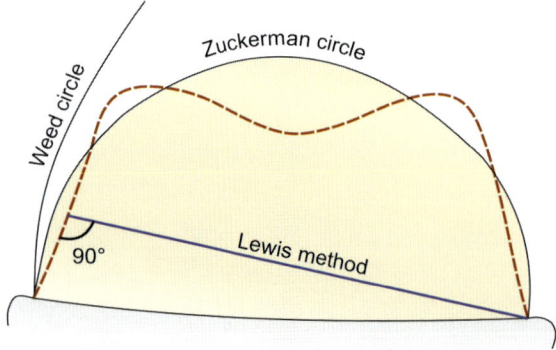

Fig. 4.11: Three methods to analyze resistance form of tooth preparation

a. *Adequate tooth reduction*

i. *Occlusal reduction:* Occlusal reduction should be uniform and planar. This ensures sufficient occlusal clearance and preservation of tooth structure.

Sufficient bulk of metal and/or ceramic provides strength to the restoration, which is achieved by providing adequate occlusal clearance. Occlusal thickness varies with different restorative materials

Gold alloys—1.5 mm (functional cusp) and 1.0 mm (non-functional cusp)

Base metal alloys—1.5 mm (functional cusp) and 1.0 mm (non-functional cusp)

Porcelain fused to metal crowns—2.0 mm (functional cusp) and 1.5 mm (non-functional cusp)

All-ceramic crowns—1.0–1.5 mm uniform thickness

The occlusal equilibration with opposing teeth is also mandatory, for example, plunger cusps should be reduced accordingly. All the line and point angles should be rounded. Any groove in the center of the occlusal surfaces should be avoided to prevent stress concentration and to distribute the forces over a larger surface area. The occlusal or incisal offset can be given on partial veneer crown preparation to provide space for the truss of metal, providing reinforcement.

ii. *Axial reduction:* Inadequate axial reduction may lead to a bulbous, over-contoured restoration which will have a disastrous effect on periodontium. Adequate axial reduction, both in depth and taper, is mandatory for sufficient resistance and structural durability.

iii. *Functional cusp bevel:* Functional cusp bevel is a bevel on the lingual inclines of the maxillary palatal cusps and the buccal inclines of the mandibular buccal cusps (functional cusps) providing space for an adequate bulk of metal in the area of heavy occlusal contact (Figs 4.12a and b). If the bevel is not placed on the functional cusp, it may lead to perforation in the casting because of thin margin or over-

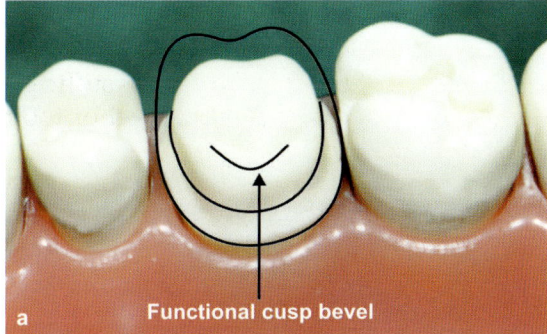

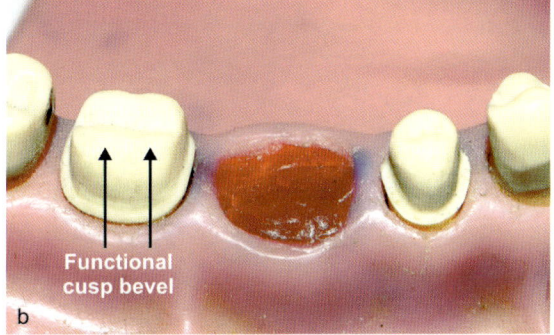

Fig. 4.12a and b: Functional cusp bevel

contouring on that surface hindering with the occlusion.

If an attempt is made to obtain space for an adequate bulk in a normally contoured preparation, it will result in over inclination of the buccal surface, which will destroy excessive tooth structure while lessening retention.

b. *Selection of the alloy:* The metal to be used as the restorative material must be selected on the basis of superior physical properties and also its strength to bear the challenges of oral environment.

c. *Metal ceramic framework design:* The minimum thickness of the metal should be 0.2–1.0 mm (Gold thickness can be 0.2–0.3 mm, base metals should be 0.5–1.0 mm). Also, the substructure must support an even thickness of the porcelain veneer (1.0–1.5 mm).

Metal should preferably be in the area of the centric stop to enhance the durability of the restoration and occlusal contacts need to be 1.5–2.0 mm away from the porcelain- metal

junction. Cut-back for porcelain-metal junction should be 90° or greater.

d. *Margin design:* The various types of margins, which can be employed in a cast restoration, are depicted in Figs 4.13a–g. The relevant indications, advantages and disadvantages are tabulated in Table 4.1. However, the bevel, chamfer and the shoulder are commonly used margins. The difference between chamfer and shoulder is that chamfer is less than 0.5 mm wide and is rounded while shoulder is 0.75 mm to 1.0 mm wide and sharp. Another form of finish line, the heavy chamfer (0.75 mm depth with obtuse angle) is also employed in certain cases of all-ceramic restorations. Chamfer is mostly given on the lingual sides while shoulder is given on the labial sides. Alternatively, the chamfer is given where less bulk is required and the metal is malleable, whereas the shoulder is given where more bulk is required and the metal is not malleable.

Knife edge/feather edge finish lines should be avoided.

3. Margin Integrity

Poor margin adaptability is considered as the main cause of failure of the restoration. It also affects the health of the underlying tooth. Since, the process of leakage of luting agents is slow at the margins, subsequently the damage of the underlying tooth; the margin adaptability is to be thoroughly analyzed at the time of placement of the restoration and also periodically. Indirect restorations with

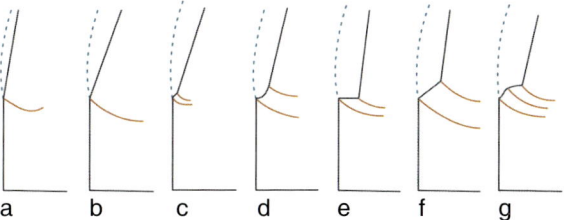

Figs 4.13a–g: Different margin designs: (a) Feather edge; (b) Chisel; (c) Bevel; (d) Chamfer; (e) Shoulder; (f) Sloped shoulder; (g) Shoulder with bevel

Table 4.1: Margin designs

	Advantage	Disadvantage	Indications
1. Feather edge	Conservative	Does not provide sufficient bulk	Not recommended
2. Chisel edge	Conservative	Location of margin is difficult to control	Occasionally on tilted teeth
3. Bevel	Removes unsupported enamel, allows finishing of metal	Extends preparation into sulcus if used on apical margin	Facial margin of maxillary partial coverage restorations
4. Chamfer	Distinct margin, adequate bulk, easier to control	Care needed to avoid un-supported lip of enamel	Lingual margin of cast metal restorations and metal ceramic crowns
5. Shoulder	Bulk of restorative material	Less conservative	Labial margins of complete ceramic crown and metal ceramic crowns
6. Sloped shoulder	Bulk of material, advantages of bevel	Less conservative	Facial margin of metal ceramic crown
7. Shoulder with bevel	Bulk of material, advantages of bevel	Less conservative, extend gingival margins apically	Facial margin of posterior metal ceramic crowns with supragingival margin

poor marginal adaptability should be repeated.

C. Esthetic Factors

The appearance of patient is assessed prior to the planning and initiating the treatment, i.e. show of teeth and gums during speech, smile and laugh. Patient's expectations are also noted and incorporated in planning. The indirect restorations, especially the anterior ones, should improve the overall esthetics of the patient. The attractiveness of the restoration is characterized by several factors including both teeth and the surrounding tissues.

Esthetic characteristics are categorized as vertical features and horizontal features. Vertical features pertain to incisor display and the gingival display. Inadequate incisor display can be because of limited lip mobility, and/or short clinical crown. The gingival margin in relation to the upper lip during smiling is also an important feature. Usually, younger patients show more teeth and gingiva during smile than do adults. The horizontal features pertain to buccal corridors (the space between facial surfaces of posterior teeth and the corners of lips during smiling).

Another feature, which should be looked into, is the 'smile arc' (relationship of the curvature of incisal edges of the maxillary incisors and canines to the curvature of the lower lip during smiling). Ideally, the maxillary incisal edge curvature is parallel to the curvature of the lower lip. A flat smile arc is considered unesthetic.

The gingival display or the gummy smile can be because of short teeth, normal teeth or long teeth.

i. In case of short teeth (worn out teeth), if the crown:root ratio is favourable, crown lengthening procedures are undertaken to reveal the teeth. If crown:root ratio is unfavourable, orthodontic extrusion should be the corrective measure. In certain cases of delayed active eruption, crown lengthening with osseous re-contouring is necessary.

ii. In case of teeth with normal height, surgical correction of gums should be sufficient; if not, orthodontic intrusion should be carried out in consultation with the patient.

iii. In case of teeth longer than usual, orthodontic intrusion, surgical correction and mucogingival grafts may be required.

The other gingival features affecting esthetics are:

a. *Gingival zenith (apical aspect of free gingival margin):* The marginal zenith position has always been an important component of a beautiful smile. The central incisors display distal gingival zenith from the vertical midline by 1.0 mm. The lateral incisor shows a deviation of gingival zenith by 0.5 mm, whereas in canines, the distal deviation is 0.3 mm. The gingival zenith vis-à-vis anterior teeth help create desired axial inclination of the tooth and the restoration.

b. *Recession:* Gingival recession is the most disturbing situation, as regards gaining esthetics in extracoronal restorations, especially in anterior teeth. Many factors lead to recession, viz. periodontal problems, iatrogenic trauma to the gingival tissues and over ambitious gingival retractions. Numerous surgical methods are employed to cover these areas of recession by free gingival grafts. Alternatively, porcelain in that particular color is applied onto the recession area (radicular margin of the restoration). To restore the normal height of the restoration in teeth with recession, an acrylic or silicone mask can be used as a removable prosthesis over elongated crowns.

c. *Height and symmetry of papilla:* The height and symmetry of papilla depends upon the contact point/area, morphology of interproximal surfaces and also the tooth form.

The maintenance of papillary height and symmetry is mandatory during tooth preparation. Care should be taken to avoid traumatizing the interproximal col during preparation. The placement of the interproximal margin below the level of col would result in loss of papilla height.

d. *Color of gingiva:* The color of gingiva varies for population of different ethnic backgrounds. The usual color ranges from coral pink to pink along with certain melanin pigmentation.

The color of gingiva is difficult to measure due to their elasticity and irregular morphology. Three main methods are used for measuring gingival color in dental studies: Visual, photometric color and spectrometric. The determination of gingival color is carried out with subjective visual observation due to its convenience and low cost. However, many factors can interfere with visual measurement such as lightning condition, experience, age and eye fatigue. Photometric method has limitations inherent to photographic procedure such as lightning control, film emulsion and film processing. The most precise color data can be obtained by using photometric measurement. But the ease of use in clinical setting makes visual method the most common choice. There are a few shade guides available for gingival color matching. Even the available shade guides have high color difference between gingival shade guide and gingiva. There has been insufficient information about distribution and classification of gingival color to develop an ideal shade guide.

Root canal treated teeth may blacken the crown as well as root of the tooth. The black or dark root color may reflect through the gums. It is advisable to bleach such teeth before placing the restoration. Usually very light shades are not preferred in dark gingival color. The color of skin should also be considered while deciding the color of the restoration.

e. *Height of gingival contour:* The gingival contour around the anterior teeth is also a feature in maintaining esthetics of the restorations of that area. The upper lip covering 1.0–2.0 mm of the gingival contour margin is considered ideal during smiling. The gingival contour can be mal-positioned in delayed eruption cases and also in certain periodontal problems. Such problems are treated by orthodontic positioning of the tooth in the arch or surgically repositioning the height of contour of the gingival tissues around the teeth.

The height and width ratio of the anterior teeth, especially the incisors, vis-à-vis the gingival contour height should also to be looked into. The ideal 78:22 ratio of height and width should be maintained in anterior restorations. Shortening or elongating the height, simulating the ideal ratio, improves esthetics of the restorations.

Summarily, not only should we be concerned with the health of the surrounding tissues, but also the esthetics as well. The margins and the contours of the restorations affect the ultimate tissue health and esthetics; utmost care necessitates achieving the esthetics in indirect restorations.

Bibliography

1. Analoui M, Papkosta E and Cochran M. Designing visually optimal shade guides. J. Prosthet. Dent.: 2004;92:371–6.

2. Blair FM, Wassell RW and Steele JG. Crowns and other extracoronal restorations: Preparations for full veneer crowns. Br. Dent. J.: 2002;192:561–71.

3. Brandau HE, Yaman P and Molvar M. Effect of restorative procedures for a porcelain jacket crown on gingival health and height. Am. J. Dent.: 1988;1:119–22.

4. Donovan TE and Chee WL. Cervical margin design with contemporary esthetic restorations. Dent. Cl. North Am.: 2004;48:417–31.

5. Donovan TE and Cho GC. Soft tissue management with metal-ceramic and all-ceramic crowns. J. Calif. Dent. Assoc.: 1998;26:107–12.

6. Dutra MB, Ritter DE, Borgatoo A, Derech CA and Rocha R. Influence of gingival exposure on the smile esthetics. Dent. Press J. Orthodont.: 2011;16:111–8.

7. Gilboe DB and Thayer KE. Beveled shoulder concept: full gold crown preparation. J. Can. Dent. Assoc.: 1980;46:519–23.

8. Goodacre CJ. Designing tooth preparations for optimal success. Dent. Cl. N. Am.: 2004;48:359–85.

9. Goodacre CJ, Wayne VC and Aquilino SA. Tooth preparations for complete crowns: An art form based on scientific principles. J. Prosthet. Dent.: 2001;85:363–76.

10. Heydecke G, Schnitzer S and Turp JC. The color of human gingiva and mucosa: visual measurement and description of distribution. Clin. Oral Investig.: 2005;9:49–57.

11. Huang JW, Chen WC and Huang TK. Using a spectrophotometric study of human gingival color distribution to develop a shade guide. J. Dent.: 2011;39:e11–6.

12. Hunter AJ and Hunter AR. Gingival crown margin configurations. A review and Discussion: Terminology and widths. J. Prosthet. Dent.: 1990; 64:548–52.

13. Hunter AJ and Hunter AR. Gingival crown margin configurations: a review and discussion. Part I: terminology and widths. J. Prosthet. Dent.: 1990;64:548.

14. Hunter AJ and Hunter AR. Gingival margins for crowns: a review and discussion. Part II: discrepancies and configurations. J. Prosthet. Dent.: 1990;64:636–42.

15. Ito M, Marx DB, Cheng AC and Wee AG. Proposed shade guide for attached gingiva—a pilot study. J. Prosthodont.: 2015;24:182–7.

16. Khera S, Goel V, Chen R and Gurusami S. Parameters of MOD cavity preparations: A 3-D FEM study, Part II. Oper. Dent.: 1991;16:42–54.

17. Kois JC. Altering gingival levels: the restorative connection part I: biologic variables. J. Esthet. Dent.: 1994;6:3–9.

18. Kois JC. The restorative-periodontal interface: biologic parameters. Periodontol.: 1996;11:29–38.

19. Langeland K and Langeland LK. Pulpal reactions to crown preparation, impression, temporary crown fixation and permanent cementation. J. Prosthet. Dent.: 1965;15:129–43.

20. Leempoel PJB, Lemmens PL, Snoek PA and van't Hof MA. The convergence angle of tooth preparations for complete crowns. J. Prosthet. Dent.: 1987;58:414–6.

21. Morimoto S. Fracture strength of teeth restored with ceramic inlays and overlays. Braz. Dent. J.: 2009;20:143–8.

22. Nevins M and Skurow HM. The inter-crevicular restorative margin, the biologic width and the maintenance of the gingival margin. Int. J. Periodontol. Rest. Dent.: 1984;3:30–9.

23. Nicholls JI. Crown retention I. Stress analysis of symmetric restorations. J. Prosthet. Dent.: 1984;31:179–84.

24. Nohl FSA and Steele JG and Wassell RW. Crowns and other extracoronal restorations: aesthetic control. Br. Dent. J.: 2002;192:443–50.

25. Orkin DA, Reddy J and Bradshaw D. The relationship of crown margins to gingival health. J. Prosthet. Dent.: 1987;57:421–4.

26. Parker MH. Resistance form in tooth preparation. Dent. Cl. N. Am.: 2004;48:387–96.

27. Peston JD. Rational approach to tooth preparation for ceramometal restorations. Dent. Cl. North Am.: 1977;21:683–98.

28. Rosner D. Function, placement, and reproduction of bevels for gold castings. J. Prosthet. Dent.: 1967;13:1160–6.

29. Sadowsky SJ. An overview of treatment considerations for esthetic restorations: a review of the literature. J. Prosthet. Dent.: 2006;96:433–42.

30. Santos DM, Moreno A, Vechiato-Filho AJ, Bonatto LR, Pesqueira AA, Laurindo MCB, Medeiros RA, da Silva EVF and Goiato MC. The importance of the lifelike esthetic appearance of all-ceramic restorations on anterior teeth. Case Report in Dentistry: Article ID 2015;704348:1–5.

31. Sarandha DL. Effects of location of gingival finish lines on periodontal integrity. J. Nepal Dent. Assoc.: 2013;13:74–7.

32. Saridag S, Sevimay M and Pekkan G. Fracture resistance of teeth restored with all-ceramic inlays and onlays: an in vitro study. Oper. Dent.: 2013;38:626–34.

33. Scoble HO and Donovan TE. Tooth preparation for indirect esthetic restorations. J.Calif. Dent. Assoc.: 1990;18:31–7.

34. Soares C, Martins L, Fonseca R, Correr-Sobrinho L and Fernandes A. Influence of cavity preparation design on fracture resistance of posterior leucite reinforced ceramic restorations. J. Prosthet.Dent.: 2006;95:421–9.

35. Syu JZ, Byrne G, Laub LW and Land MF. Influence of finish-line geometry on the fit of crowns. Int. J. Prosthodont.: 1993;6:25–30.

36. Witwer DJ, Storey RJ and von Fraunhofer JA. The effects of surface texture and grooving on the retention of cast crowns. J. Prosthet. Dent.: 1986;77;116–21.

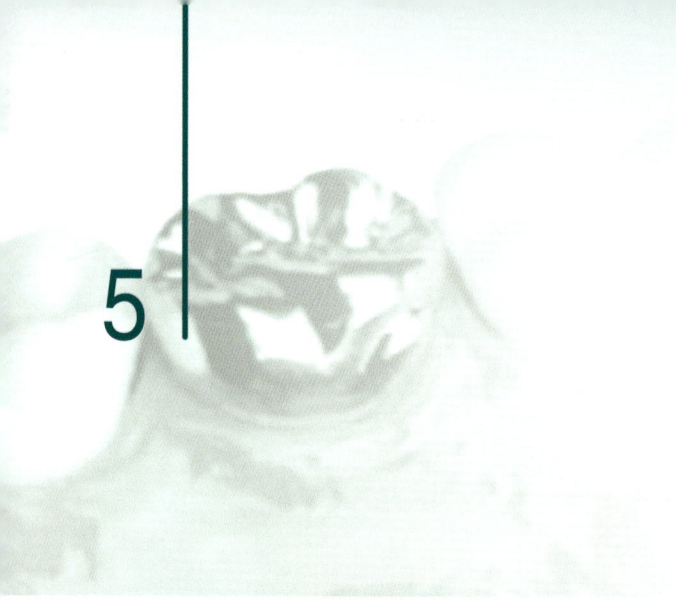

5

Inlays and Onlays

The choice of the restorative material depends upon the amount of remaining tooth structure that can be utilized for gaining resistance and retention form. The direct restorations are usually not advisable in teeth where more than half the tooth structure is lost, especially the dentin support. The success of direct restorations is also doubtful where wider proximal area is involved. The indirect restorations provide the requisite resistance and retention form and also support the remaining tooth tissue, especially onlays and the full crowns.

Indication for Inlays and Onlays

Indirect inlays and onlays are indicated in cases such as:

- Large cavities where remaining tooth structure is not sufficient for achieving retention form in direct restorations
- Requiring better strength and longevity of the restoration
- Need for better anatomical details, especially, cuspal planes and contact areas
- In case, the anatomy is to be modified (cusps, contours and embrasures)
- For patients who do not afford long chairside time (systemic or social reasons)

METAL INLAYS AND ONLAYS

Various metals and their alloys are used for fabrication of cast inlays and onlays. The commonly used alloys are as follows:

1. *Gold alloys:* The gold alloys and other noble metals such as palladium, platinum and rhodium are rarely used these days (palladium gaining some popularity). The gold alloys are further divided into four types depending upon the amount of gold and the other added elements. Type 1 (83% Au, 10% Ag, 6% Cu) and type 2 (77% Au, 14% Ag, 7% Cu) are used for inlays and onlays, whereas type 3 (75% Au, 11% Ag, 9% Cu) for crown and bridge prosthesis and type 4 (69% Au, 25% Ag, 10% Cu) are used for partial dentures. Many gold based alloys contain small amount (1.0–5.0%) of palladium to improve resistance to tarnish and corrosion without significant change of color. Silver and zinc are added in traces to improve upon the physical properties. Silver is usually more reactive to air/oxygen and not considered as a noble metal.

2. *Palladium alloys:* The palladium alloys are mostly preferred in metal-ceramics. Generally, palladium alloys are 'white'. Most of these alloys have silvery appearance unless the gold contact is greater than 40% and the palladium 6%.

Both palladium and silver absorb oxygen when molten, which may result in porous castings. Silver-palladium alloys usually contain 75% silver and 25% palladium, whereas the reverse concentration is for palladium-silver alloys. Copper has also been added to palladium–silver alloys. Palladium has excellent tarnish/corrosion resistance and biocompatibility in oral environment. The high melting point (1170–1190°C) of palladium facilitates high firing temperature of porcelain (950–1000°C) for palladium fused to porcelain restorations.

3. *Base metal alloys:* The metals, which are reactive to air/oxygen, are designated as base metals. These metals are also referred to as non-noble or non-precious alloys (nomenclature not used in routine). The commonly used base metal alloys are nickel and/or cobalt with approximately 15–20% chromium. The chromium imparts the passivating effect on base metals, making them corrosion resistant.

Beryllium and Molybdenum have also been added to improve upon the properties of the base metals. Beryllium controls the castability and surface oxidation at high temperature. Molybdenum decreases the coefficient of thermal expansion. 'Progold' (containing mainly copper and zinc) has also been used. These alloys show poor physical properties and tarnish easily.

4. *Titanium and its alloys:* Titanium is considered as the most biocompatible metal used for dental castings. This does not fall in the category of noble and base metals, but considered as a separate entity. Titanium is available in pure form and also along with traces of iron, oxygen and carbon. Titanium is resistant to tarnish and corrosion. The corrosion protection is derived from a thin passivating film. The coefficient of thermal expansion is 9.0–11.8 $\times 10^{-6}$, (ideally required) and the density is 4.51 g/cm^3. The low density of titanium provides for high strength, lightweight castings. The elastic modulus of pure titanium is comparable to tooth enamel and noble alloys.

Titanium has the highest melting temperature (1668°C) of all the metals used in casting. The titanium must be melted in a vacuum or inert gas to prevent oxidation. The incorporation of oxygen can lead to brittle castings and also significant loss of ductility. However, oxide layer helps in bonding and also provides biocompatibility. Pressure vacuum casting machine along with compatible investment material is required to ensure acceptable castings.

Aluminium, tin and vanadium have been added to pure titanium to improve upon its qualities. The widely used alloy is Ti-6Al-4V is stronger than pure titanium and less biocompatible. Addition of 1.0–10.0% copper in Ti-Al-V alloy increases the hardness and decreases the tensile strength.

Hafnium has also been added to titanium alloys, resulting in stronger alloy without compromising other physical properties.

The marginal gap width in titanium restorations are 10–15%, which is higher than gold; however, it can be successfully used for inlays and onlays. The physical and mechanical properties of commonly used casting alloys are given in Table 5.1.

Requirements of Dental Casting Alloys

The dental casting alloys should have the following properties:

1. *Biocompatibility:* The alloy should be biocompatible, i.e. it should tolerate oral fluids and should not release any harmful products in the oral cavity.
2. *Coefficient of thermal expansion:* The coefficient of thermal expansion should be close to that of tooth (11.4×10^{-6}/°C).
3. *Melting range:* The melting range should be low. Low melting range metals form smooth surfaces with the investment (mold wall) of the casting. The compensation of the casting shrinkage from the solidus

Table 5.1: Physical and mechanical properties of commonly used casting alloys

Property	Titanium alloys	Gold alloys	Palladium alloys	Base metal alloys
Density (gm/cm^3)	4.43–4.51	18.0–19.5	10.6–10.9	4.40–9.5
Hardness (VHN)	130–210	125–240	140–150	270–350
Melting point (0°c)	1660–1668	875–1000	1170–1190	1250–1475
Elongation (%)	15–24	10–18	10–11	1.0–2.5
Coefficient of thermal expansion (in/°C × 10^{-6})	9.0–11.0	14.0–15.6	14.5–15.0	14.0–16.5

temperature to room temperature must be achieved through controlled mold expansion. However, higher melting range casting alloys are preferred for porcelain fused to metal restorations.

4. *Tarnish and corrosion resistance:* The alloy should resist tarnish (thin film of surface deposit or an interaction layer adhering to metal surface) and corrosion (physical dissolution of metal in oral environment).

5. *Modulus of elasticity:* The alloys should have sufficient elastic modulus to prevent excessive elastic deflection from functional forces. The strength should be more as the number of teeth being replaced, increases. For example, the alloys for bridgework require higher strength than alloys for single crown.

6. *Castability:* The molten metal should exhibit low contact angle so as to wet the investment mold completely. The alloy should not form any oxide layer or interact chemically with the mold wall during casting process. The alloy after casting should be easily separated from the investment.

7. *Finishing and Polishing:* The alloys should be conveniently polished and finished. (Hardness and ductility of the alloys; for example, base metal alloys being harder are difficult to finish and polish as compared to noble metals).

8. *Esthetics:* The finished and polished cast alloy should be pleasing to eyes.

CAVITY PREPARATION

The principles of tooth preparation for any type of indirect restorations are described in Chapter 4. The cavity preparation for gold inlays is described.

Before starting with cavity preparation, the tooth must be evaluated carefully for the following factors that influence the design of the cavity.

- Anatomic/morphological characteristics of the clinical crown
- Position of tooth in the arch (configuration of contact areas)
- Occlusal and proximal relations
- Recession, if any
- Condition of soft tissues around
- Extent and location of carious lesions

Principles of Cavity Preparation

The principles of cavity preparation are described following the sequence as given by Dr GV Black. The cavity shape to be followed for cast gold restorations is as under (the modifications required for composite and ceramic inlays are described in subsequent pages). The differences in cavity preparations of silver amalgam and cast gold are described in Table 5.2, refreshing basic knowledge of cavity preparation.

1. Outline form

i. External Outline Form

The external outline form of the cavity preparation for inlay should consist of straight

Table 5.2: Differences in cavity preparation for silver amalgam and cast restorations

Silver amalgam	Cast restorations
i. Intercuspal width is 1/4th of intercuspal distance (outline form is narrow).	Intercuspal width is 1/3rd of intercuspal distance (outline form is wide).
ii. Cavity depth is more.	Comparatively less depth.
iii. Cavity walls are kept convergent occlusally (minor undercuts)	Cavity walls are kept parallel (no undercuts)
iv. Buccal and lingual proximal walls are convergent occlusally.	Buccal and lingual proximal walls are parallel.
v. Cavosurface bevel is contraindicated (butt joint is preferred).	Cavosurface bevel is given.
vi. All line angles and point angles are rounded and axiopulpal line angle is bevelled	All line angles and point angles are well defined and axiopulpal line angle is slightly rounded
vii. No reverse bevel is given	Reverse bevel is indicated
viii. Grooves are not given, only locks are given	Grooves are given, locks are not given

lines and smooth flowing curves, avoiding any sharp angles. The finishing line should be extended on the occlusal surface to include retentive fissures and on to the proximal and cervical areas until the carious lesion is removed and the margins are convenient for finishing of the preparation. Enamel rods at the cavosurface margin should be supported by dentin and laterally by rods that lie within the preparation. Enamel that has been undermined by caries must be removed. The cavosurface margin is placed in sound tooth tissue in order to obtain a well-fitted casting.

The long axis of bur (169 L and 271) is kept parallel to the long axis of the tooth crown at all times. For mandibular molars and premolars whose crowns tilt slightly lingually, the bur should be tilted 5–10 degrees lingually to conserve the lingual cusps.

In case, a fissure extends onto the marginal ridge, it may be treated either by enameloplasty if the defect is shallow; or the outline form is extended by creating a cavosurface bevel. This procedure protects the enamel at the cavosurface margins.

After preparation of the occlusal outline form, the cavity is extended proximally as in Black's Class II preparations.

The occlusal cutting is extended towards the contact area through the marginal ridge. The cutting is then extended bucco-lingually. With the bur so positioned that it rests two-third on dentin and one-third on the enamel, a proximal ditch is made with a slight pressure. Since, width of the bur is 0.8 mm, it cuts 0.3 mm of enamel and 0.5 mm into the dentin. The proximal ditch is carried gingivally with the intent of keeping the gingival seat just below the contact area. The gingival extension can be checked with the length of the bur.

Ideal extension of the proximal box should be such that the buccal and lingual walls project perpendicular to the proximal surface, clearing the adjacent tooth. The gingival extent of the cavity should remove caries and also provide

0.5 mm clearance of the un-bevelled gingival margin with the adjacent tooth (Figs 5.1a and b).

The axial wall should follow the contour of the tooth bucco-lingually at a depth of 0.2–0.5 mm in the dentin (Fig. 5.2). Reverse bevel is placed on the cervical wall (Fig. 5.3).

The external outline form for the gold inlay follows a similar external form as that for the amalgam cavity. Application of the concept of taper will necessitate a change in the proximal outline form, from that used in the amalgam cavity (Fig. 5.4). The placement of bevel makes the outline form slightly wider for cast restorations.

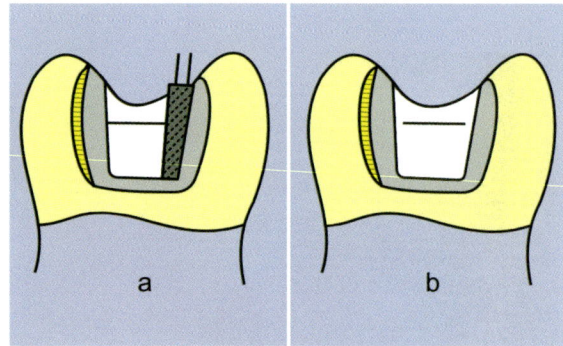

Fig. 5.1: Extent of gingival margin with adjacent tooth. a. extending gingival margin, b. prepared gingival margin

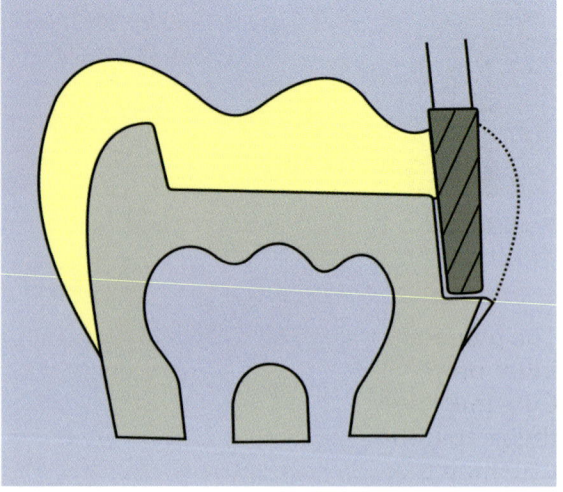

Fig. 5.2: Placing axial wall 0.2–0.5 mm inside dentin

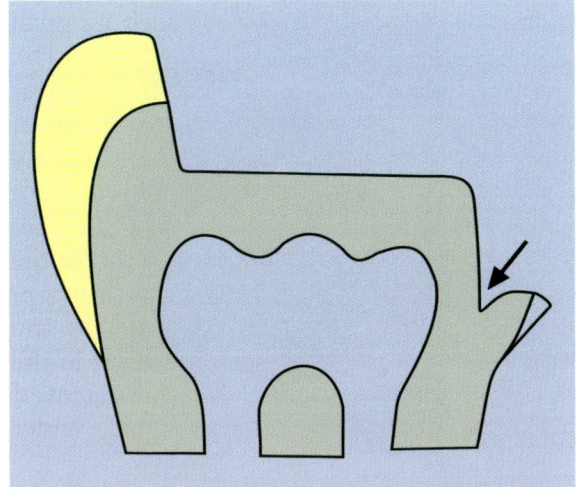

Fig. 5.3: Reverse bevel placed on cervical wall (arrow)

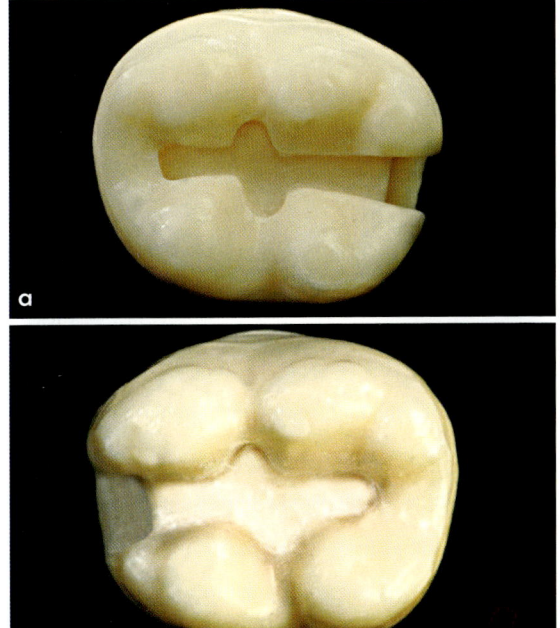

Figs 5.4a and b: Outline form a. amalgam b. gold inlays

ii. *Internal Outline Form*

The pulpal floor and the axial wall of the gold inlay preparation must be placed in dentin. Care must be taken to protect the pulp. When the preparation has to be taken beyond its usual internal limits because of the extent of the lesion, the additional loss of dentin is substituted with an appropriate cement base. The amount of taper required varies with the depth or length of the preparation from the occlusal to cervical aspect. In shallow preparations, parallelism enhances the resistance and retention form of the preparation. Deep cavities require taper to facilitate seating of the restoration.

While it is difficult to establish an exact measurement for the length of the occlusal walls, owing to the anatomic variations of teeth, the pulpal floor will usually be positioned 0.5 mm into dentin below the central groove (1.75 to 2.00 mm) (Fig. 5.5).

The cervical floor should be in sound tooth tissue. When a cement base is placed to form a portion of this floor, it is necessary to maintain at least one-half of the area in sound tooth tissue to support the restoration. Ragged enamel edges at the gingival and proximal areas may be removed with hand instrument such as chisel or a flame-shaped diamond point. However, it is better to postpone finishing of the walls till the remaining caries and/or old restorative material is completely removed and the base is applied. This facilitates visibility of the gingival area, which otherwise remains obscured, may be because of haemorrhage following beveling of the gingival margin (Figs 5.6a and b)

Line angles in both the occlusal and proximal portions of the preparation should be well defined. The axio-pulpal line angle is slightly rounded. The flare of the proximal

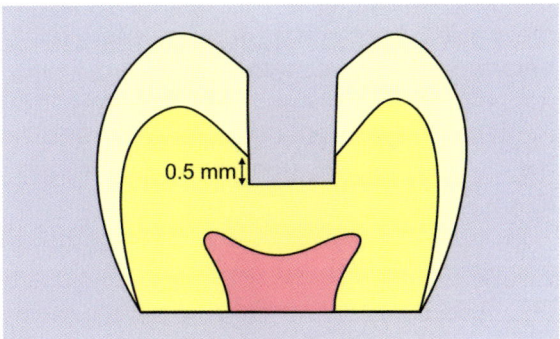

Fig. 5.5: Placing pulpal floor 0.5 mm inside dentin

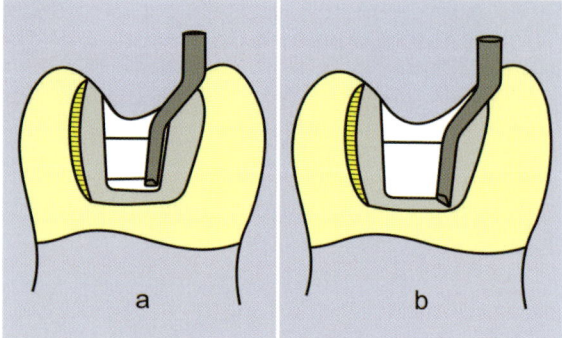

Figs 5.6: a. finishing of cervical wall. b. placing gingival bevel

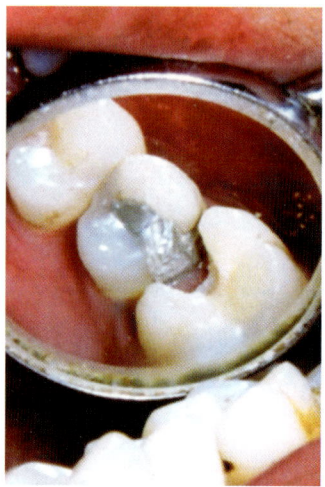

Fig. 5.7: Overcontoured silver amalgam restoration in second premolar

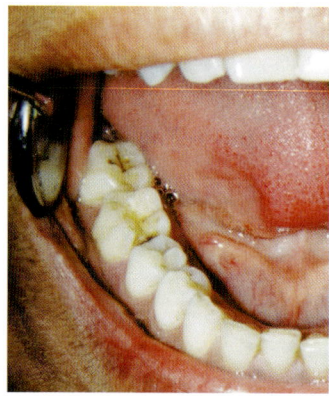

Fig. 5.8a: Distal surface of second premolar flattened

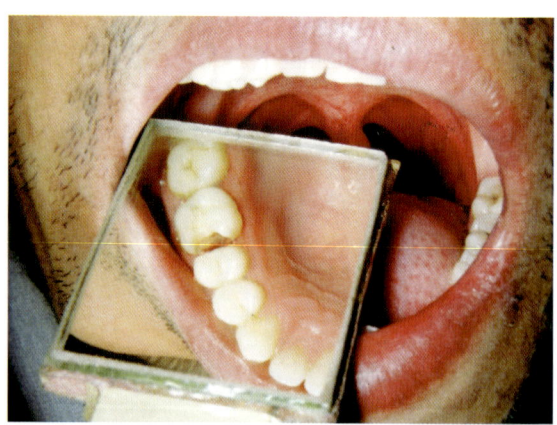

Fig. 5.8b: Walls of proximal box widened to accommodate flat adjacent tooth

walls should form axio-proximal angles of 100 to 110 degrees.

The width of the cavity should be such that one-third of the cuspal inclines are included on both sides of the central groove. The equal cutting of cuspal inclines, sometimes is to be modified keeping in view the altered anatomy of the teeth. For example, the mandibular premolar has a prominent buccal cusp and a very small lingual cusp with the central groove positioned lingually from the midline. When preparing the occlusal portion of this tooth, about two-thirds of the occlusal width should be removed from the buccal incline plane and only one-third from the lingual incline plane.

The proximal contour of the adjacent tooth should be corrected, especially when already restored (Fig. 5.7).

In case, the proximal surface of the adjacent tooth is flat, it is to be corrected before final finishing of the preparation (Figs 5.8a and b).

The dissimilar height of the cusps dictate the pulpal floor to be slightly tilted to the lingual side. The cervical floor may or may not be parallel to the pulpal floor, depending upon the inclination of the coronal portion of the tooth and the relationship of the soft tissue at the cervical area.

Another modification is accomplished during mesio-occlusal cavity preparation of maxillary premolars and first molars. In such cases, the mesio-buccal margin is minimally extended buccally away from the contact area so that the margin is barely visible from the buccal side. To achieve this, the secondary flare is omitted and the margins are finished with enamel hatchet.

During restoration of maxillary first molars, if both mesial and distal surface are carious, but the oblique ridge is strong and unaffected, consideration should be given to restore both the proximo-occlusal surfaces independently. The distal carious lesion should be restored with a disto-occluso-palatal onlay, capping the disto-palatal cusp, which protects the cusp from subsequent fracture.

Occasionally, a buccal groove on the occlusal surface is continuous with a buccal surface groove. This may indicate extension of the cavity outline to include the fissure to its termination. The gingival extension of the cavity in this groove considerably enhances retention form of the restoration.

FLARES

The flares are of following types:
a. *Primary flare:* As per the old concept of inlay cavity preparation, the proximal walls were divided into two halves. The axial half was placed at 90° to the axial wall and proximal half had an angulation of 45° to the axial half. This proximal half that helped to bring the proximal wall into self-cleansing areas was known as the primary flare. It was believed that the axial wall should be at 90° to the proximal box wall to provide resistance and retention form to the cavity but later it was found that flaring of the walls right from axiofacial or axiolingual line angles till the cavosurface margin did not alter the resistance and retention form. This implies that the flaring of lingual wall and buccal wall of proximal box from the axial wall (axiolingual and axiofacial line angles respectively) to the proximal cavosurface margins is known as primary flare (Figs 5.9a and b).
Functions: The function of the primary flare is to keep the proximal, buccal and lingual walls in the self-cleansing areas.

b. *Secondary flare:* The secondary flare is a flat plane superimposed peripherally to a primary flare. It is as good as the occlusal bevel given to create a circumferential tie in gold inlays to take the advantage of malleability of gold alloys (Figs 5.9a and b). In case of broad contact, the primary flare is extended till proximal cavosurface margin is in the embrasure area (Fig. 5.9 c). If one-third of incline plane is involved, cusp coverage is planned.
Functions: A secondary flare creates the needed obtuse angulation of the marginal tooth structure given exclusively for gold inlay preparations.

2. Resistance and Retention Form

The preparation of the tooth for cast restoration should be so designed that it must resist the dislodging forces that may cause fracture of the tooth or the restoration. The preparation should also retain the restoration bearing all types of functional forces (Figs 5.10 and 5.11).

Parallelism of the opposing walls aid in frictional retention of the cast restorations. Flat pulpal and cervical floors provide adequate resistance against functional forces. The cavity form should have well-defined angles without any undercuts. The cutting instruments are oriented along the long axis of the tooth crown. The tapering fissure bur is preferred so as to achieve occlusal divergence of 2–3°. The divergence can accordingly be increased depending upon the depth of the cavity. The occlusal divergence enables removal of wax pattern and placement of the finished cast restoration.

The design of the proximal box and its margins depend upon the following factors:
- The extent of caries in that area
- Configuration of the tooth vis-à-vis the adjacent tooth
- The relationship with adjacent teeth (contact area/embrasures)
- Occlusion with opposing tooth
- Choice of material.

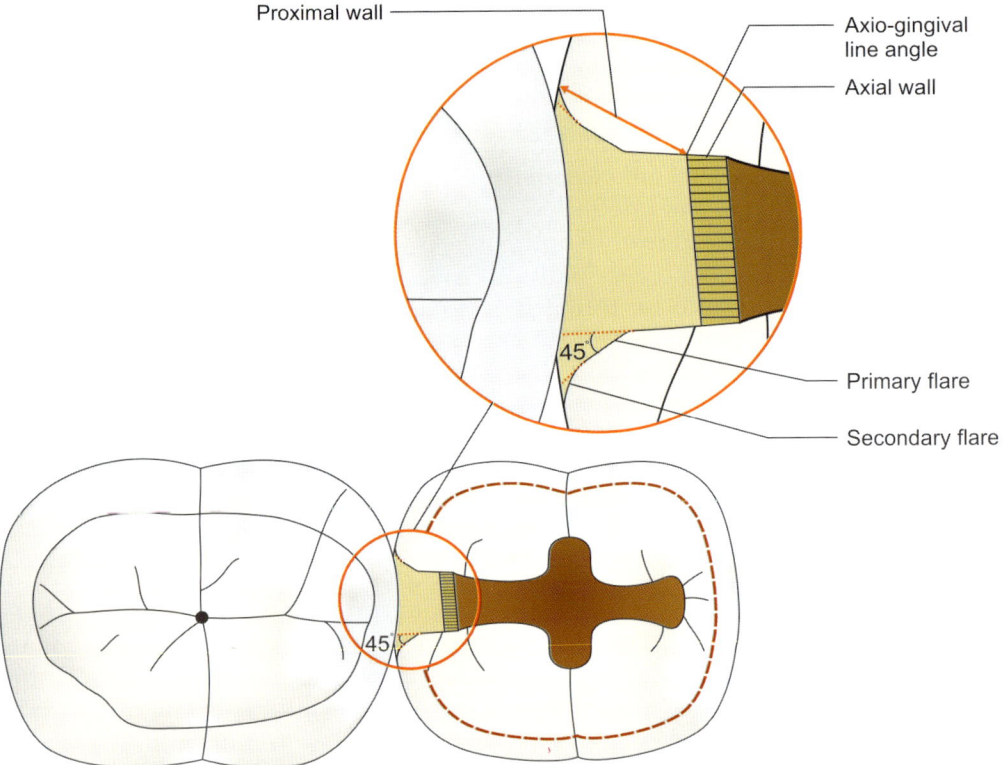

Proximal wall —

Axio-gingival line angle

Axial wall

45

Primary flare

Secondary flare

45

Fig. 5.9a: Old concept: primary and secondary flare

The axio-pulpal line angle is rounded for uniformly dissipating occlusal stresses. The occlusal dovetail prevents proximal displacement of the restoration.

In case, the depth of cavity or the required parallelism of the walls cannot be achieved, secondary retentive features should be incorporated. Slots and pinholes may be placed parallel to the line of draw to increase retention.

Retentive Grooves

Retentive grooves may be given in the bucco-axial and linguo-axial line angles. The grooves should be in sound dentin near dentino-enamel junction. The depth of the groove (0.3 mm) should be more than the width (1.5 mm). The grooves should preferably be given after placing the base (Figs 5.12a and b).

Bevels

The weakest link in any cast restoration is the tooth-cement-cast interface. Even an accurate casting does not accept precisely with the tooth surface, leaving some discrepancies. Bevels help overcome discrepancies and improve adaptation.

The peripheral marginal anatomy of the preparation (relation with the casting and luting cement) is known as the *circumferential tie*. The mandatory features for circumferential tie are:

- Enamel must be supported by sound dentin.
- Enamel rods forming the cavosurface margin should be continuous with sound dentin.
- Angular cavosurface angles formed by the enamel rods should be trimmed.

The cavosurface bevels create obtuse angled marginal tooth structure, which is bulkiest and strongest. Such type of marginal tooth

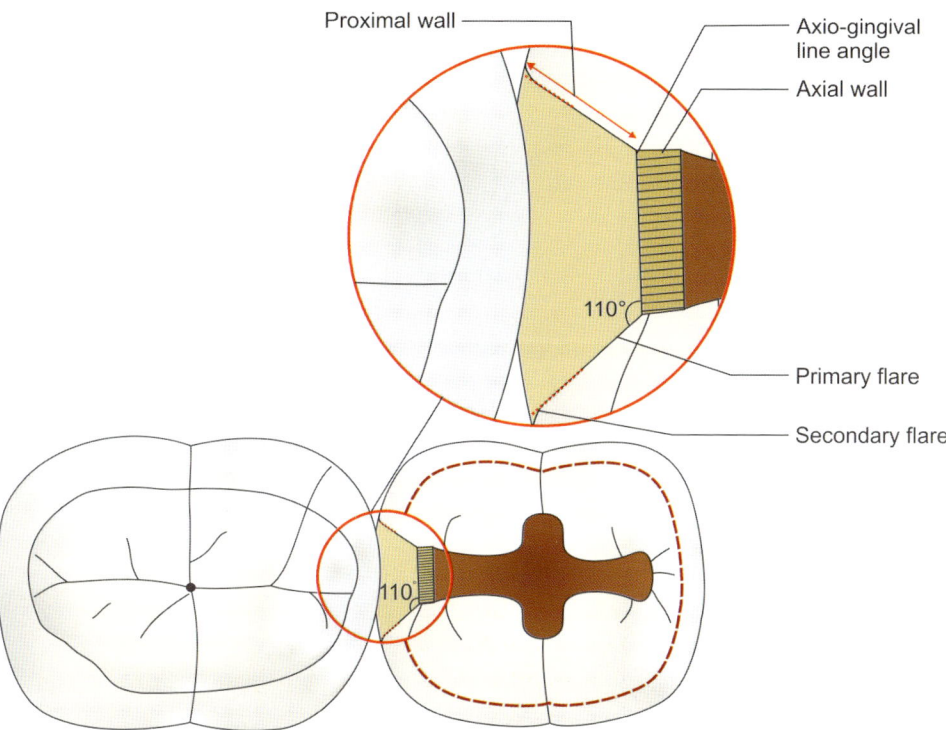

Fig. 5.9b: New concept: primary and secondary flare

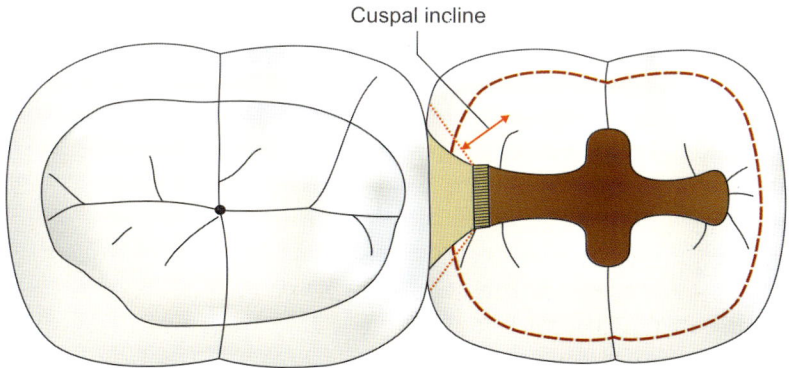

Fig. 5.9c: Flares in broad contacts

structure produces an acute angled casting, suitable for adaptation. In case of onlays, covering the tooth structure overcomes this feature.

The bevels reduce error factors of the marginal discrepancy between cast and the tooth margin and indirectly improve retention form, decreasing the frictional component between tooth and the casting.

The cervical bevel, after the cavity preparation is usually placed with the flame shaped extra fine finishing burs or gingival marginal trimmers. These instruments provide a steeper bevel required for an effective adaptation of the metal margin.

The greater bulk of the cervical margin produced by the flame shaped instrument is advantageous since impression making and

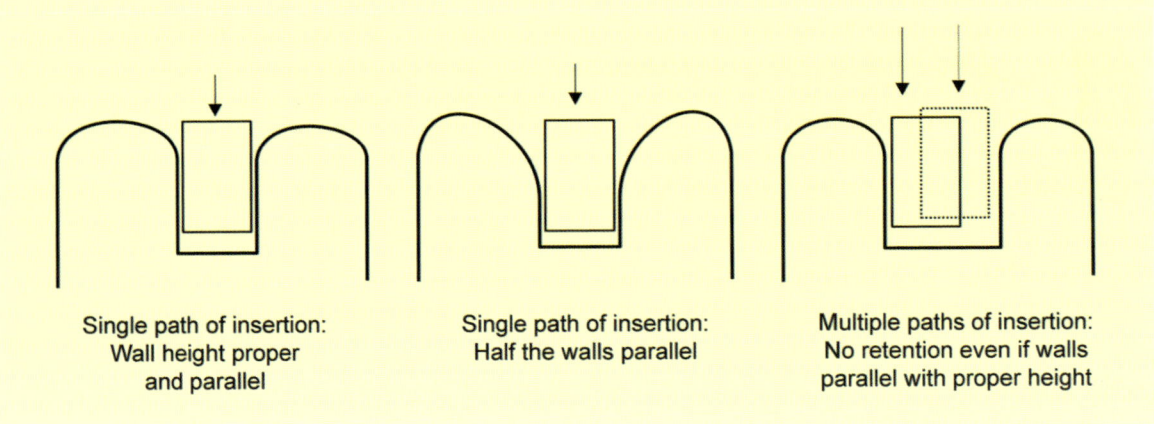

Single path of insertion:
Wall height proper
and parallel

Single path of insertion:
Half the walls parallel

Multiple paths of insertion:
No retention even if walls
parallel with proper height

Fig. 5.10: Path of insertion and retention

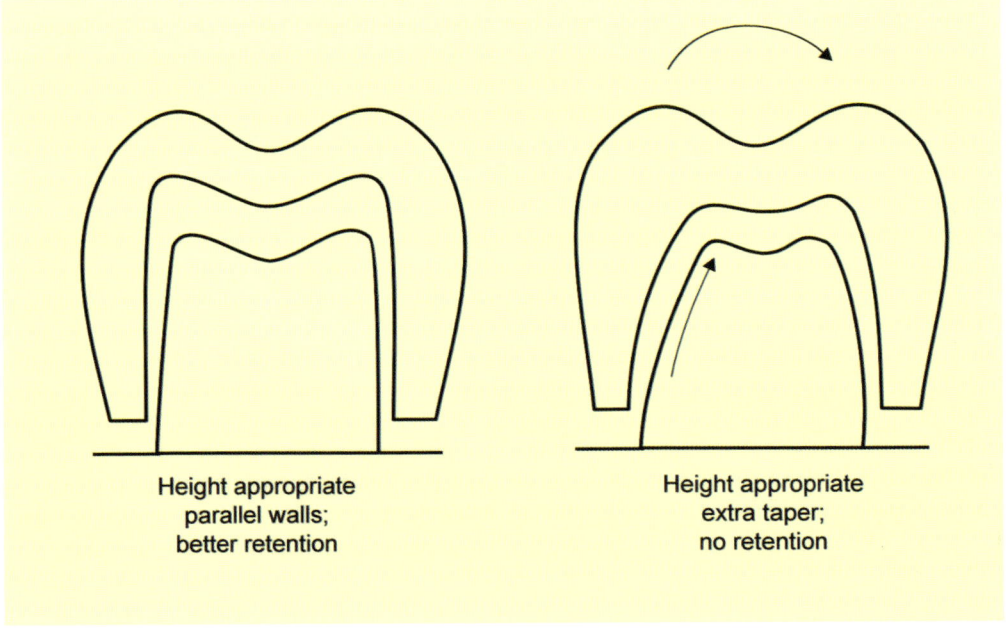

Height appropriate
parallel walls;
better retention

Height appropriate
extra taper;
no retention

Fig. 5.11: Height of walls, taper and retention

finishing the casting becomes easier. The use of disc is not recommended since the disc may slice the whole cervical area.

Whenever, a direct wax pattern is to be formed, the bevel used is of greater bulk and extends a greater width across the cervical floor. The bevel on the cervical margin for the direct technique should be about one-fourth to one-third of mesio-distal width of the cervical floor and includes the proximal cervical cavosurface angles. Such a bevel is placed with a gingival marginal trimmer prior to finishing the proximal enamel walls.

The depth of the cavosurface bevel on the occlusal margin should be approximately one-fourth the depth of the respective wall. This should produce an occlusal marginal enamel of 140° and occlusal marginal metal of 40°. If

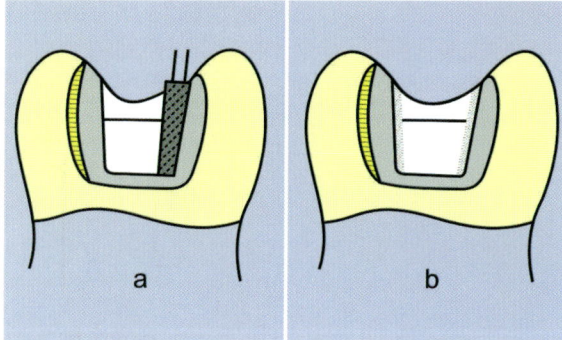

Figs 5.12a and b: a. Placing proximal grooves, b. proximal grooves (shadow)

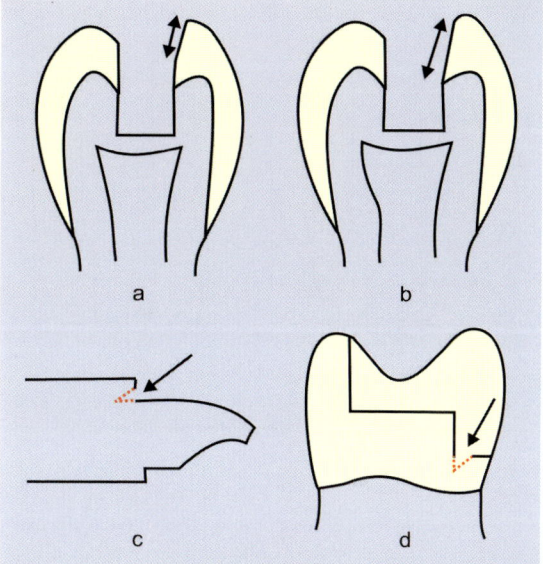

Figs 5.13a–d: a. Partial (direct filling gold), b. short (gold inlays), c. inverted (porcelain fused to metal crowns—labial shoulder), d. reverse bevel (gold inlays—in cervical wall)

the cuspal inclines are so steep that the diamond point at a 40° angle to the external enamel surface is parallel with the enamel cavity wall, then no bevel is indicated.

The axio-pulpal line angle is rounded using the appropriate diamond points to avoid concentration of stresses at this junction.

Bevels indirectly improve retention forms for a cast restoration, since bevels decrease the direct frictional component between the tooth and the casting. The circumferential tie of tooth-casting interphase is a susceptible friction zone and if left to direct contact will lead to less retention of the restoration.

The different types of bevels are:

1. *Partial:* It involves part of enamel wall (Fig. 5.13a). This is indicated in direct filling gold.
2. *Short:* It involves entire enamel wall (Fig. 5.13b). This type of bevel best suited in cast gold inlays.
3. *Inverted:* It is given on the labial shoulder of metal ceramic crowns to effectively improve the esthetics at the margins (Fig. 5.13c).
4. *Reverse bevel:* This bevel is placed at the dentinal portion of the cervical wall towards the axio-pulpal line angle. This is indicated in cast gold inlay preparations (Fig. 5.13d). The earlier concept of long bevel (Fig. 5.14a–d) was discarded over the years.

3. Convenience Form

The convenience form provides accessibility and visibility to carry out the operative procedures. Proper access is mandatory for removing the carious dentin/old restorative materials, flaring buccal and lingual wall of proximal box in the embrasure areas, creating secondary flare if need be and finishing of cavosurface margins. All these features aid in retention and better adaptation of the restorative materials.

4. Removing Residual Caries

The remaining caries, if any, should be removed using small round burs or with hand excavators.

The excavated regions can be filled with the base material to the level of the required depth of the cavity. The base material is the choice of the operator keeping in mind the clinical conditions.

Deep caries with residual dentin thickness of less than 1.0 mm should be excavated slowly. Only 'infected dentin' and not the

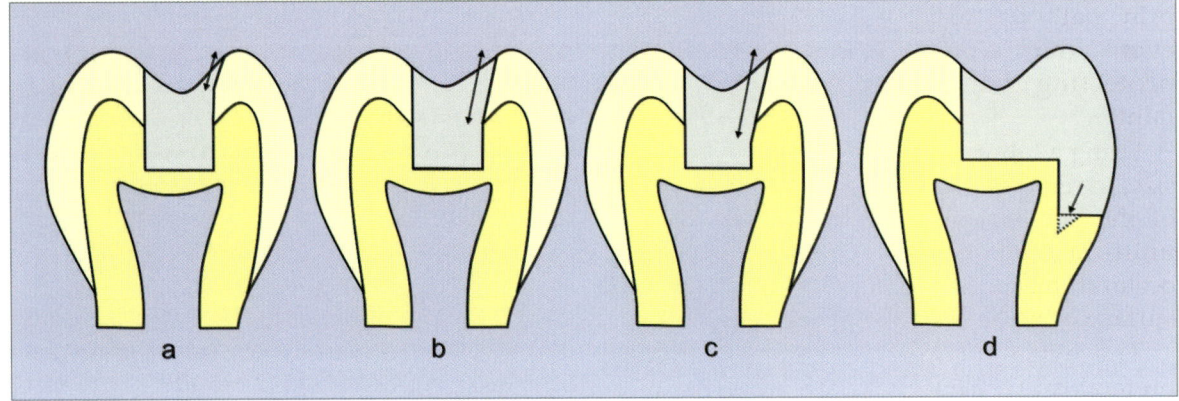

Figs 5.14a–d: Bevel. a. partial; b. short; c. long or full d. reverse

'affected dentin' should be removed. Calcium hydroxide is preferred as sub-base followed by a base of suitable cement. The cement base should be thick enough to protect the underlying dentin and calcium hydroxide liner from functional stresses.

5. Finishing Enamel Walls and Margins

The marginal fit of a cast restoration depends upon the approximation of cast metal to tooth tissue surfaces. The walls should be smooth and even for proper withdrawal of wax pattern.

Conventional diamond points and cross-cut fissure burs leave roughened tooth surfaces. Hand instruments may also leave notched irregularities. These notches and irregularities need to be finished properly.

If coarse or medium grit diamond points have been used during cavity preparation, the walls and margins should be finished with 16–24 fluted carbide-finishing burs followed by plain carbide bur.

6. Cleaning the Preparation

The preparation should finally be thoroughly rinsed with water or saline and gently air dried. The preparation is evaluated for undercuts, if any. A trial impression with gutta-percha stick is helpful to evaluate undercuts, taper and the line of draw of the preparation. In case of discrepancy, the preparation can be modified accordingly.

Inlay or Onlay

The amount of the remaining tooth structure and the occlusal load over the potential restoration must be evaluated thoroughly. When the isthmus of the preparation involves half or more than half of the buccal/palatal cusp, especially the functional cusp(s), cusp covering (onlay) should be considered. In areas of low stress and/or the non-functional cusps, the undermine dentin and/or minor undercuts, if any, should be filled with glass-ionomer cement or composite resin.

Onlay Preparation

The inlay, being an intracoronal restoration, may not protect the remaining weak tooth structure, if any. Such restorations, depending upon their bucco-lingual width, usually exert a wedging pressure outward from the center of the tooth. If more than one-third of cuspal incline planes are involved, the concerned cusp(s) should be covered (onlay preparation). The onlays protect the remaining weaker tooth structure from occlusal, laterally and apically directed forces.

The onlay/coverage of one, two or three cusps minimizes the potentially damaging effects of stress in an intra-coronal restoration. The onlay exhibits less stress than the inlay, principally by distributing the occlusal load evenly over a wide surface; subsequently protecting the tooth from biomechanical failure.

Using a tapering fissure bur of appropriate size, the cusp is reduced following the contour of the occlusal surface so as to achieve a uniform thickness of 1.5 mm of metal for occlusal surface and 1.0 mm for buccal/lingual surface of posterior teeth (Fig. 5.15).

The extra-coronal margins are placed preferably at the enamel and the design of the finish line can be selected depending upon the restorative material (chamfer is indicated in cast gold and shoulder in base metal) (Fig. 5.16). Shoulder is also preferred in all-ceramic and porcelain fused to metal preparations. Because of ductility and malleability of the gold, the margins can be burnished and well adapted to the tooth surface.

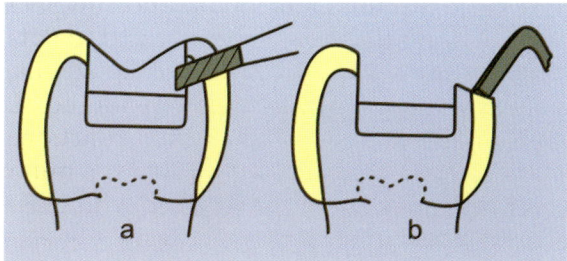

Figs 5.15a and b: a. Cusp reduction, b. reduced cusp

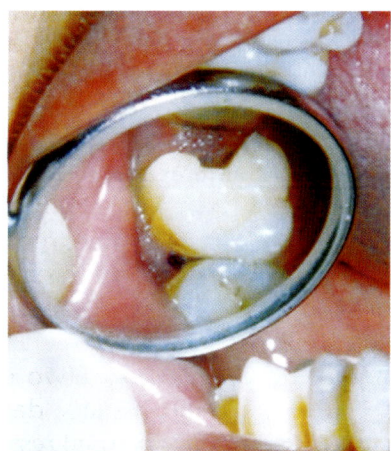

Fig. 5.16: Placement of shoulder or chamfer

Many a times, the onlays are preferred where re-contouring of the proximal surface (mesial or distal) is indicated. In such cases, both the cusps of that proximal area is included. In case, the proximal width between two teeth is more, onlays covering both the cusps of adjacent teeth, is indicated; rather than over-contouring by covering one tooth only.

When functional cusps are capped, it is advisable to place a contra-bevel on the opposing tooth surface. For example, if both the buccal cusps of mandibular molars are capped, lingual extension of the cavity is mandatory as is followed in lingual complex of class I cavities. Even if non-functional cusps are capped, contra-beveling on opposing tooth surface is advisable. Such preparations help bear the occlusal forces in a better way.

COMPOSITE INLAYS AND ONLAYS

Indirect resin restoration is one of the most rapidly growing treatment modality for teeth requiring esthetic restorations. As the physical properties of the indirect composite materials have substantially improved, the composite inlay now is the preferred choice of the operator. The physical properties of composite restorations are improved when the composite is free of voids and the resin matrix is completely polymerized. The complete polymerization of the composite may not be feasible in direct techniques. This can be accomplished in the laboratory by polymerizing the composite under pressure, vacuum, intense light, heat, inert gas or a combination of these conditions.

The direct composite, though routinely used, are having certain limitations, such as:
• Despite the incremental techniques being used for direct restorations, the polymerization shrinkage of the resin during curing may lead to marginal defects, cuspal distortion and crack formation/propagation within the tooth tissues, subsequently resulting in post-operative sensitivity.

- Adequate bond may not be achieved in areas where the cavosurface margin is situated on dentin.
- The polymerization in deep inter-proximal areas may not be properly achieved, leading to partly cured resin at the interface.
- Increase wear in excessive load bearing areas.
- Water sorption resulting in hydrolytic instability.
- Proper contours and contacts may not be achieved.

To overcome these clinical problems, the composite inlay system was introduced. It has been established that heat treatment enhances the resin hardness and wear resistance and reduces microleakage.

A composite resin inlay is defined as 'a restoration that has been fabricated from composite resin with a form established either by an indirect or direct procedure outside the oral cavity and cemented into the prepared cavity'.

Evolution of Composite Inlay Material

The system and materials used in composite inlays were introduced in early eighties. Over the years, plenty of systems have evolved using composite resins. The evolution proceeds as:

a. First Generation Composite Inlays

i. *SR Isosit system:* SR Isosit (microfilled composite) is a homogeneously filled composite containing 55% by weight colloidal silica plus 20% lanthanium fluoride. The composite is available in seven shades (not matching vita shades).

ii. *Coltene-Brilliant:* The Coltene-Brilliant system is fine hybrid composite containing 78.5% by mass glass fiber (particle size 0.5 mm). The composite inlay is cured on a fabricated die and further polymerized in the Coltene DI500 light/heat curing oven for 7 minutes at a temperature of 120°C. The composite is available in four vita shades.

iii. *Kulzer inlay:* Kulzer system is coarse hybrid composite containing 80% glass ceramic filler by mass. The composite inlays are light cured and then tempered for three to six minutes in light units.

iv. *Visio Gem:* Visio Gem was initially introduced as a material for anterior composite veneers, but its use was expanded to include indirect composite inlays. The inlays are initially light cured followed by a 15-minute curing under vacuum.

b. Second Generation Composite Inlays

i. *Sculpture:* Sculpture is advanced light, heat and vacuum cured polymer glass restorative material. 1.0 mm diameter ceramic fillers are incorporated for achieving better strength.

ii. *Herculite:* Herculite is BisGMA micro-hybrid light activated composite along with 0.6 mm ceramic fillers. The filler particles reduce the polymerization shrinkage while increasing the modulus of elasticity.

iii. *Art glass:* Art glass contains Barium glass (0.7 mm radiopaque filler) and a moderate amount of colloidal silica for the purpose of enhancing handling characteristics.

The material is photocured in a special unit using a xeno stroboscopic light (emission of 4.5 watts power in the range of 320 and 500 nm). This range is significant because excitation of camphoroquinone (initiator) is optimized at about 470 nm.

iv. *Belleglass HP and NG:* The resin matrix in Belleglass HP is chemically similar to that of the BisGMA restorative systems. Belleglass HP is polymerized under pressure at an elevated temperature (138°C) and in the presence of nitrogen.

The use of nitrogen during polymerization helps increasing the wear resistance of the material. Nitrogen produces an oxygen-free environment, which results in higher level of polymerization.

Belleglass NG incorporates advanced nano-particles and submicron filler particles providing improved physical properties.

The composition and properties of indirect composite inlay system is tabulated in Table 5.3.

Table 5.3: Indirect composite inlay system: Composition and properties

Brand name (Manufacturer)	Composition	Polymerization	Key points
Art glass (Heraeus-Kulzer)	70 wt% filler of barium silicate glass (0.7 μm). 30 wt% organic resin matrix. Art glass contains four to six functional groups facilitating more double-bond conversions.	Photocuring is carried out in a special unit using a xenon stroboscopic light. The system emits 4.5 watts luminous power, initially for only 20 milliseconds, followed by rest of 80 milliseconds. The short excitation time followed by a longer period of non-exposure allows the already cured resin molecules to partially relax, allowing non-reactive double-bond carbon groups for reaction.	Used to fabricate inlay, onlays and crowns with/without metal substrate.
Belleglass HP and NG (Kerr Sybron Corporation) (Belleglass NG incorporates advanced nano-particles and submicron filler particles providing improved physical properties)	The base (dentin) composite has barium glass fillers (78.7% wt) and resin matrix; (BisGMA), whereas surface (enamel composite) has borosilicate fillers (74% wt) which provide enhanced optical characteristics. The resin matrix of enamel composite contains saturated methacrylate diure-thane of TEGDMA and aliphatic dimethacrylate.	The base (dentin) composite is light cured, with a conven-tional light curing unit. The surface (enamel) composite is heat cured. The complete polymerization is carried by light curing followed by heating in an oven at 140°C at 80 psi for 20 minutes. The atmosphere is maintained oxygen free and under nitrogen gas pressure.	• The reduction in size of the filler improves the polishability and smoothness of the material. • Provides high flexure strength. • Excellent wear resistant • High translucency • Shrinkage approximately 0.9%
Sinfony (3M ESPE)	Polyfunctional metha-crylate monomers, as resin matrix along-with Ultra-fine glass ceramic powder (strontium aluminium	Two polymerising units: Visio alpha is equipped with a halogen lamp and Visio beta is equipped with four fluorescent tubes. The polymerization wavelength	Used for full veneers, inlays/onlays, glass fibre reinforced bridges and for the customiza-tion of prefabricated teeth. Pyrogenic silica, having large surface area provides thicke-

Contd...

Table 5.3: Indirect composite inlay system: composition and properties (*Contd...*)

Brand name (Manufacturer)	Composition	Polymerization	Key points
	borosilicate glass—40% wt)—0.5 μm size as filler and as a microfiller. Pyrogenic silica as a microfiller.	ranges from 400 to 500 nm.The polymerization mode for alpha source is 40°C for 15 seconds; whereas, beta source is 40°C for 15 minutes.	ning effect and also controls the rheological properties of the composite. Two sources of polymerization improves physical properties.
Targis-Vectris (Ivoclar Vivadent)	Resin matrix—conventional BisGMA and filler. Filler—77wt%, barium glass (1.0 μm). Along with spheroid silica (0.25 μm) and colloidal silica (0.05 μm).	Targis is coated with glycerine gel (Targis Gel) to prevent formation of oxygen-inhibited surface layer. Polymerized in 450–500 nm halogen light unit for 10 minutes followed by tempering in heat (95°C) for 25 minutes and cooling for 5 minutes.	The material can be used with and without metal framework to fabricate adhesive inlays/ onlays/ veneers and crowns.
SR Adoro (Ivoclar Vivadent)	The components include SR Link (to bond to metal frame-work), a liner, dentin material, stains, incisal material and Opaquer. SR Link comprises a monomer that contains a highly hydrophobic hydro-carbon chain. The resin matrix consists of UDMA and TEGDMA along with fillers (63% by weight and 10–30 μm size). Upon polymeri-zation, the copolymers get integrated into the composite and a homogeneous composite with a high filler content is obtained.	Polymerization is similar to Targis; Halogen light followed by heating.	SR Adoro is improved version of Targis. The phosphoric acid reacts with the metal or the metal oxide, forming a phos-phate layer. The passivating phosphate layer on the metal surface soon becomes inert. The methacrylate group of the phosphoric acid reacts with the monomer components of S R Link, forms a copolymer, and provides a bond to the veneering resin.
Solidex (Shofu)	Light cured composite. Resin matrix is co-polymer of multi-functional (25%) and conventional (22%) along with fillers (53%,	Polymerization is carried out by halogen lights, curing for 1–5 minutes at a temperature of 55°C.	Available in 16 shades, used for inlays/onlays, veneers, crowns and temporary prosthesis. Provides high abrasion resistance and is cost effective.

Contd...

Table 5.3: Indirect composite inlay system: composition and properties *(Contd...)*

Brand name (Manufacturer)	Composition	Polymerization	Key points
	1.0 µm size silicone dioxide and aluminium - oxide and micro-ceramic fillers)		
Sculpture Plus (Pentron)	Nano-hybrid composite for indirect restorations. Resin matrix is poly-carbonate dimethacry-late (PCDMA) along-with nano particle fillers such as borosilicate glass, alumina, zirconium silicate and initiators.	Polymerization is two way curing; 5 minutes of pressure curing followed by 3 minutes of curing under high intensity light.	Available in 16 shades, used for inlays/onlays, veneers crowns, etc. Esthetically much better.
Paradigm and Paradigm MZ 100 (3M ESPE)	Nano hybrid composite (ceramic blocks added to make Paradigm MZ 100) Resin matrix is cross-linked BisGMA and TEGDMA along with fillers (85% ultrafine zirconia-silica)	Conventional polymerization (cross-linking ensures thorough polymerization)	Available in 12 shades; wear resistance is superior (similar to enamel). Used for indirect restorations, core build-up, etc.
Vita Zeta (Vita Zahnfabrite)	Light curing composite. Resin matrix is UDMA, TEGDMA along with 44% fillers of silicone dioxide.	Polymerization is carried out with curing unit of wavelength 300–500 nm, at a temperature of 40°C.	Used for indirect restorations; has high abrasion resistance.
Pearleste EZ (Tokuyama–Tokyo)	Nanosized indirect composite. Resin matrix is combination of TEGDMA, UDMA and Bis-MPEPP (methylacryloxy polyethoxy phenyl propane) along with fillers (0.04–0.08 µm) zirconia-silica.	Polymerization is carried out by curing at high pressure mercury lamp (350–500 nm) for two minutes followed by heating for 15 minutes in an oven under pressure.	Nano-sized fillers provide high level of translucency and esthetics.

Indications

The indications for indirect composite restorations are by and large same as for metallic restorations. The main indications are:

i. *Esthetic:* Replacement of existing metallic restorations for esthetic reasons is considered as the main indication.

ii. *Large defects:* These restorations are indicated for large defects or replacement of large compromised restorations. The contours so developed are more durable than direct composites.

iii. For improvement in contacts and contours (minor modification of proximal anatomy).

Contraindications

i. *Heavy occlusal forces:* Composite inlay is not preferred in patients who have bruxism and other clenching habits. Heavy wear facets or a lack of occlusal enamel are good indicators of bruxism and clenching habits.

ii. *Inability to maintain dry field:* Perfect moisture control is pre-requisite for successful adhesion of composite inlays.

iii. *Deep sub-gingival preparation:* Composite inlay is not indicated in preparations with deep sub-gingival margins, since these margins may not be recorded properly and are also difficult to finish.

iv. Patients who do not maintain oral hygiene.

Advantages

- The physical properties of indirect composites are much better than direct ones.
- They wear less than direct composites.
- The polymerization shrinkage is substantially reduced with indirect techniques.
- The weakened tooth structure can be strengthened by adhesively bonding the indirect restorations.
- Provide better contours (especially proximal contours) and occlusal contacts than direct restorations. Also, the adaptation at the cavosurface margins, especially the gingival margins, is better in indirect restorations.
- The biocompatibility is much better than direct composites.
- The indirect techniques allow for fabrication of the restoration in the dental laboratory. The chairside time is saved.

- Cross-splinting of the compromised tooth.
- Easy removal, if replacement is mandatory.

Disadvantages

- Indirect techniques require a high level of competency. Any compromise during preparation, impression making, cementation and finishing the restoration may lead to failure.
- Laboratory processed resins are highly cross-linked, therefore, very few double bonds remain available for chemical adhesion of the composite cement. The restoration must be mechanically abraded and chemically treated to facilitate adhesion of the cement. The bond between the indirect composite restoration and the composite cement is a weak link in the system.
- Indirect restorations are relatively difficult to repair.
- Indirect composite restorations are costlier than conventional cast metal restorations.

Cavity Preparation

The cavity preparation is by and large same as for gold inlays. Certain modifications are required for adhesive preparations. The important modifications are:

1. 2.0 mm isthmus width at the occlusal aspect.

2. No less than 2.0 mm cavity depth at its most shallow point.

3. The axial wall depth should be minimum 1.0 mm (1.0–1.5 mm).

4. The primary flare angle (90–100°) of exit in the proximal walls (may not be in the embrasure areas).

5. 10–12° occlusal taper exiting from the most gingival aspect to the occlusal cavosurface to allow passive seating of the restoration.

6. All internal line angles should be rounded.

7. Gingival margins should be a flat butt joint with no bevel.

Using fine diamond points, refine all margins to a smooth butt finish, particularly at the gingival floor and proximal walls. If the cusps require protection from occlusal load, they will need to be reduced in height by at least 2.0 mm at angle to the vertical, which is parallel to the original occlusal cuspal incline. This will ensure an even thickness of composite over the cusp and avoid acute angles within the restoration, which may become stress points leading to initiation of fractures. Do not provide bevels at the margins, because bevels will lead to fine fragile margins in the resin restoration.

The differences in cavity preparations in Gold, Base metals and Composite/porcelain are described in Table 5.4 and Fig. 5.17.

Classification of Composite Inlays

Composite inlays can be classified according to the method of curing.

a. *Inlays cured under heat and pressure:* The composite employed for such inlays is heat

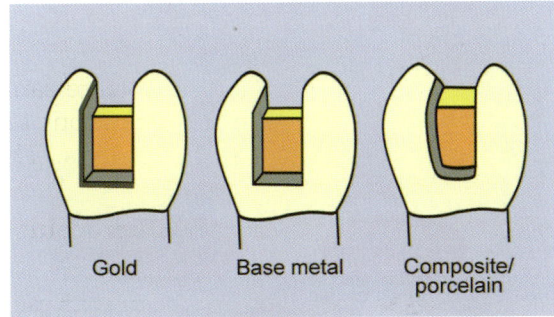

Fig. 5.17: Difference in cavity: Gold, base metal and composite/porcelain

cured. The inlays are cured at high temperature (120°C) and under pressure (SR Isosit system).

b. *Light cured inlays:* These inlays are cured by light (Dentacolor, Visio Gem).

c. *Secondary cured inlays:* These inlays utilize initial curing at room temperature by light followed by additional curing by heat (120°C) and light (5–7 minutes) (Brilliant Aesthetic System).

Method of Fabrication

The composite inlays can be fabricated either in office or in laboratory.

a. In-office Fabrication

The fabrication of composite inlay in office involves following steps:

- The prepared cavity is isolated preferably using rubber dams. The cavity walls are painted with a lubricant compatible with the hybrid composite material, which facilitates easy removal of inlay. [Examples: Brilliant Direct Inlay System (Coltene - Whaledent) and True Vitality System (Den-Mat Corp.)].

- A retainerless, contoured, clear matrix is adjusted around the proximal area of the prepared cavity. A clear reflecting wedge is placed at the inter-proximal gingival margins. The wedge is firmly placed to create rapid separation of the teeth (wedge compensates for thickness of the mylar matrix band facilitating developing contact area with the adjacent tooth).

Table 5.4: Difference in cavity preparation		
Gold	*Base metal*	*Composite/porcelain*
Narrow outline	Narrow outline	Wider outline
Depth less	Depth less	Depth more
Bevels given	No bevel	No bevel
Less taper (2–6° depending upon depth)	Less taper (2–6° depending upon depth)	More taper (10–12°)
Definite line angles	Definite line angles	Rounded line angles

- The hybrid composite material is placed into the prepared cavity starting with the proximal box. The material is gently condensed with a ball burnisher. The occlusal portion of the preparation is also filled and gently condensed. The ball burnisher used for condensation should be coated with a resin adhesive to avoid sticking of the material.
- The pressure of the wedges helps rapid separation of the teeth and also do not allow excess material at the gingival area. The inter-proximal area is cured for 30 seconds both from facial and the lingual aspects; followed by curing of occlusal surface for 30 seconds (soft polymerization).
- After the completion of light curing, the inlay is gently teased out of the prepared cavity (a gentle lift from the proximal area using hand instruments is usually required). If the inlay resists removal, a loop of dental floss along with a small increment of the composite material is placed in the central fossa area of the inlay and light cured. The inlay is then pulled along the path of withdrawal.
- Fresh lubricant is painted on the inlay surfaces. The lubricant excludes air and allows the inlay to completely cure without an air-inhibited layer. The air-inhibited layer is the softest layer of composite resin and should be excluded. The inlay is light cured for an additional 60 seconds, followed by tempering in an oven at 110°C for 7 minutes. (The combined light and heat curing ensures complete polymerization of the material, provides increased hardness and wear-resistance. Polymerization shrinkage is also minimized.)

b. Laboratory Fabrication

The fabrication of composite resin inlay, carried out in the laboratory, involves the following steps:

- The rubber base material is used to make impression of the prepared cavity (Fig. 5.18a). A stone die is also prepared accordingly

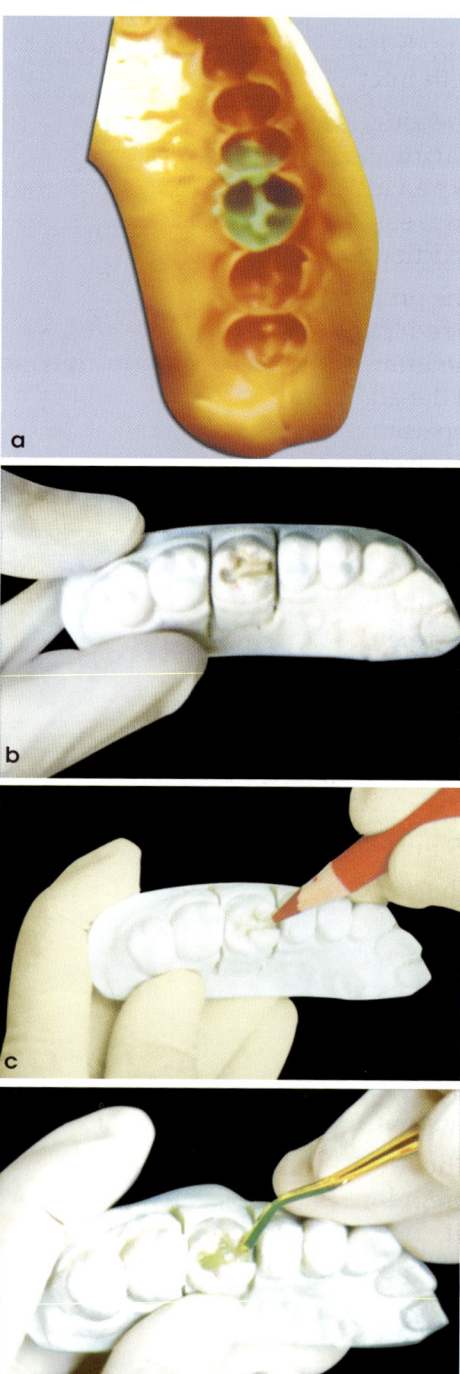

Figs 5.18a–d: Fabrication of composite resin inlay. a. impression of the prepared cavity, b. stone die of the prepared cavity. c. marking the margins, d. filling the cavity

(Fig. 5.18b). The prepared cavity is filled with interim materials.

- The gingival contacts should remain intact during sectioning the cast even at the expense of the adjacent tooth. The impression can be poured again if an additional cast is required.

- The preparation margins are outlined with a red pencil (Fig. 5.18c). A separating medium is applied to the internal surface of the die and also to the adjacent tooth. The separating medium is dried with a gentle air stream.

- The composite material of better viscosity and the correct shade is selected. Initially, the proximal area followed by occlusal area should be filled by gently condensing the material. The occlusal and proximal anatomy is carved simulating functional anatomy (Fig. 5.18d). Each surface is light cured for 60 seconds. The inlay is then removed from the die.

- The inlay is heat treated in an oven for 15 minutes at 100°C (Fig. 5.18e).

- The inlay is thoroughly cleaned ultra-sonically in a water bath and dried. The characterizing stain is applied to pits and fissures with a brush and light cured for 40 seconds (Fig. 5.18f). Stain may also be applied when the composite resin is being layered into the preparation to develop internal characterization.

- The inlay is tried in the die for any irregularities, if any, and also the marginal fit. If the proximal surface needs to be adjusted, a 5.0 × 5.0 mm square piece of double-sided articulating film, held in an articulating forceps, placed against the proximal surface of the tooth that is next to the prepared tooth. The inlay is seated and then removed to evaluate the mark on the proximal surface. This area can be adjusted using sof-lex disks (Fig. 5.18g).

- The temporary filling material is removed from the cavity using hand instruments.

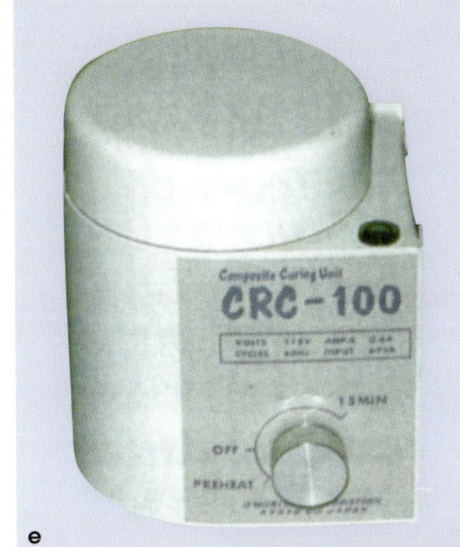

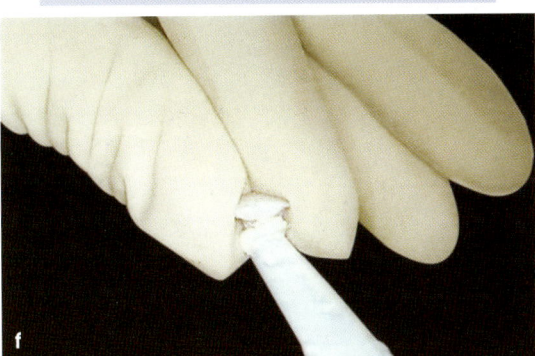

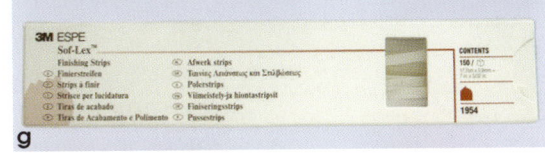

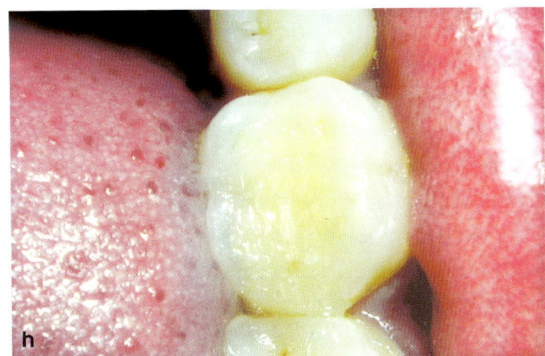

Fig. 5.18e–h: Fabrication of composite resin inlay contd. e. oven for curing inlay, f. cleaning the inlay and curing, g. sof-lex discs, h. inlay placed in the cavity

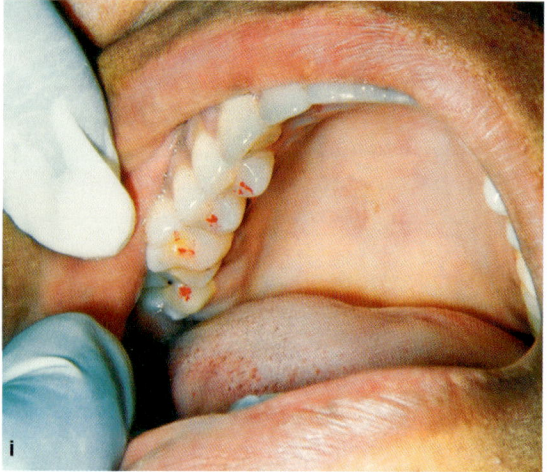

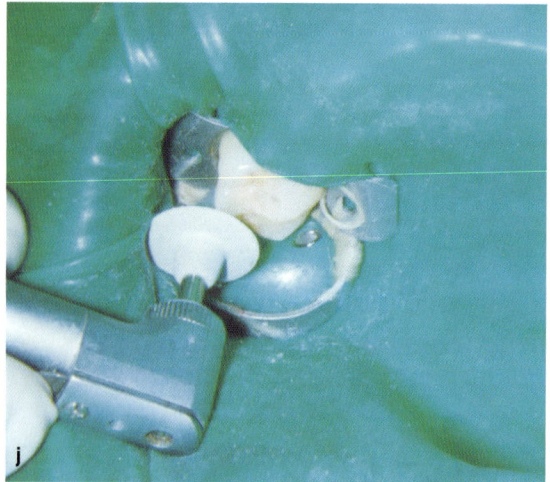

Figs 5.18i and j: Fabrication of composite resin inlay contd. i. verifying occlusal relations, j. finishing and polishing of cavity

area of the tooth. A heavy-weight rubber dam should be used to afford optimal gingival retraction during cementation.

- After seating the inlay, verify that the margins of the inlay coincide with the cavosurface margins of the tooth preparation. The excess material is trimmed off using safe-sided abrasive points.

- The occlusal relationships both in centric occlusion and in lateral movements are verified (Fig. 5.18i). If occlusal adjustment is necessary, the surface can be re-characterized. The final polish of the restoration and refinement of the margins should be carried out after bonding.

- Each restoration needs to be evaluated for marginal integrity, proximal contact relationship with adjacent teeth, occlusal relationship with the opposing arch and color. The color of the cement should be compatible with the selected shade for the inlay.

- The inner surfaces of the inlay are roughened to allow for chemical cross-linking between the cementing agent and the composite.

- The cavity is thoroughly cleaned using slurry of pumice powder. The enamel margins are etched for 20 seconds, and washed with a gentle water spray. The dentin and etched enamel are pretreated with an aluminum oxalate dentin conditioner for 30 seconds. The dual-cured cement is mixed in accordance with the manufacturer's instructions and applied to the tooth preparation and the internal surface of the inlay. Alternatively, the ultrasonics are used to place and bond the inlays. The ultrasonic technique takes advantage of the thixotropy of the composite resin. As soon as ultrasonic energy is applied, a highly viscous composite turns into a low viscous material. The clinicians can identify and remove the overhangs easily, because the excess composite gets as viscous as it was before

The residual temporary filling material is further cleaned with a prophylaxis brush and slurry of pumice powder.

- The inlay is then placed in the prepared cavity and evaluated clinically (Fig. 5.18h). A pack of gauge must be placed around the teeth to protect the patient from aspirating the inlay.

- The tooth should be isolated before placing the inlay, preferably with rubber dam. It is advisable to isolate at least two teeth distal to the tooth being restored. This facilitates inlay seating since the clamp jaws might impinge on the gingiva or inter-proximal

as soon as the ultrasonic energy is discontinued. The restoration is light cured from all aspects; proximal, facial, lingual, and occlusal, for 60 seconds each.

After polymerizing the cement, the margins of the restoration are finished with multifluted finishing burs using in sequence. The restoration is then finished and polished with an aluminum oxide polishing disk. The final polish is accomplished with a composite resin polishing paste (Fig. 5.18j). The rubber dam is removed and the occlusion is verified with articulating film in centric occlusion and excursive movements. If the occlusion is adjusted, then the restoration is re-polished.

CERAMIC INLAYS

The composites and ceramics have improved with the passage of time and both are indicated in large restorations. The physical properties of composite resin are such that it can neither withstand heavy occlusal loads nor is strong enough to be used in thin sections. The ceramics provide better properties than resin composites. Ceramics exhibit superior esthetics; better wear resistance and exceptional bond strength (with adhesive cements). The decision whether to opt for indirect composite or indirect ceramic is difficult. Ceramics are best suited as substitute for lost tooth structure since these restorations restore the tooth rigidity and strength. A few authors are of the view that size of the isthmus is important in selecting ceramic or composite as indirect restorative material. In case, the isthmus is less than two-third of the inter-cuspal width, composite is indicated and if the area is more than two-third of the inter-cuspal width, the ceramics are indicated.

Ceramic inlays/onlays are contraindicated for patients with poor oral hygiene, teeth with insufficient tooth structure left for bonding, or the cases where moisture control could not be achieved. These are also contraindicated in patients with para-functional habits such as bruxism, clenching, etc.

Types of Materials

The criteria for selection of ceramic material for inlays/onlays depend upon following characteristics.

a. *Marginal adaptation:* The longevity of the indirect restoration depends upon marginal adaptation, wear resistance of the luting cement, the cavity design and modulus of elasticity of the base, etc. There is definite and direct relationship between poor marginal adaptability and dissolution of the cement. It is established that a gap of 50–100 µm is always present at the tooth-restoration interface irrespective of the material choice. This gap, especially with the use of adhesive cements, may not cause much damage to the restoration in terms of discoloration and secondary caries. The materials which have the potential to adapt with the tooth surfaces, are preferred.

b. *Esthetics:* All ceramic restorations are esthetically pleasing. Castable ceramics produce highly translucent structure after de-vitrification. Surface staining can be used to obtain requisite stains. The color stains can be lost or weakened during occlusal adjustments.

c. *Strength:* The ceramic material should be able to resist initiation and propagation of the fracture. The structural inbuilt of the ceramic material control these two factors.

Ceramics, which are fired and sintered, usually exhibit porosities. This inherent weakness can partially be overcome by cast ceramics. The subsequent heat process and surface pigmentation do not encourage porosities. The process rather increases the strength.

Earlier, ceramic inlays were fabricated whereby ceramic was incorporated over the metal as in porcelain fused to metal restorations (Figs 5.19 a–e). However, with the advent of improved ceramic materials, all-ceramic inlays are fabricated (Figs 5.20 a–c).

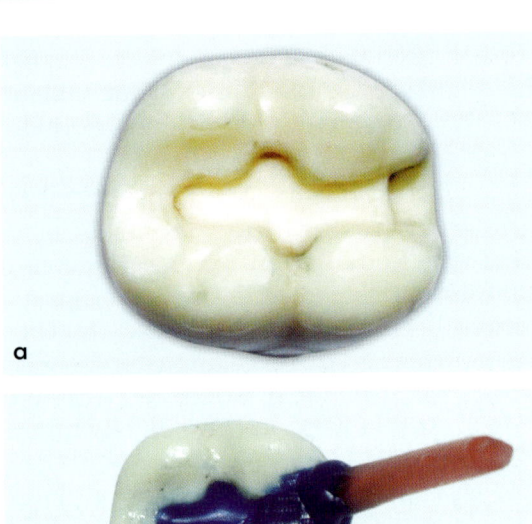

a

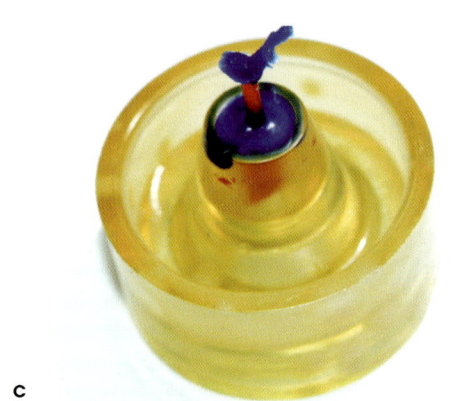

b

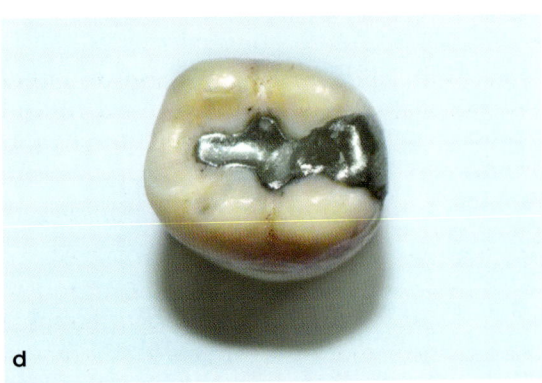

c

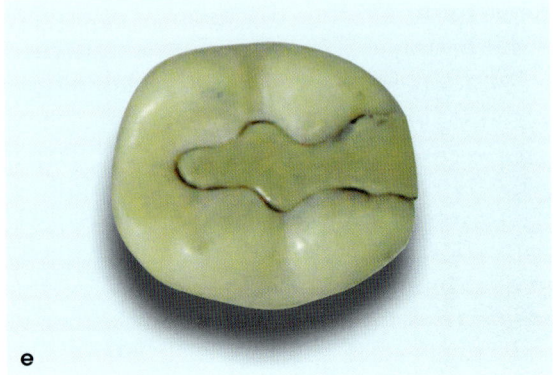

d

Figs 5.19a–d: Earlier concept of ceramic inlays. a. cavity prepared, b. wax pattern, c. casting of wax pattern, d. metal casting.

e

Fig. 5.19e: Ceramic over the metal

Cavity/Tooth Preparation

The basic principles of cavity preparation for ceramic restorations are by and large same as for cast restorations.

Since ceramic is very fragile and liable to fracture during insertion and adjustments, certain features are incorporated for ceramic restorations, modifying the cavity preparation. The modified features are:

a. *Adequate thickness of ceramic:* The strength of ceramic is directly proportional to its thickness, however, greater thickness is avoided, which may jeopardize the pulpal health. A uniform thickness of 2.0 mm is considered ideal for ceramic inlays and onlays; however, axially 1.5 mm reduction is preferred.

b. *Avoidance of internal stress concentration areas:* The internal line angles are rounded and the undercuts are filled prior to final impression making. The sharp angles create stress concentration areas.

c. *Creating positive path of insertion:* The positive path of insertion is determined by the inclination of the adjacent walls. Though, the preparation walls are kept divergent occlusally even in cast gold restorations, but in ceramics the divergence of 10–12° is mandatory. The ceramic restorations are very fragile and during seating or try-in procedures may fracture. The greater divergence of walls allow proper seating of the restoration.

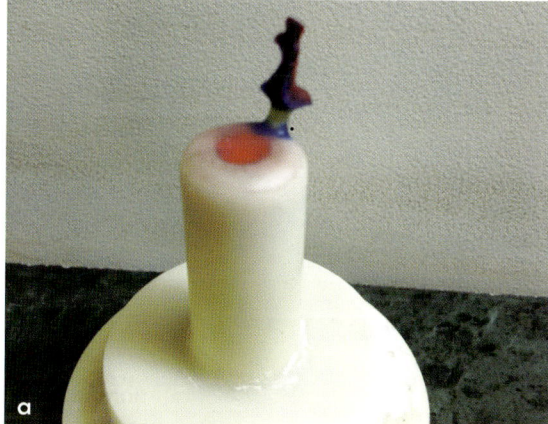

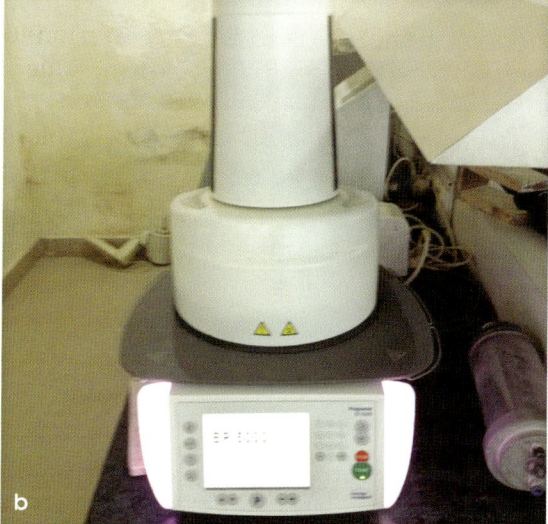

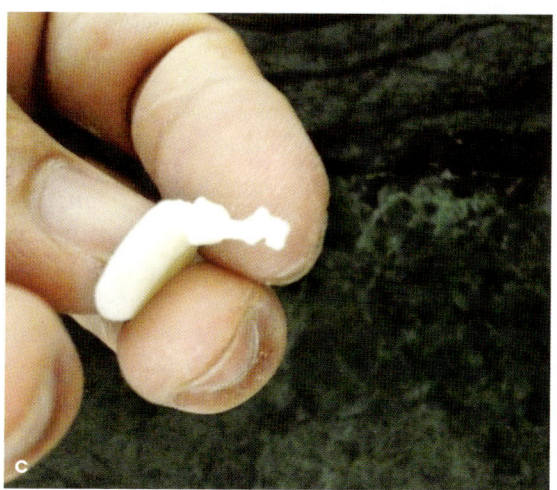

Figs 5.20a–c: All ceramic inlay preparation. a. inlay mould, b. curing the inlay, c. cured inlay

d. *Avoiding bevels of any kind:* The cavosurface angles are kept at 90° without any bevel. The bevels reduce porcelain thickness at the edges and weaken the restoration; subsequently, the restoration may fracture at the edges.

The Base

The base is placed to protect the pulp and also to act as substitute for lost dentin. The base material under the ceramic restorations should have sufficient rigidity and strength. The ceramics being brittle must be bonded to a substrate capable of supporting functional stresses. In a given system, when stress is applied to different materials showing different modulii of elasticity, the material of greatest rigidity absorbs the higher part of the stress. In case the base is weak, the stresses will be borne by the ceramic only, which might lead to its fracture.

When the compression load is generated on the occlusal surfaces, it turns into tensile load on to the inferior surface of the restoration. In case, the substrate fails to bear the load and yield, the restoration fails. The flexible substrate allows early failure of ceramic restorations.

The glass-ionomer cement, owing to its low compressive strength is not preferred as a base under ceramic restorations. However, glass-ionomer cement can be used in the correction of minor irregularities and undercuts.

It is established that resin composite should be used as base under ceramic restoration owing to their greater modulus of elasticity.

Cementation of Ceramic Inlays/Onlays

The ceramic restorations, as emphasized, are weak and fragile; therefore, the potential stresses on to the restoration are to be taken care of. The cements which have no adhesive properties such as zinc phosphate, etc. are likely to create stress concentration areas during function, leading to fracture of restorations or even the tooth. The adhesive cements are preferred, which can make bond with the tooth as well as the restoration.

The commonly used cements for luting of ceramic restorations are glass-ionomer cements and resin-based cements. The glass-ionomer cement has the advantage of bonding to enamel and dentin, fluoride release and low solubility in oral environment; however, it is established that ceramic restorations cemented with glass-ionomer cements are weak and exhibit poor fracture resistance. Resin modified glass-ionomer cement was also as good as conventional GIC (the cohesive strength of resin modified glass-ionomers is much lower than composites).

The resin luting cements are routinely used luting agents in ceramic inlays/onlays. These cements exhibit better strength, insolubility in oral environment, biocompatibility and esthetic potential. The light cured agents when used in posterior restorations might not be cured fully because of limitation of the light penetrating more distally. This may lead to poor hardness of the cement and also more solubility.

The dual cure cements are preferred. These cements can polymerize in inaccessible areas. These cements also provide better working time and adhesion to the substrate.

Procedure for Cementation

The steps followed for cementation of ceramic inlays/onlays are:

- The cavity is thoroughly cleaned before try-in (The restoration is cleaned, placed in the cavity and analyzed for any discrepancy).
- The cavity is isolated using rubber dam.
- The inner surface of the restoration is etched with 8–12% hydrofluoric acid for 1–3 minutes depending upon the ceramic material used. Acid treatment dissolves the glass material creating micro-porosities. Feldspathic porcelain needs more time than others. After etching, the inner surface is thoroughly cleaned with air-water rinses.

- The silane-coupling agent is then applied without touching the inner surface of the restoration. Silane enhances the porcelain-resin bonds by promoting the wetting of ceramic surfaces and allowing the resin to flow into the microporosities.
- The cavity/preparation is also etched with 30–35% phosphoric acid for 10–15 seconds. The preparation is rinsed with air-water spray. The excess of water is removed using slow air.
- A thin layer of adhesive is applied to the tooth surface and also the restoration. The resin-based cement is painted to the restoration and the cavity and seat the restoration with a little pressure.
- The patient is asked to close in functional occlusion.
- Excess cement is removed from the margins. The cervical area is cleaned.
- The margins are light cured for 40–60 seconds from all the directions.
- The glycerin-based gel may be applied to all accessible margins to prevent the occurrence of oxygen inhibited resin layer.
- The final polishing usually is not required in ceramic restorations. In case, polishing is required, it should be carried out by diamond impregnated finishing points and polishing gels.
- Intra-oral adjustments after cementation should be avoided.

Bibliography

1. Ahlers MO, Morig G, Blunck U, Hajto J, Probster l and Frankeberger R. Guidelines for the preparation of CAD/CAM ceramic inlays and partial crowns. Int. J. Compu. Dent.: 2009;12:309–25.
2. Albers HF. Ceramometal bonded inlays and onlays. J. Esthet. Dent.: 2000;12:122–30.
3. Arnetzl GV and Arnetzl G. Design of preparations for all-ceramic inlay materials. Int. J. Comput. Dent.: 2006;9:289–98.
4. Aspros A. Inlays and onlays: clinical experiences and literature review. J. Dent. Health Oral Disord. Ther.: 2015;2:1–7.

5. Banks RG. Conservative posterior Ceramic restorations: a literature review. JPD: 1990;63:619–26.

6. Beier US, Kapferer I, Bustscher D. Giesinger JM and Dumfahrt H. Clinical performance of all-ceramic inlay and onlay restorations in posterior teeth. Int. J. Prosthodont.: 2012;25:395–402.

7. Blatz MB, Sadan A and Kern M. Resin-ceramic bonding: a review of the literature. J. Prosthet. Dent.: 2003;89:268–74.

8. Borba M, Bon AD and Cecchetti D. Flexural strength and hardness of direct and IRC. Braz.Oral Res.: 2009;23:5–10.

9. Boushell LW and Ritter AV. Ceramic inlays: a case presentation and lessons learned from the literature. J. Esthet. Rest. Dent.: 2009;21:77–87.

10. Brackett MG, Kious AR and Brackett WW. Minimally retentive gold onlays: a six-year case report. Oper. Dent.: 2009;34:352–5.

11. Cai Z, Bunce N, Nunn ME and Okabe T. Porcelain adherence to dental cast and titanium: Effects of surface modification. Biomaterials.: 2001;22:979–86.

12. Carvalho RM, Pereira JC, Yoshiyama M and Pashley DH. A review of polymerization contraction: The influence of stress development versus stress relief. Oper. Dent.: 1996;21:17–24.

13. Chabouis HF, Faugeron VS and Attal JP. Clinical efficacy of composite versus ceramic inlays and onlays: a systematic review. Dent. Mater.: 2013;29: 1209–18.

14. Chabouis HF, Prot C, Fonteneau C, Nasr K, Chabreron O, Cazier S, Moussally C, Gaucher A, Jaballah IK, Boyer R, Leforestier JF, Prim AC, Chemla F, Maman L, Nabet C and Attal JP. Efficacy of composite versus ceramic inlays and onlays: study protocol for the CECOIA randomized controlled trial. Biomed. Central: 2013;14:278.

15. Conrad HJ, Seong WJ and Pesun IJ. Current ceramic materials and systems with clinical recommendations: a systematic review. J. Prosthet. Dent.: 2007;98:389–404.

16. Cramer NB, Stansbury JW and Bowman CN. Recent advances and developments in composite dental restorative materials. J. Dent. Res.:2011;90: 402–16.

17. Daronch M, Rueggeberg FA and De Goes MF. Monomer conversion of pre-heated composite. J. Dent. Res.: 2005;84:663–7.

18. Dejak B, Mlotkowski A and Romanowicz M. Strength estimation of different designs of ceramic inlays and onlays in molars based on the Tsai-wu failure criterion. J. Prosthet. Dent.: 2007;98:89–100.

19. Edlehoff D and Sorensen JA. Tooth structure removal associated with various preparation designs for posterior teeth. Int. J. Periodontics Restroative Dent.: 2002;22:241–9.

20. Ereifej N, Silikas N, Watts DC. Edge strength of indirect restorative materials. J. Dent.: 2009;37: 799–806.

21. Eriksson M, Andersson M and Carlstrom E. Titanium for prosthodontic applications: A review of the literature. Quint. Int.: 1996;27:401–8.

22. Esquivel-Upshaw JF, Anusavice KJ, Yang MC and Lee RB. Fracture resistance of all-ceramic and metal-ceramic inlays. Int. J. Protho.: 2001;14:109–14.

23. Fages M and Bennasar B. The Endocrown: a different type of all-ceramic reconstruction for molars. J. Can. Dent. Assoc.: 2013;79:140.

24. Fasbinder DJ. Clinical performance of chairside CAD/CAM restorations. J. Am. Dent. Assoc.: 2006;137:22S-31S.

25. Fasbinder DJ, Neiva GF, Dennison JB and Heys DR. Clinical performance of CAD/CAM-generated composite inlays after 10 years. J. Cosmetic Dent.: 2013;28:134–45.

26. Fennis WM, Kuijs RH, Barink M, Kreulen CM, Verdonschot N and Creugers NH. Can internal stresses explain the fracture resistance of cusp-replacing composite restorations? Eur. J. Oral Sci.: 2005;113:443–8.

27. Filho AM, Vieira LC, Ara-yo E and Baratieri LN. Ceramic inlays and onlays: Clinical procedures for predictable results. J. Esthet. Rest. Dent. 2003; 15:338–51.

28. Fliger J. Preparation design and considerations for direct posterior composite inlay/onlay restoration. Int. Dent.: 2008;12:6–15.

29. Frankenberger R, Reinelt C, Perschelt A and Kramer N. Operator vs. material influence on clinical outcome of bonded ceramic inlays. Dent. Mater.: 2009;25:960–8.

30. Galip Gurel. Porcelain inlays and onlays. Dental Clin. North Am.: 2001;45:177.

31. Gilboe DB and Teteruck WR. Fundamentals of extra-coronal tooth preparations. Part I. Retention and resistance form. JPD: 2005;94:105–7.

32. Giordano R and McLaren EA. Ceramics overview: Classification by microstructure and processing methods. Compend. Contin. Educ. Dent.: 2010;31: 6582–5684, 686–8.

33. Gonzaga CC, Cesar PF, Miranda Jr WG and Yoshimura NH. Slow crack growth and reliability of dental ceramics. Dent. Mater.: 2011;27:394–406.

34. Goodacre CJ. Palladium silver alloy: A review of the literature. J.Prosth. Dent.:1989; 62:34–7.

35. Gracis S, Thompson VP, Ferencz JL, Silva NRFA, Bonfante EA. A new classification system for All-ceramic and ceramics-like restorative materials. Int. J. Prosthodont.: 2015;28:227–35.

36. Guess PC, Schultheis S, Bonfante EA, Coelho PG, Ferencz JL and Silva NR. All-ceramic systems: Laboratory and clinical performance. Dent. Clin. North Am.: 2011;55:333–52.

37. Hannig M and Schmeiser R. Esthetic posterior restorations utilizing the double inlay technique: a novel approach in esthetic dentistry. Quint. Int.: 1997;28: 79–83.

38. Hagg P and Nilner. Questions and answers on titanium-ceramic dental restorative system. A literature study. Quint. Int.: 2007;38: e5–13.

39. Hayashi M, Wilson NHF, Yeung CA and Worthington HV. Systematic review of ceramic inlays. Clin. Oral Investig.: 2003;7:8–19.

40. Helvey GA. Classifying dental ceramics: Numerous materials and formulations available for indirect restorations. Compend. Contin. Educ. Dent.: 2014;35:38–43.

41. Holberg C, Rudzki-Janson I, Wichelhaus A and Winterhalder P. Ceramic inlays: Is the inlay thickness an important factor influencing the fracture risk? J. Dent.: 2013;41:628–35.

42. Homsy F, Eid R, Ghoul WE and Chidiac JJ. Considerations for altering preparation designs of porcelain inlay/onlay restorations for non-vital teeth. J. Prosthodont.: 2015;24:457–62.

43. Hopp C and Land M. Considerations for ceramic inlays in posterior teeth: a review. Clin. Cosmet. Investig. Dent.: 2013;5:21–32.

44. Kadowaka A, Suzuki S and Tanaka T. Wear evaluation of porcelain opposing gold, composite resin and enamel. J. Prosthet. Dent.: 2006;96:258–65.

45. Kakaboura A, Rahiotis C, Zinelis S, Al-Dhamadi YA, Silikas N and Watts DC. In vitro characteriza-tion of two lab-processed resin composites. Dent. Mater.: 2003;19:93–8.

46. Kelly J and Benetti P. Ceramic materials in dentistry: Historical evolution and current practice. Aust. Dent. J.: 2011;56:84–96.

47. Kelly J and Rose T. Nonprecious alloys for use in fixed prosthodontics: a literature review. J Prosthet. Dent. 1983;49:363–70.

48. Krifka S, Anthofer T, Fritzsch M, Hiller KA, Schmalz G and Federlin M. Ceramic inlays and partial ceramic crowns: influence of remaining cusp wall thickness on the marginal integrity and enamel crack formation in vitro. Oper. Dent.: 2009;34:32–42.

49. Leinfelder KF. Indirect composite resins. Compend. Contin. Educ. Dent.: 2005;26:495–503.

50. Mahart J, Kunzelmann KH, Chen HY and Hickel R. Mechanical properties of new composite restorative materials. J. Biomed. Mater. Res.: 2000; 53: 353–61.

51. Martin N and Jedynakiewicz NM. Clinical performance of CEREC ceramic inlays: a systematic review. Dental Mater.: 1999;15:54–61.

52. McLaren EA and Phone TC. Ceramics in dentistry–Part I: Classes of materials. Inside Dent.: 2009;5:94–103.

53. Mendonca JS, Neto RG, Santiago SL, Lauris JR, Navarro MF and De Carvalho RM. Direct resin composite restorations versus indirect composite inlays: One-year results. J. Contemp. Dent. Pract.: 2010;11: 25–32.

54. Meyer A, Cardoso LC, Araujo E and Baratieri LN. Ceramic inlays and onlays: clinical procedures for predictable results. J. Esthet. Restor. Dent.: 2003;15:338–51.

55. Milleding P, Ortengren U and Karlsson S: Ceramic inlay system: Some clinical aspects. J. Oral Rehab. 1995;22:571–80.

56. Miranda CP, Pigani C, Bottino MC and Benetti AR. A comparison of microhardness of IRC Restorative materials. J. Appl. Oral Sci.: 2003;11, 157–61.

57. Nandini S. Indirect resin composites. J. Cons. Dent.: 2010;13:184–94.

58. Ona M, Watanabe C, Igarashi Y and Wakabayashi N. Influence of preparation design on failure risks of ceramic inlays: a finite element analysis. J. Adhesive Dent.: 2011;13:367–73.

59. Petropoulou A, Pantzari F, Nomikos N, Chronopoulos V and Kourtis S. The use of indirect resin composites in clinical practice: A case series. Dentistry: 2013;3, 1–6.

60. Pol CW and Kalk W. A systematic review of ceramic inlays in posterior teeth: an update. Int. J. Prosthodont.: 2011;24:566–75.

61. Qualtrough AJE, Wilson NHF and Smith GA. The porcelain inlay: A historical view. Oper. Dent.: 1990;15:61–70.

62. Rechenberg DK, Gohring TN and Attin T. Influence of different curing approaches on

marginal adaptation of ceramic inlays. J. Adhes. Dent.: 2009;12:189–96.

63. Reiss B. Clinical results of CEREC inlays in a dental practice over a period of 18 years. Int. J. Comput. Dent.: 2006;9:11–22.

64. Ritcher J and Mehl A. Evaluation for the fully automatic inlay reconstruction by means of biogeneric tooth model. Int. J. Comput. Dent.: 2006;9:101–11.

65. Ritter AV and Baratieri LN. Ceramic restoration for posterior teeth: guidelines for the clinician. J. Esthet. Dent.: 1999;11:72–86.

66. Rocca GT and Krejci I. Bonded indirect restorations for posterior teeth: From cavity preparation to provisionalization. Quint. Int.: 2007;38:371–9.

67. Rueggeberg FA, Daronch M, Browning WD and De Goes MF. In vivo temperature measurement: tooth preparation and restoration with preheated resin composite. J. Esthet. Restor. Dent.: 2010; 22:314–22.

68. Samran A, Nassani MZ, Aswad M and Abdulkarim A. A modified design for posterior inlay-retained fixed dental prosthesis. Case Reports in Dentistry: Art. ID 2015;576820: 1–5.

69. Sato K, Matsumura H and Atsuta M. Relation between cavity design and marginal adaptation in machine-milled ceramic restorative system. J. Oral Rehabil.: 2002;29:24–7.

70. Scotti N, Coero Borga FA, Alovisi M, Rota R, Pasqualini D and Berutti E. Is fracture resistance of endodontically treated mandibular molars restored with indirect onlay composite restorations influenced by fibre post insertion? J. Dent.: 2012;40:814–20.

71. Shenoy A and Shenoy N. Dental ceramics: An update. J. Cons. Dent.: 2010;13:195–203.

72. Sorensen JA and Martinoff JT. Intracoronal reinforcement and coronal coverage: a study of endodontically treated teeth. J. Prosth. Dent.: 1984;51:780–4.

73. Stappert CF, Guess PC, Chitmongkolsuk S, Gerds T and Strub JR. All-ceramic partial coverage restorations on natural molars. Masticatory fatigue loading and fracture resistance. Am. J. Dent.: 2007;20:21–6.

74. Terry DA, Leinfelder KF and Maragos C. Developing form, function, and natural aesthetics with laboratory-processed composite resin–Part I. Pract. Proced. Aesthet. Dent.: 2005;17:313–8.

75. Terry DA and Touati B. Clinical considerations for aesthetic laboratory fabricated inlays/onlays restoration: a review. Pract. Proced. Aesthet. Dent.: 2001;13:51–8.

76. Thompson SA. An overview of Nickel-titanium alloy used in dentistry. Int. Endod. J.: 2000;33:297–310.

77. Thompson MC, Thompson KM and Swain M. The all-ceramic, inlay supported fixed partial denture. Part 1. Ceramic inlay preparation design: a literature review. Aust. Dent. J.: 201;55:120–7.

78. Tsitrou EA and van Noort R. Minimal preparation designs for single posterior indirect prostheses with the use of the Cerec system. Int. J. Comput. Dent.: 2008;11:227–40.

79. Van Dijken JWV. All ceramic restorations: Classification and clinical evaluation. Compendium: 1999;20:1115–24.

80. Veneziani M. Adhesive restorations in the posterior area with subgingival cervical margins: new classification and differentiated treatment approach. Eur. J. Esthet. Dent.: 2010;5:50–76.

81. Vohra F, Rashid H and Ab Ghani S. Modern adhesive ceramic onlays, a predictable replacement of full veneer crowns: a report of three cases. J. Dow. Univ. Health: 2014;8:35–40.

82. Wagner WC, Aksu MN, Neme AM, Linger JB, Pink FE and Walker S. Effect of pre-heating resin composite on restoration microleakage. Oper. Dent.: 2008;33, 77–8.

83. Wassel RW, Walls AWG and Steele JG. Crowns and extracoronal restorations: Material selection. British Dent. J. 2002;192, 199–211.

84. Wolf BH, Walter MH, Boening KW and Schmidt AE. Margin quality of titanium and high gold inlays and onlays—a clinical study. Dent. Mater.: 1998;14:370–4.

85. Zaruba M, Gohring TN, Wegehaupt FJ and Attin T. Influence of a proximal margin elevation technique on marginal adaptation of ceramic inlays. Acta. Odont. Scand.: 2013;71:317–24.

86. Zaruba M, Kasper R, Kazama R, Wegehaupt FJ, Ender A, Attin T and Mehl A. Marginal adaptation of ceramic and composite inlays in minimally invasive MOD cavities. Clin. Oral Invest.: 2014; 18:579–87.

87. Zhang Y, Chai H and Lawn BR. Graded structures for all-ceramic restorations. J. Dent. Res.: 2009;89: 417–21.

88. Zhang Y and Ma L. Optimization of ceramic strength using elastic gradients. Acta. Mater.: 2009;57: 2721–9.

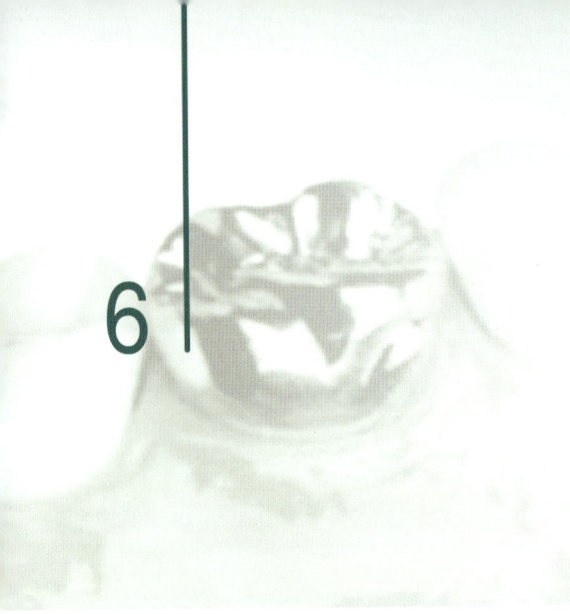

6

Post and Core Restorations

One of the major objectives of restorative dentistry is to preserve the vitality of the pulp. Repeated restorations may invite the need of endodontic intervention. In case, endodontic intervention becomes unavoidable, then the care should be taken to preserve the remaining tooth structure. The remaining tooth structure is important in planning and executing the restoration in such teeth. The factors, which should be considered by the operator, are the strategic position of the tooth in the arch, the occlusal load, which the tooth will be bearing, overall occlusal pattern and also the oral hygiene of the patient.

The restoration of endodontically treated tooth involves replacement of missing tooth structure along with protection of the remaining tooth. To replace the missing tooth structure, the operator should decide whether the retention is to be achieved through root canals or the remaining tooth structure. Already structurally weakened, such teeth are often further weakened by endodontic procedures involving access cavity and root canal preparation. Ensuring resistance and retention features for final restoration being challenging along with other problems, have resulted in the development of various materials and techniques.

Effect of Endodontic Treatment on the Tooth

After the endodontic treatment or precisely the root canal treatment, the tooth exhibits certain morphological and physical changes, which are:

i. *Loss of tooth structure:* The tooth structure might have been lost prior to the treatment because of caries and fracture, etc. The endodontic procedures such as access cavity preparation or involuntary cutting during negotiating root canals also lead to loss of tooth structure. The bulk of the remaining dentin is important since the strength of the tooth is proportional to it. As the bulk of the dentin is decreased, the stiffness of the tooth is decreased. It is established that even the conservative access cavity preparation decreases the stiffness of the tooth by 5%; whereas in class II preparation, there is 40% loss of stiffness and 60% stiffness is lost in mesio-occluso-distal preparation.

ii. *Physical changes:* It is believed that root canal treatment leads to dehydration, consequently, weakening the tooth. A few authors, however, do not favour this notion, claiming that dentin hardness is not altered after endodontic treatment.

iii. *Altered appearance:* The root canal treated tooth may show altered appearance because of presence of residual pulp remnants and even medicaments. The chemically altered dentin reflects light differently, which modifies appearance.

iv. *Proprioception:* Sense of proprioception is lost in root canal treated teeth. Neuro-sensory feedback mechanism is impaired because of loss of pulpal tissues.

The restoration of endodontically treated teeth is planned following the guidelines as:

- The root canal treatment should be of good quality. Only clinically asymptomatic tooth will not suffice. Radiological assessment is acceptable, though computer aided radiography can be preferred in evaluating the quality of obturation.

- It is a common notion that endodontically treated teeth fracture easily because of increased brittleness; however, the amount of remaining tooth structure controls the fracture resistance of the tooth. The operator should take extra care so that the loss of tooth structure during cavity preparation, especially the post-preparation be minimized. The root canal treated tooth with sufficient amount of dentin can conservatively be restored without the need of extra retentive devices.

- The reinforcement of remaining tooth structure with bonded materials can also be planned. The long-term validity of this reinforcement with time is questionable; however, the treatment is effective in teeth with less surface area remaining (for example, premolars).

- The operator should analyze all factors before placing post, especially in the posterior teeth. The post in posterior teeth is avoided as far as possible. The post is placed only to retain core. A few authors are of the view that the post and core should be built using the same material. It minimizes the vertical stresses and is also time saving.

- Length of the post depends upon the configuration of the core required and the length of the root. The amount of stresses, which destabilize the restorations, should also be considered.

- The removal of gutta-percha always disturbs the apical seal. Early or delayed removal of gutta-percha might not be significant in disturbing the apical seal. Quick removal with heated instruments, however, is considered better method. Guttacut, a recently developed instrument, utilizes this principle.

Prior to restoration, a decision is to be taken whether the support from root is required or not. The substitution of the crown portion may be with or without the help of pins, is referred to as 'core'. The root canal support of the core, may be metallic or plastic, is referred to as 'post' or 'dowel'. Collectively, the system is known as 'post and core' or 'post-core" system. By and large, care should be taken to achieve resistance and retention form from the core only without the root canal support. In case this is not feasible, the root(s) should be thoroughly assessed before planning the post preparation.

The root/root canal should be assessed for following features:

- The remaining coronal/incisal tooth structure present along the root

- The quantum of occlusal load, which the restored tooth will be bearing

- Number of root canals required for resistance and retention form

- Configuration of the root canal

- The thickness of dentin around the root canal

- The amount of dentin, which can be utilized in preparation of post

- Caries/resorption inside the root, if any

- Periodontal support

- Possibility of extra retentive devices, if any

- Sufficient length of the post, which can be achieved from the root canal

Functions of Post

The post serves the following functions:

- It retains core, which further helps in restoration of the lost tooth structure.
- It resists the tensile forces, which tend to pull the restoration away from the tooth.
- It distributes occlusal forces along the length of the roots to the periodontium (crowns of endodontically treated teeth are usually damaged to an extent that the remaining tooth structure cannot distribute the forces along the natural ways).
- It maintains the marginal integrity of the final restoration by providing sufficient rigidity at the margins, which further prevents the breakdown of cement medium.

Classification of Posts

For convenience, the posts are classified into four classes:

Class I   Self-retentive metal posts (post with self-cutting threads or different types of screws)

Class II   Metal posts with passive retention (no direct contact between the post and the root canal wall. The post needs luting cement for the space present between the post and the root canal wall)

Class III Non metal posts with passive retention (fiber reinforced posts and ceramic posts along with adhesive cement)

Class IV   Biological posts (dentin posts along with adhesive cement)

Types of Posts

- Custom cast posts
- Pre-fabricated posts
  A. Passive posts
     a. Tapered
        - Smooth
        - Serrated
     b. Parallel
        - Smooth
        - Serrated
  B. Active posts
     a. Tapered
        - Self-threaded
     b. Parallel
        - Self-threaded
- Fiber reinforced posts
  A. Carbon fibers
     - Mirafit carbon
     - Endo post
     - Carbonite system
     - Composi post
  B. Silica fibers
     a. Quartz fibers
        - Aesthetic post
        - Aesthetic post plus
        - Style post
        - Light/light DT post
     b. Glass fibers
        - Snow post
        - Mirafit white
        - Luscent anchor
        - Fiberkov post
        - Fiber white parapost
     c. Polyethylene fibers
        - Ribbond/Ribbond THM
        - Construct
- All-ceramic posts
- Dentin posts (Biological posts)
- Miscellaneous post systems
- Light transmitting post (intra-radicular rehabilitation)

The fiber reinforced posts are categorized clinically as 'generation', based on radiopacity and their esthetic appearance. The generations are:

1. *Generation I* (neither radiopaque nor esthetic)
   - Composi post
   - C post
2. *Generation II* (esthetic but not radiopaque)
   - Esthetic post

- Light post
- Fiber white
- Fiberkov
- Dentatus luscent anchor

3. *Generation III* (Esthetics and radiopaque)
   - DT light post
   - DT light post illusion
   - Snow light
   - Rely-X post
   - FRC postec plus

I. Custom Cast Posts

Custom cast posts are fabricated from a negative reproduction of the prepared root canal. Wax or cold cure resins are usually used to obtain the patterns, which are then invested and cast using an appropriate alloy. Type III and type IV gold alloys are commonly used; however, the base metals and titanium alloys are also being used.

The custom cast posts conform to the configuration of the prepared canal and are significant in flared canal. The characteristic features of these posts are:

- The custom cast posts conforming to the root canal configuration (usually taper) are less retentive than parallel posts (may be custom cast or prefabricated)
- The posts do not induce any stress during installation
- The posts may act as wedge during load transfer
- Venting is required during cementation

II. Prefabricated Posts

The different shapes and sizes of the post are prefabricated and designed to fit in a prepared canal space. This differs from the custom cast post because the canal is prepared according to the available post. The resulting fit may or may not be exact but it is usually clinically acceptable.

The prefabricated posts are made of metal or plastic. The plastic prefabricated posts are usually preferred. The plastic posts are available in tapered and parallel configuration. Further, the shapes can be smooth or serrated; the serrated ones offer better retention.

Prefabricated posts are mainly divided into following two types.

A. Passive Posts

The passive posts achieve retention mostly by adherence of the cementing medium with post and the dentin. The types of passive posts are:

a. *Tapered posts:* The taper designs are preferred, since they simulate the root canal configuration, thereby lessening the chance of a lateral perforation. Tapered posts exhibit least stresses during cementation; however, they may create a wedging effect inside the root.

The currently available tapered plastic posts exhibit taper ranging from 1.1 to 6.2°. The tapered plastic posts are selected according to the size of the reamer or file. The size at the apex is usually 1.0, 1.2, 1.3 and 1.6 mm and correspondingly the diameter is increased coronally. Two numbers in each set are indicated one, the diameters at the tip and second, 10.0 mm from the tip.

The different tapers and sizes are available suitable to different root canal configurations. The commonly available tapered passive (smooth sided) posts are Kerr endopost and Mooser post. These are the least retentive of all post designs.

b. *Parallel posts:* The parallel posts may have a serrated or smooth surface. Smaller diameter of such posts are also used as accessory retentive devices (pin into periapical dentin of root canal). It is also necessary to evaluate the tooth structure available for placing post as well as pin, if required. If there is insufficient available dentin, keyways can be prepared at the cervical end of the post. The para-post (serrated parallel post) is manufactured with a groove running its entire length, which acts as a cement vent.

The use of a serrated parallel plastic post is preferred in straight bulky canals.

The post should be large enough to accommodate as far the coronal portion of the canal as possible, but small enough to leave an adequate thickness of dentin at the apical end.

The parallel posts provide greater retention and create less stress than tapered posts, e.g. Whaledent para post, the Boston post and the Parkell parallel post. A modified design of parallel-sided post with tapered apical end is also available (Schanker's design).

i. *Whaledent parapost system:* This post system provides the most equitable distribution of masticatory forces. It has three designs; viz. Parapost, Parapost plus and Unity system. All are passive, parallel and vented (Figs 6.1a–d).

These are usually made of either stainless steel or titanium. The vertical channels on the Parapost, spiral flutes and/or grooves on Parapost plus and a raised diamond pattern of Unity posts provide extra retention when used with luting cements.

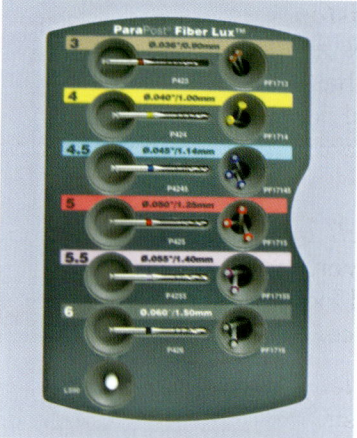

Fig. 6.1b: Parapost (inner)

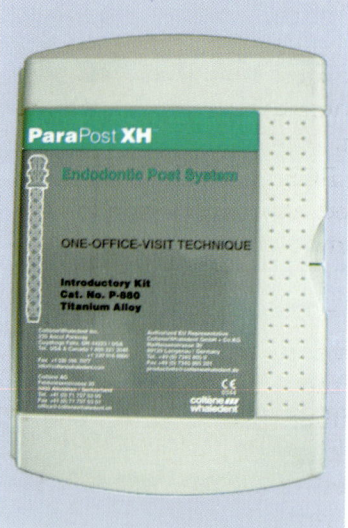

Fig. 6.1c: Parapost XH (outer)

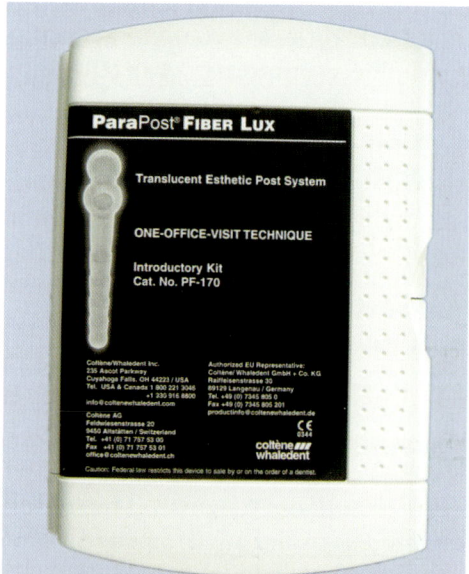

Fig. 6.1a: Parapost (outer)

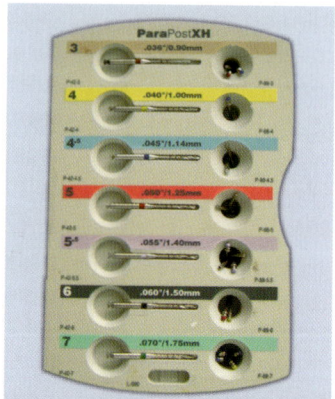

Fig. 6.1d: Parapost XH (inner)

ii. *The Boston post system:* The Boston post resembles a Parapost without the vertical venting channel. It is made of titanium with horizontal non-engaging serrations. These are also available with deeper grooves and rough surfaces.

iii. *Parkell parallel post system:* This is a passive, vented, serrated post with an anti-rotational lock that fits into the prepared root canal space.

iv. *Parallel post with tapered apical ends:* These posts were designed to provide better retention achieved by parallel posts (coronal half) along with tapered post conforming to the tapered apical half of the canal. It is of two types:

- *Degusa:* The straight and tapered portions are generally of equal lengths and are smooth.
- *Unitek BCH system:* Fine serrations are provided along parallel sides of the post and a smooth apical taper of 2.0 mm.

B. Active Posts

The active posts depend primarily on engaging the dentin directly. The threads on the post either screw into the dentin, or fit into threaded channels (prepared in the dentin) and 'tapped' much like a bolt (Fig. 6.2). These are more retentive than passive cemented posts. The self-threading posts produce the greatest stresses when installed in the root. These posts, not only act as a wedge, but may

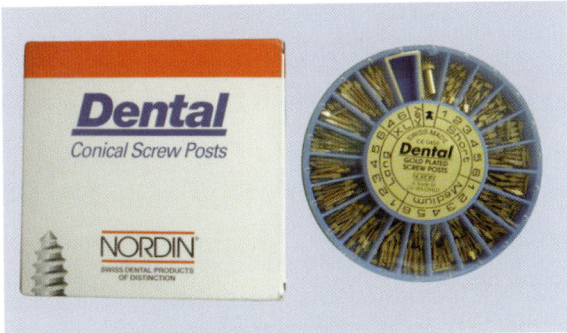

Fig. 6.2: Screw posts

also induce fracture lines into the dentin. These are of following types:

a. *Tapered self-threaded:* The simplest of all the threaded posts, these are available in different sizes, diameter and lengths. The overall taper varies from 3.0 to 30° (taper for the tip is 1.0 to 3.0°). Because of bulky head (head size 2.6 mm long and 1.6 mm across), it is preferred in molars. It is frequently used on teeth having minimum of coronal tooth structure and multiple divergent canals. Post-core can be fabricated in single appointment; for example, Dentatus screw posts.

The threads cut into dentin by 0.1–0.2 mm. The channel to receive the post is prepared by a drill sized 0.1 mm larger than the diameter of the shaft of the post. The blades (threads) extend beyond the shaft by 0.2 mm and engage into dentin. The retention is reinforced by cementing the post using any dual-cure resin cement.

b. *Parallel self-threaded:* The parallel self-threaded posts are more retentive than serrated posts (offer maximum retention).

These posts produce stresses in the root, both at the apical end and the coronal half of the root. It is recommended to 'back off' or reverse the post by half turn to minimize the stresses when slight resistance to threading is felt.

These posts are of three types. The first two have sharp threads and are vented to reduce stresses due to hydraulic cementation. They differ only in their length of threads along the shaft. The types are:

   i. V-Lock Posts

   ii. Radix-Anchor system

  iii. Post with pre-tapped channels

i. *V-lock posts:* These posts have 'micro-threads', extending 0.5 mm from the shaft and continue its full length. V-lock posts are supplied with precise drills that prepare a parallel walled canal just slightly larger than the shaft. They can be cemented with appropriate cement. V-lock posts are less retentive, comparable to passive para-posts.

ii. ***Radix-Anchor system:*** It differs from V-lock posts by the quality of threads (sharp threads extend only partly down the shaft). It is vertically vented and fits along the root surface.

iii. ***Post with pre-tapped channels:*** These posts employ threads on their sides for retention and are inserted into the canal whose walls are pre-threaded with a specially designed instrument. The luting cements are utilized for placement of posts in the root canal (Kurner anchor post). These are two to three times more retentive than parallel-serrated posts.

These posts are parallel in design with no vertical vent. They have rounded high frequency threads that fit into counter threads 'tapped' into the dentin with a manual thread cutter. The unique feature of these posts is the Kurer root facer, which prepares a flat seat in the root into which the coronal portion fits perfectly. This feature overcomes the problem of Radix Anchor system (fitting against an uneven root surface).

The disadvantage with this type of system is that there is a potential for root fracture because of inherent stresses. Frequent cleaning of the root canal walls is required for better adaptations.

The specifications of various post systems are elaborated in Table 6.1.

Factors affecting Selection of Posts

The factors guiding the selection of posts are:

a. *Root selection:* Wider roots are best suited for post preparation, e.g. distal roots of mandibular molars and palatal roots of maxillary molars. However, additional retention (reinforcing post) can be achieved from adjacent smaller canals.

b. *Root morphology:* The contours and the shape of the prepared root canal affects post selection. The narrow roots, especially in the apical third (mandibular incisors) are not indicative of parallel posts. The requisite dentin around the post may not be available with these root canals. A tapered post should be preferred. When the outline of the canal is oval, it is difficult to prepare a circular post channel to receive a parallel post. In such cases, a custom post fabricated according to the shape of the canal.

c. *Remaining coronal tooth structure:* The 'thumb rule' says, when more than half the crown structure is lost, post and core should be considered. The use of a post should be considered for anterior teeth, when one or both proximal walls are missing and for posterior teeth, when two adjacent proximal walls are missing.

d. *Occlusal forces:* The occlusal forces on individual tooth are influenced by various factors, viz. tooth type, presence or absence

S.no.	Post	Taper	Type	Surface
			Table 6.1: Specifications of various post systems	
1.	BCH	0 degree	Stainless steel	Serrated
2.	Colorama	0–6 degree	Stainless steel	Smooth
3.	Dentatus	Variable	Gold plated/Brass	Threaded
4.	Enpost	1.1 degree	Precision plastic pattern	Smooth
5.	Endopost	1.1 degree	Prefabricated precious metal	Smooth
6.	Kurer anchor	0 degree	Pre-tapped steel	Threaded
7.	Parapost	0 degree	Stainless steel/Precious plastic pattern	Serrated
8.	Radix anchor	0 degree	Steel	Threaded

of adjacent teeth, function of tooth in the arch and oral habits of the patient, etc.

Factors affecting Post Retention

The following factors affect the retention of post:

1. Post Length

The accepted principle regarding the post length is 'more the length, more the retention'. It is established that increase in length increases retention (3.0 mm increase in post length enhances 40% of the retention). The practical limitations, however, restrict the clinician to remain in the space properly covered by dentin. The length of the post can be increased as far as possible, provided the post all around its length, should be encircled by a minimum of 1.0 mm of dentin (Fig. 6.3).

The remaining gutta-percha length at the apical end should be 3.0–7.0 mm, depending upon the length of root. During removal of gutta-percha, as the apex is approached, the possibility of dislodging the root canal filling increases. The probability of uncovering the unfilled accessory/lateral canal increases, leading to re-infection. Above all, the post should be encircled by at least 1.0 mm of dentin, which may not be available at the apical end. A short post, besides providing poor retention, can also lead to fracture of the root.

It is generally accepted that the length of post should be more than the crown, preferably one and a half times the length of the crown. The post can be kept halfway between alveolar crest and root apex. If the end of the post is at or above the alveolar crest of bone, the part of the root investing the post uncovered by bone will not be able to transmit forces from post to tooth. The occlusal forces can produce stresses in the unsupported root, fracturing it diagonally from tip of the post down to the crest of bone.

2. Post Taper

The parallel posts are approximately twice more retentive than tapered posts (Fig. 6.4). The tapered posts tend to produce greater stress in the shoulder area of the restoration, while the parallel post causes more stress in the apical area, especially during cementation. In an effort to minimize the splitting potential of a tapered post, a flat surface is created at the occlusal end of the preparation, which will resist apically directed forces and prevent

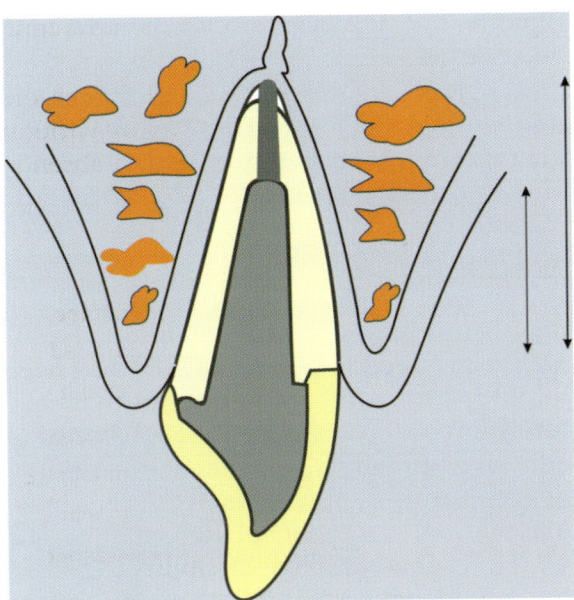

Fig. 6.3: Adequate length of post

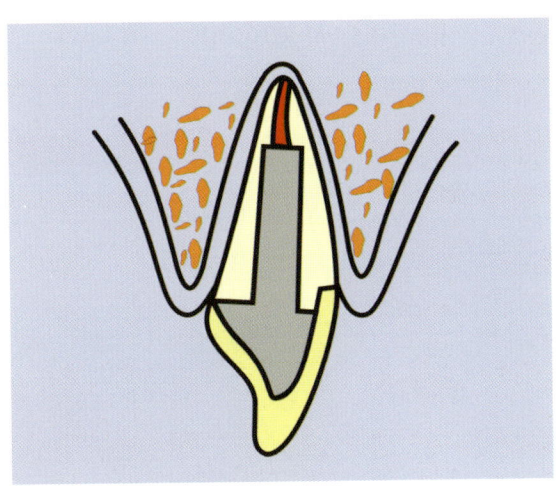

Fig. 6.4: Parallel post

wedging. The proximity of the apical end of a parallel post to the periphery of root canal may increase the danger of a lateral perforation, since the amount of dentin at the periphery of apical end of post would be much less. A combination of parallel and tapered posts (cervical half of the post parallel and the apical half tapering) is designed to take advantage of the parallel post and to minimize the complications at the apical end (Fig. 6.5).

3. Post Diameter

The diameter affects both resistance and retention of the restoration. The smaller diameter post may get displaced or fracture. Enlarging the diameter is not the safest way of improving retention because it does destroy dentin and weakens the remaining root. The width of the post should not exceed one-third the diameter of root. 1.0 mm of dentin thickness around the post (The mesio-distal diameter of an average root is 3.0–4.0 mm at the apex) should always be preserved.

4. Surface Texture

The surface texture of the post (smooth, serrated or threaded) plays an important role in the retention. Threaded posts have been reported to be the most retentive. The pre-tapped, parallel-sided threaded posts are approximately twice as retentive as a parallel-sided serrated post and approximately six

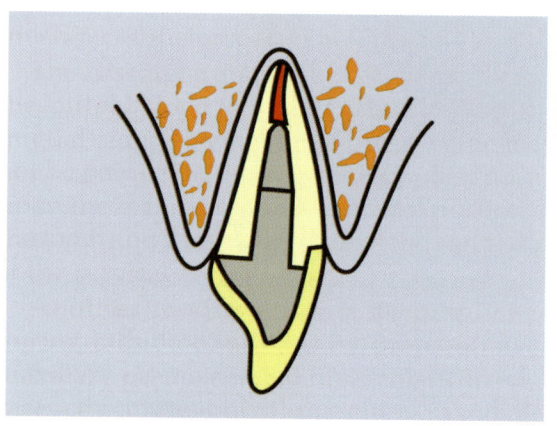

Fig. 6.5: Combined parallel and tapered post

times as retentive as a smooth sided tapered post.

Threaded posts, however, do generate stresses. Tapered threaded posts are more damaging because of the combination of taper and threads. Posts with serrated walls, which may and may not engage the sides of the canal are more retentive than the smooth surface post. Surface treatment of posts such as sandblasting, cleaning with hydrofluoric acid do aid in retention. Pre-sandblasted prefabricated posts provide better retention than non-treated posts.

5. Cementing Medium

Several types of luting cements have been used for the placement of posts in the canal. Zinc phosphate cement, polycarboxylate cement and glass-ionomer cement are being used in routine. All cements are good in compressive strength, fairly good in shear strength but poor in tensile strength. However, resin cements are available with improved tensile strength property.

It is established that there is hardly any significant difference in retentive ability amongst routinely used cements. The resin cements are however more retentive than other cements.

A vent is given on one side of the post to relieve hydrostatic pressure. This may be in the form of a V-shaped groove or a flat side on the round post (Fig. 6.6). Hydrostatic pressure can lead to bouncing of post or even lead to fracture of root.

The new adhesive bonding agents are now being used for post retention. The 4-META product, C & B Metabond has been found to be significantly superior in tensile retention as compared to other bonding adhesives (Panavia, Gluma, Mirage Bond, Scotchbond, Tenure) as well as glass-ionomer and zinc phosphate cements. The 4-META adhesives have the ability to adhere to tooth structure as well as metals, resins and porcelain.

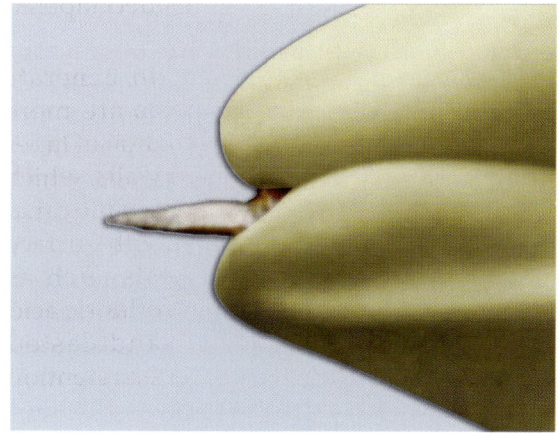

Fig. 6.6: Venting on post

The smear layer should be removed from the walls of the canal to open the dentinal tubules so that the cementing medium could flow into the tubules aiding mechanical lock. It is recommended to use 17% EDTA (chelates the calcium/phosphate salts from the dentin) followed by irrigation with 5.25% sodium hypochlorite to flush away the decalcified dentin and the remaining organic material.

Clinical Procedures

The clinical steps involved in preparation of post-core are:

1. Removing the Gutta-percha

The first step in post preparation is precisely removing the gutta-percha up to the predetermined length without disturbing the apical seal. Obturation techniques with gutta-percha include cold lateral compaction, compaction of heat-softened gutta-percha, injecting thermoplasticized gutta-percha (Obtura) placing gutta-percha in the canal and softened by mechanical means (Mc-Spadden) and heated gutta-percha surrounding a plastic/metal carrier (Thermafil). Gutta-percha can be safely removed from the root canal in every technique, except in Thermafil, the disruption of apical seal is must; therefore, such a technique is avoided in cases where post placement is anticipated. The pertinent

question is whether gutta-percha should be removed immediately after the obturation or after a gap of some time. A few authors observed no difference in immediate or delayed removal of the gutta-percha; however, it is advisable to remove the gutta-percha on the same day of obturation or within 24 hours. The gutta-percha becomes brittle as the time passes and the removal is difficult. More so, the apical seal is less disturbed during removal of gutta-percha. The gutta-percha removal is facilitated by following methods:

i. ***Thermo-mechanical removal:*** The gutta-percha removal is initiated using small round burs. The coronal/cervical 2.0–3.0 mm of gutta-percha should be removed rotating the round bur in slow motion. After the initial removal, burs should not be used in the root canal; otherwise the direction of the bur may lead to deviated track. A gently warm file is inserted in the gutta-percha and allowed to stay till it cools down. The file is then rotated anticlockwise removing the entangled gutta-percha. The process is repeated till the required length is achieved (Figs 6.7a–f).

ii. ***Chemical removal:*** In case the gutta-percha is brittle, gutta-percha dissolving agents can be used to soften the same. The commonly used solvents are Eucalyptol, Halothane and Turpentine oil. The chloroform being carcinogenic is not used these days. Turpentine oil is less toxic but there is a concern that it may lead to dimensional

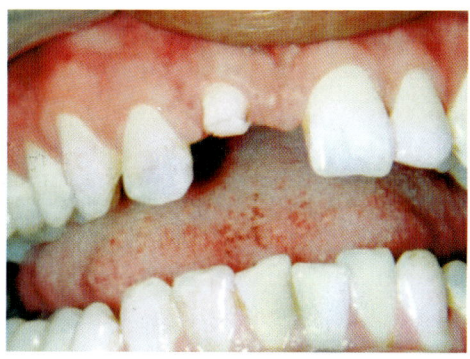

Fig. 6.7a: Preoperative

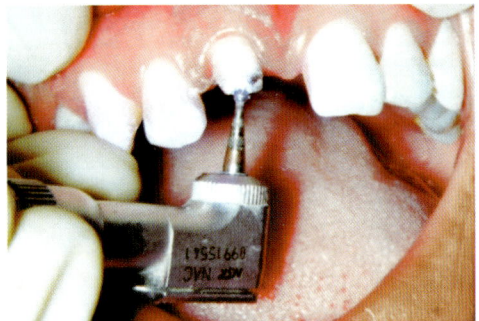

Fig. 6.7b: Initial use of round bur

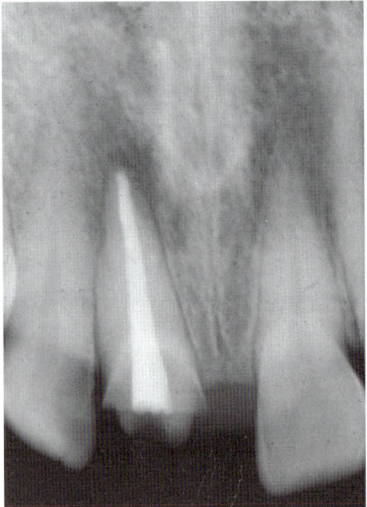

Fig. 6.7c: Preoperative radiograph

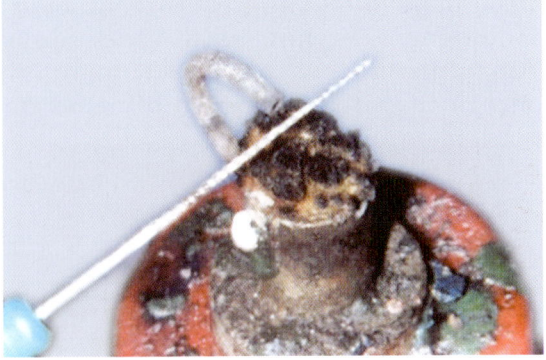

Fig. 6.7d: Warming the file

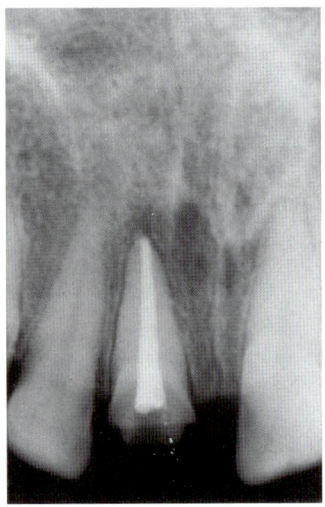

Fig. 6.7e: Radiograph after removing coronal gutta-percha

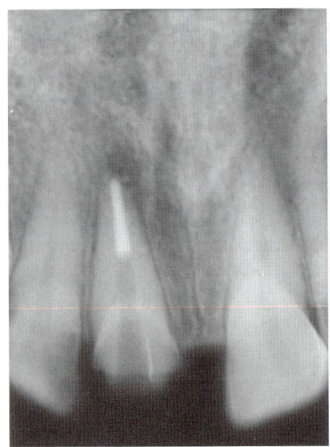

Fig. 6.7f: Removal of gutta-percha

changes in the gutta-percha, subsequently increased microleakage. Commercial preparations as Endosolv-R is used where the sealer used is resin based and Endosolv-E is used where the sealer is eugenol based. The softened gutta-percha is removed following the same method.

iii. ***Thermal removal:*** A heated instrument (say plugger) is inserted into the root canal in a pre-determined length; it softens and removes the gutta-percha. A system B spreader/plugger with a stopper is inserted into the root canal at pre-determined length, heated (up to 200°C) and kept for 3–5 seconds. The plugger is then twisted facilitating removal of gutta-percha. Another plugger

(Buchanan plugger) can be used to compact the gutta-percha at the apical end. The thermal technique, though good for wider canals, pose difficulty for narrow canals. In case of silver cone obturation, the cutting of cones inside the root canal is avoided. In such cases, retreatment using gutta-percha is advisable.

2. Preparation of Canal Space

Various instruments are being used for preparing the canal space for a post. The long shank burs and reamers are preferred initially. Non-end cutting slow speed instruments are preferred. Care should be taken not to disturb the apical seal while using rotary instruments. The use of rotary instruments should be avoided especially in apical-third area. Iatrogenic perforations generally arise from use of end-cutting burs, failure to appreciate root anatomy and use of incorrect angulations.

The Gates Glidden drills (size 0.6–1.5 mm; No. 1–6) are used in straight and small canals. The final preparation should be completed with Peaso reamers (size 0.7–1.7 mm; No. 1–6).

In order to distribute stresses properly and also to avoid counter sinking of the post, a keyway is prepared in the root canal (Figs 6.8a–d). In case of posterior teeth, two root canals should be taken to avoid rotation and to distribute the stresses properly (Figs 6.9a–e).

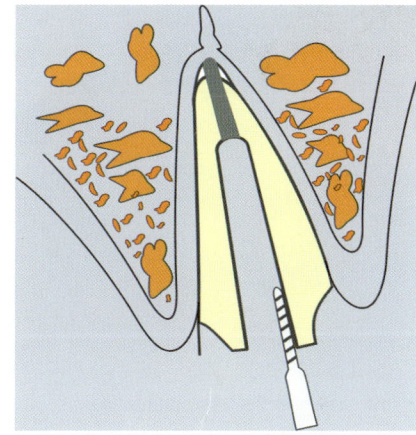

Fig. 6.8b: Diagrammatic view—preparing keyway

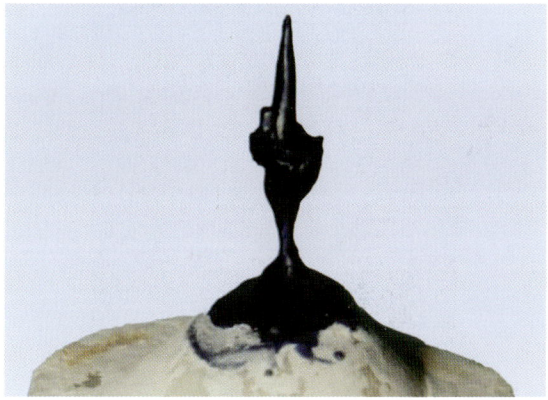

Fig. 6.8c: Wax pattern showing keyway

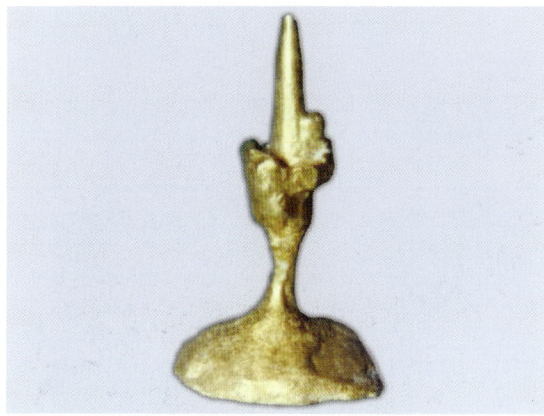

Fig. 6.8d: Cast showing keyway

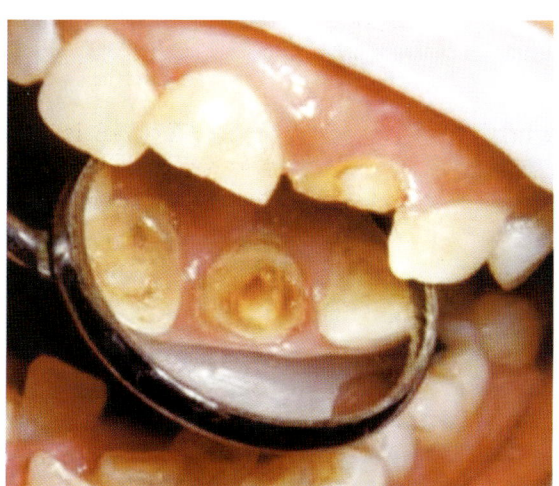

Fig. 6.8a: Preoperative

The prepared post space is washed thoroughly using 3.0% hydrogen peroxide followed by normal saline.

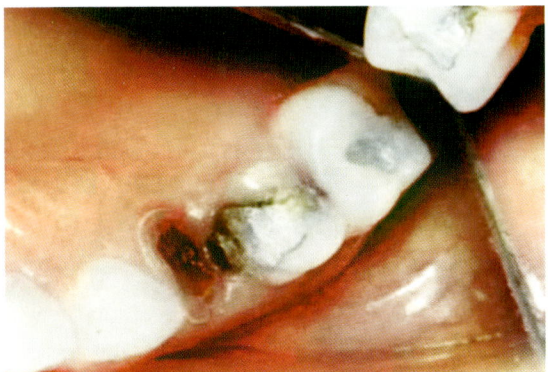

Fig. 6.9a: Preoperative

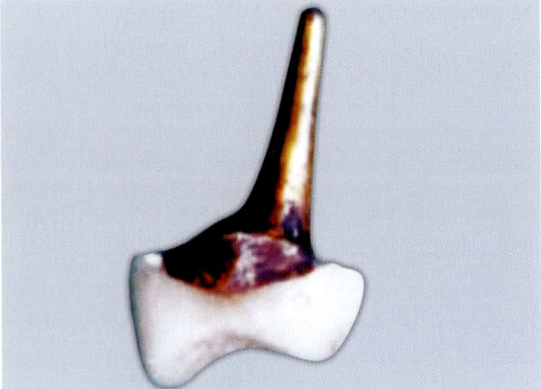

Fig. 6.9b: Single post

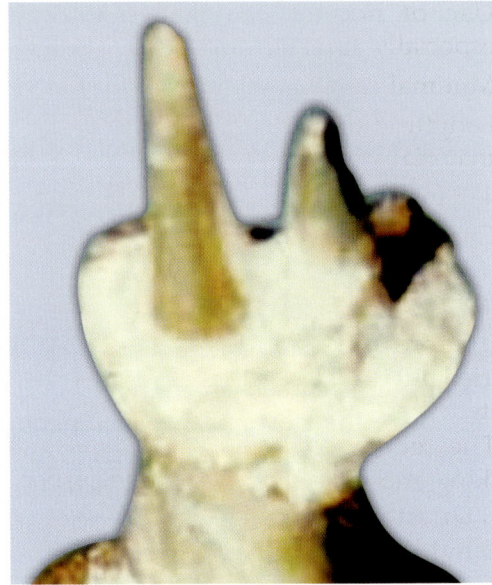

Fig. 6.9d: Two posts

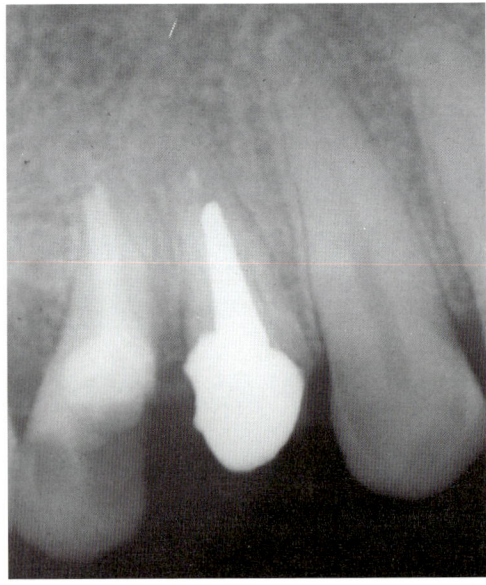

Fig. 6.9e: Postoperative radiograph

The prepared post space should not be left empty for long. This may result in accumulation and reactivation of micro-organisms in the post space. In case the impression making procedure is to be delayed, the said space should be properly closed as is followed in root canal dressings. Optimal post space preparation implies:

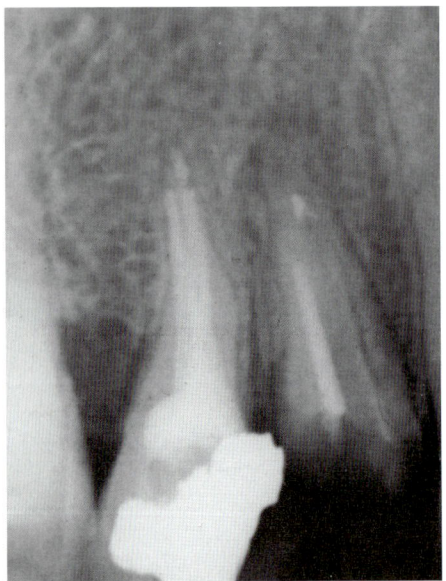

Fig. 6.9c: Radiograph showing one canal prepared

- Use of non-end-cutting instruments, especially rotary.
- Minimal canal enlargement
- Length to be decided on the basis of post material
- 4–5 mm gutta-percha is kept at apical end
- Care should be taken not to lose the path.

3. Impression making of the Post Space

The impression making of the post space is carried out to fabricate cast in custom cast post system.

The techniques utilized in impression making are:

    i. Direct method
    ii. Indirect method

i. **Direct method:** The custom post-core is fabricated directly from the prepared space using resin or wax pattern.

For making an impression, the selected pin (may be plastic or metal) is roughened with carborundum disc. Alternatively, an old file or reamer can be used. A thin layer of sticky wax is applied over the pin. The apical end should be properly covered by sticky wax. The pin with sticky wax is tried in the root canal. The instrument should be free in the root canal including the apical end. If not, the smaller diameter instrument is tried following the same protocol. After selection, the instrument is coated with blue inlay wax, gently warm and inserted into the root canal. Keep it in the root canal for 60 seconds and then gently withdraw the instrument. The 'post' impression is ready. Check carefully for any voids, breakage and also the apical end. The process can be repeated, if need be. The post is inserted back and the core is built in patient's mouth using blue inlay wax. While using blue inlay wax during core preparation of maxillary anterior teeth, care should be taken not to injure patient's tongue, as melted wax can fall over the tongue. Either a piece of cotton or operator's left thumb should be kept under the core during manipulation (Figs 6.10a–h).

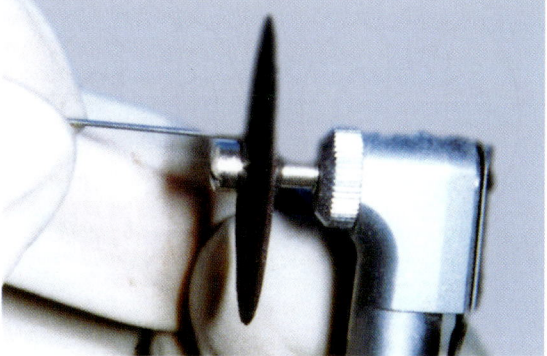

Fig. 6.10a: Roughening the needle

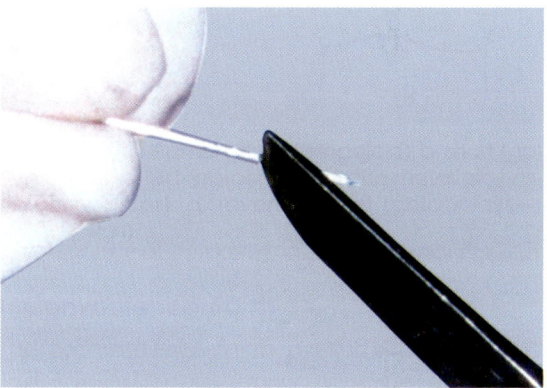

Fig. 6.10b: Applying sticky wax

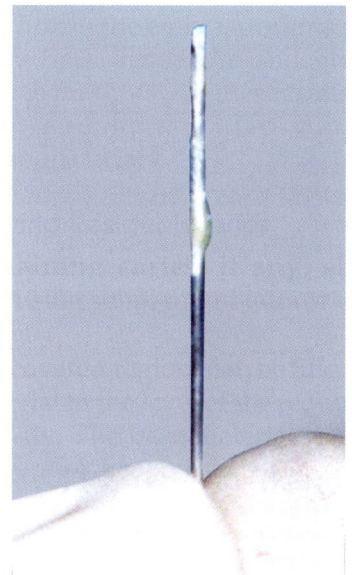

Fig. 6.10c: File with wax

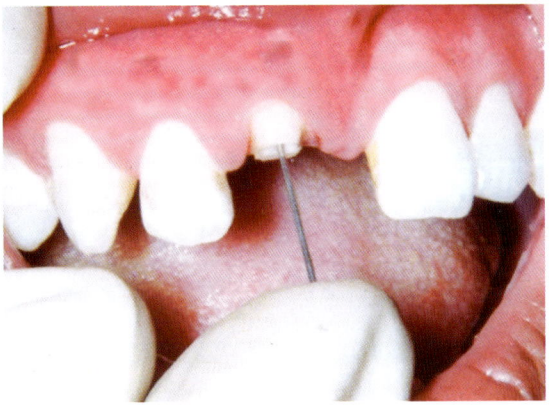

Fig. 6.10d: Inserting into canal

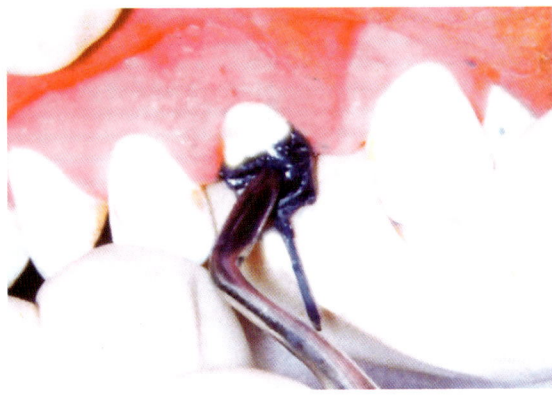

Fig. 6.10g: Core build-up

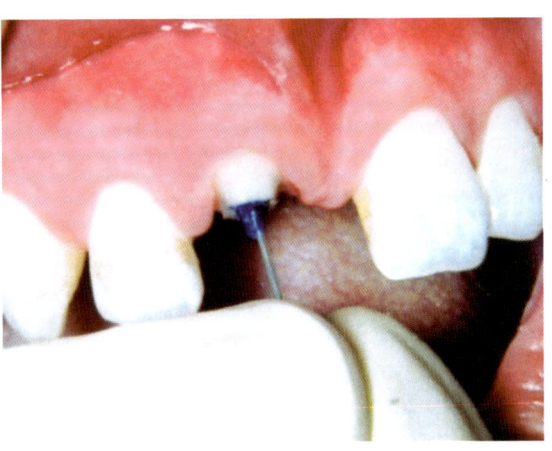

Fig. 6.10e: Pushing the pattern out

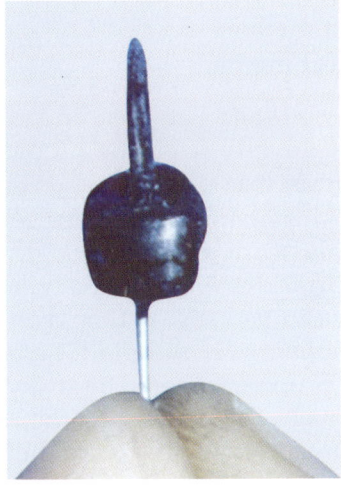

Fig. 6.10h: Final impression of root canal

In case the impression is made in resin, the plastic pin is preferred. Readymade plastic pins are available; alternatively, a blade of comb can be guided to make it round which can also be used. Acrylic resin is coated over the plastic pin and inserted into the canal. Make the pin stable for a couple of minutes and then the pin along with the resin is taken out (Fig. 6.11a–c). It is checked for any voids or discrepancies and if found so, the process is repeated. The resin can be manipulated easily in the mouth without being distorted.

The 'splint-fiber' used for splinting periodontally involved teeth, is also being tried in impressing making at post space.

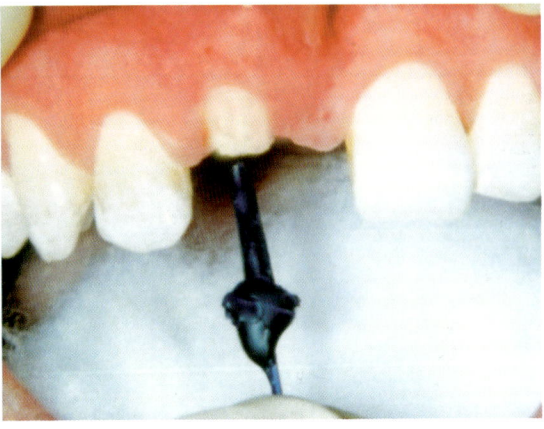

Fig. 6.10f: Take out the pattern

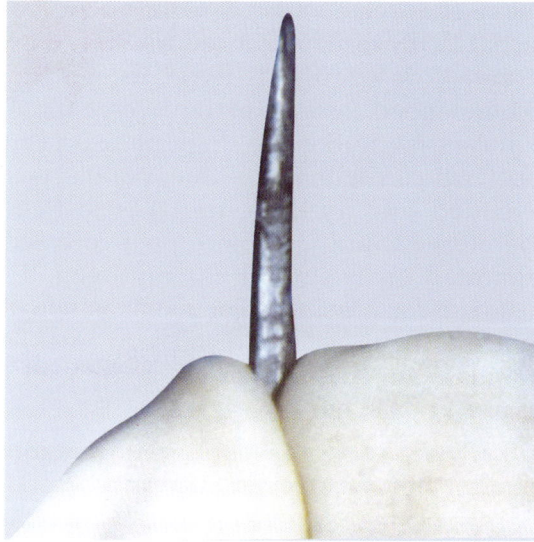

Fig. 6.11a: A plastic pin

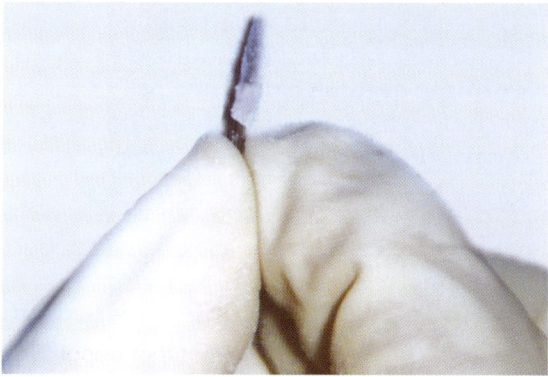

Fig. 6.11b: Applying acrylic

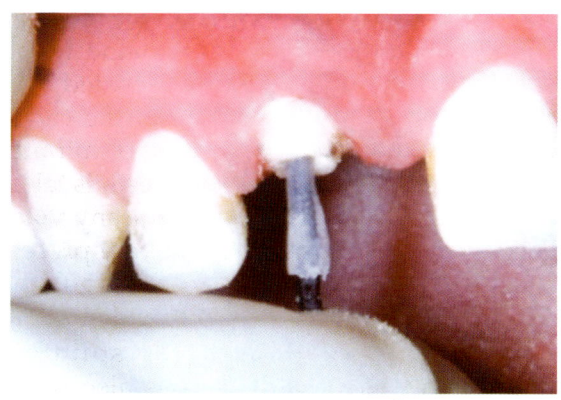

Fig. 6.11c: Taking pattern

Splint fiber coated with composite is used to make the post. It is cured partially inside the root canal and finally cured outside the oral cavity. Similarly, plastic pin coated with composite can be utilized for post space impression. The fit can be tried repeatedly adding more composite.

ii. *Indirect method*

A custom post-core can be fabricated in vitro by making the impression on a cast.

To prepare the cast, the impression material (preferably rubber base) is injected into the canal. The use of lentulo-spiral ensures the elimination of entrapped air in the impression material inside the canal. The impression should be reinforced with some type of rigid material, viz. steel wire, plastic pin or a root canal instrument (Figs 6.12a–d). The reinforcing devices not only strengthen the impression during fabrication, but also during pouring and separation.

The cast with prepared space for post is lubricated by applying machine oil or cocoa butter. The impression is made using blue inlay wax along with metal pin as described for direct methods. The indirect method saves time of the operator since the impression can be made by some assistant in the clinic or laboratory.

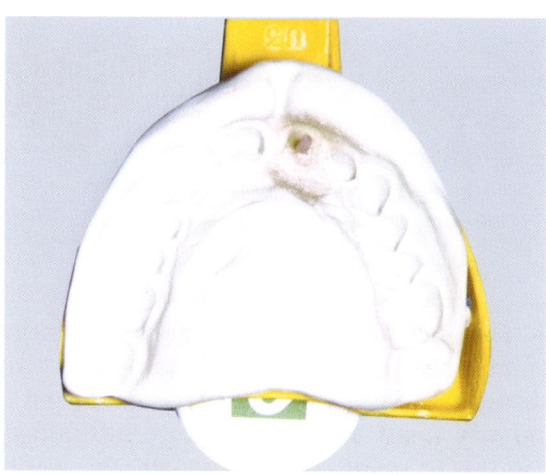

Fig. 6.12a: Impression of root space

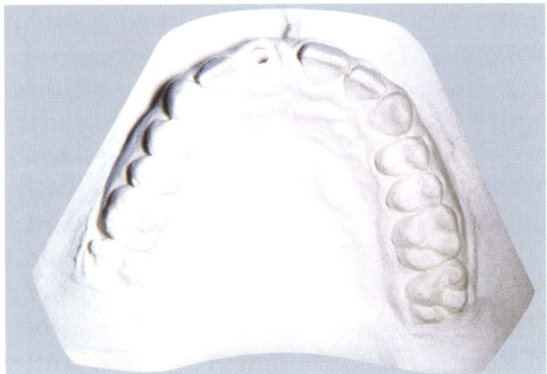

Fig. 6.12b: Impression of root space on cast

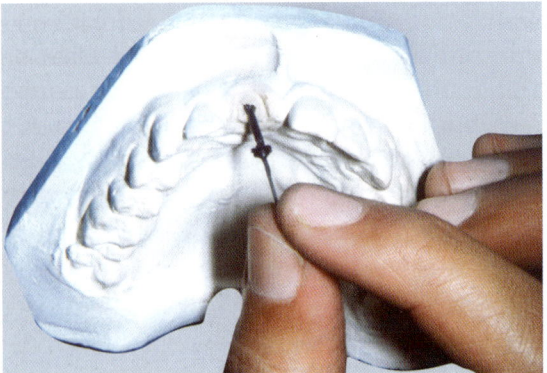

Fig. 6.12c: Making impression with blue inlay wax

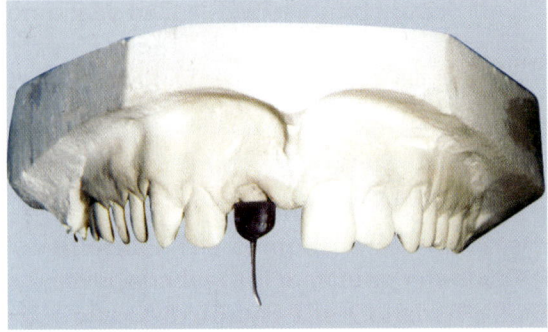

Fig. 6.12d: Final impression

iii. *Two piece custom post:* For the restoration of anterior teeth and premolars having straight canals, a single piece cast post is usually used along with an amalgam or composite resin core. However, in case of molars or if a tooth is severely damaged and

also the key teeth which is required for fixed partial denture where more resistance and retention is required, two piece post is recommended. Because of the divergent roots in molars, fabrication of a single piece post and core (post-core with two or three parallel posts extended into multiple roots) is difficult. Therefore, a multiple piece post-core with separated posts should be employed. The post-core for a mandibular molar is usually divided into mesial and distal segments. The maxillary molar post-core is composed of facial and palatal components.

For a two-piece post-core, the pieces must be rigidly bound together after insertion. The core can be made in two halves held together by interlocking plugs, which can be made by cutting a keyway or dovetail in one-half of core pattern.

The core can be fabricated in two halves with pinholes in first half and interlocking pins in the second half. The core is pinned together when both halves have been cemented in the tooth.

iv. *Post-inlay system:* Many a times, teeth that have been restored with crown may require endodontic treatment later. Removing the crown may lead to fracture of the coronal portion of tooth or the crown or both. Even in long span bridges, removal is difficult. Under the circumstances, it becomes mandatory to initiate root canal treatment through the cast restoration.

An endodontic access through a crown is often larger because the crown obscures the morphology of the tooth and makes it difficult to locate the root canal.

After completion of the root canal treatment, the remaining un-restored part can be restored with cast posts with an attached inlay to close the access opening. A prefabricated post with a composite resin or with an amalgam seal can also be used. This repair process has been referred to as a 'secondary retention post'.

If a post with an attached inlay is fabricated, the combined restoration is retentive and is also able to withstand laterally directed forces.

Because this restoration is a combination of a post and an inlay, it is designated as post inlay system.

Ferrule Effect

The common failure of the post-restored tooth is fracture of the root. The post core should be so designed, that it minimizes the chances of root fracture.

A 'ferrule'is a metal ring or covering around the coronal part of the root intended for increasing the resistance form. The word originates from combination of two latin words 'ferrum' (iron) and 'viriola' (bracelet). A dental ferrule is an encircling band of cast metal round the coronal surface of the tooth. It can also be defined as 'the 360° metal collar of crown surrounding the parallel walls of the dentin extending coronal to the shoulder of the preparation'. The ferrule resists stresses such as functional lever forces, the wedging effect of tapered posts and the lateral forces exerted during the post insertion.

During functional movements the forward movement of mandibular anterior teeth (Fig. 6.13), the forces put on the core portion of the post and core creates pressure on the palatal surface of the root at the apical end of post. This process may lead to fracture of the root (Figs 6.14a and b). To increase resistance of the root to such fractures, the core portion is made to encircle the root/remaining crown, so as the forces generated on core may dissipate within the total root. This covering of the core portion on to the root is known as 'Core ferrule'. The full veneer crown over the core having sufficient length of the coronal tooth provides ferrule effect, known as 'crown ferrule'. In case the length of the remaining crown is sufficient and the core portion is minimal, there is no need to have additional core ferrule effect (the coronal portion of the remaining tooth would bear the forces

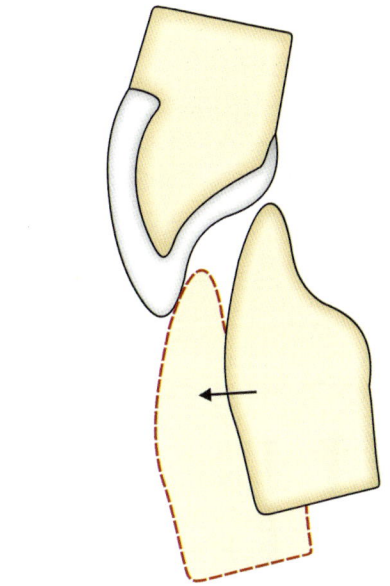

Fig. 6.13: Forward movement of mandibular incisors in relation to maxillary incisors

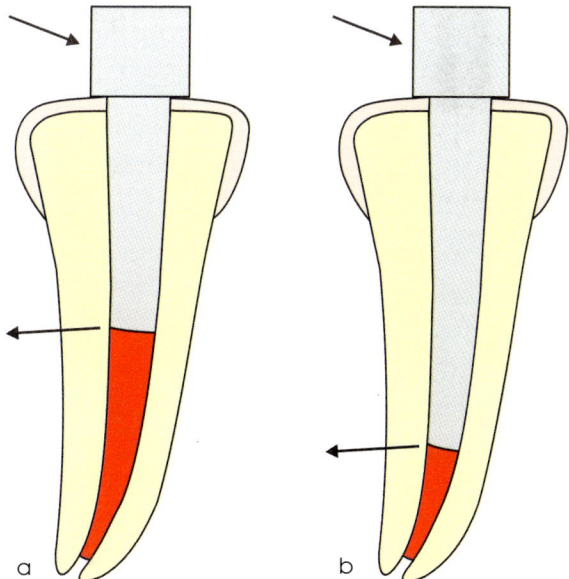

Fig. 6.14a and b: Forces on core portion can lead to fracture of root

generated by the functional movements as in normal tooth). The restored crown in such cases will be sufficient to provide ferrule effect.

The cervical collar along the post increases the resistance of the post and core to torsional forces. The length/height of this covering is also important. The minimum ferrule length/height should be 1.0–1.5 mm while restoring maxillary anterior teeth (Fig. 6.15); however, 1.5–2.0 mm is considered adequate. The fracture resistance is increased with the increase in ferrule length/height.

Ferrule width is also an important parameter. 2.0 mm width of the remaining dentin thickness is considered adequate ferrule width.

Ferrule is classified as 'crown ferrule' and 'core ferrule'; although the main ferrule effect is provided by full veneer crown (Fig. 6.16). The dislodging forces vary in anterior and posterior teeth. In case, the dislodging forces are severe in nature, additional core ferrule is required. The combined effect provides the requisite resistance to fracture of the post core restorations. Ideally, the ferrule is divided into two: 'Complete ferrule' and 'Partial ferrule'. In case, it is practically feasible to encircle 1.5–2.0 mm of the coronal tooth structure with the core, it provides 'complete ferrule' effect (Fig. 6.17). Alternatively, covering only the side walls with core may provide 'partial ferrule' effect (Fig. 6.18).

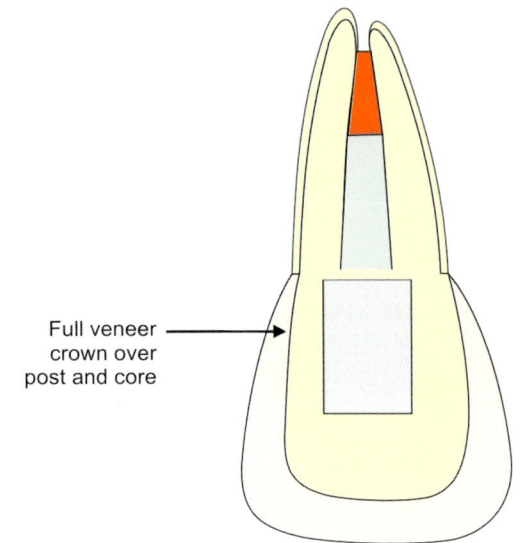

Fig. 6.16: Full veneer crown over core, providing crown ferrule effect

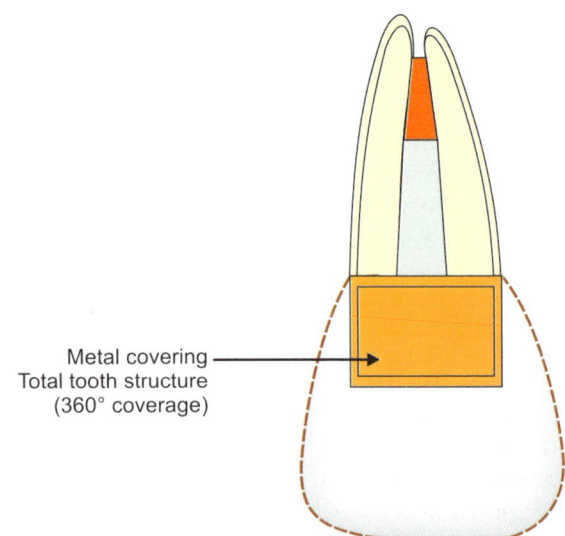

Fig. 6.17: Metal covering all the surfaces of tooth (360 degree coverage): complete ferrule effect

Many a times, clinical conditions warrant thinning of dentin wall around the root canal and the remaining crown portion. It is established that walls are considered 'too thin' when they are less than 1.0 mm in thickness. Covering of metal core over this thickness might not be practicable. In such cases, ferrule effect is achieved only by the full veneer crown.

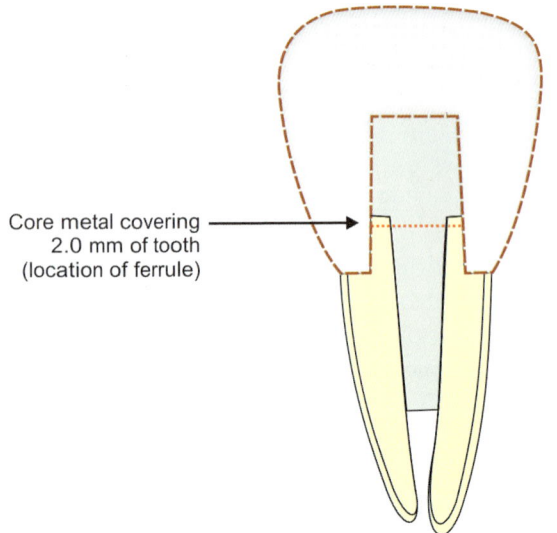

Fig. 6.15: Ferrule height: 2.0 mm covering of the tooth structure

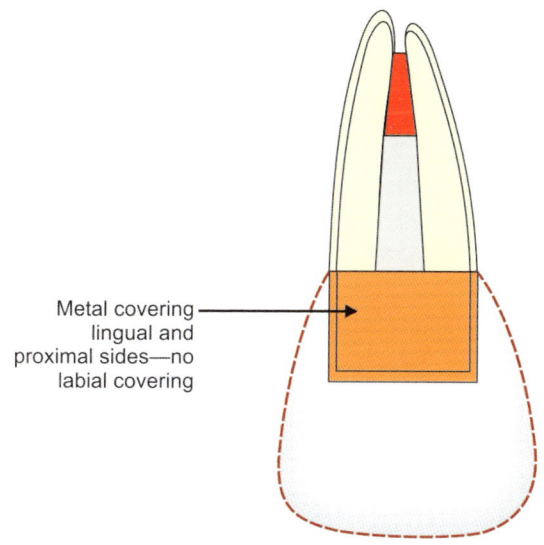

Metal covering lingual and proximal sides—no labial covering

Fig. 6.18: Metal covering lingual and sides, without labial: Partial ferrule effect

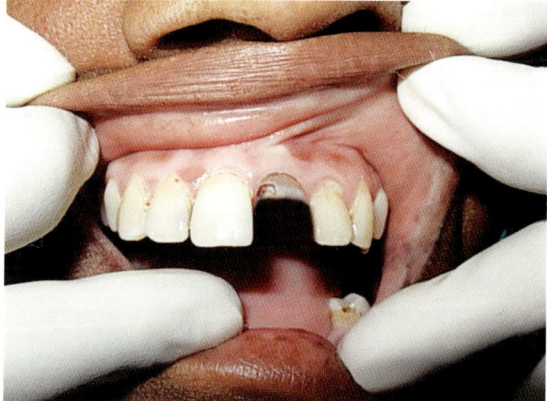

Fig. 6.19a: Preoperative

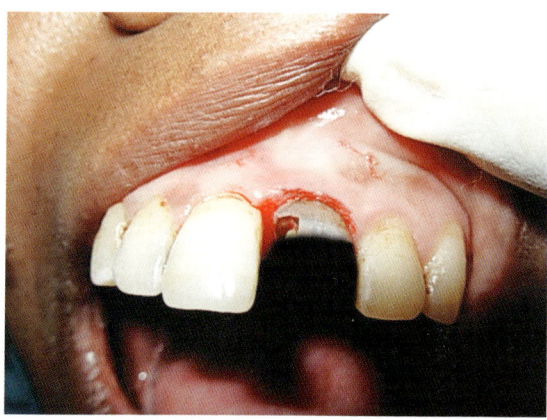

Fig. 6.19b: Crown lengthening procedure

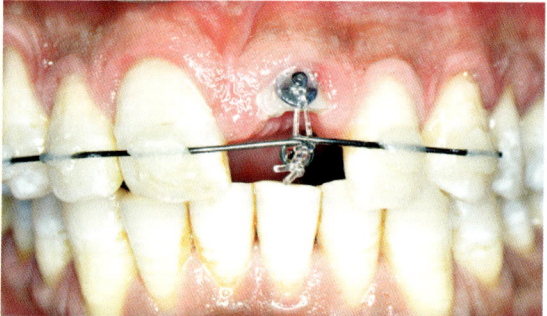

Fig. 6.20: Orthodontic extrusion

The following features are important:
- The remaining dentin thickness should be 1.0 mm
- The number of remaining dentin thickness walls (preferably three or at least two wall must be present; if only one wall is left, alternative treatment planning, such as crown lengthening or orthodontic extrusion is planned)
- Amount of lateral forces (excessive forces need more of remaining tooth structure)

Thus, in critical conditions where there is insufficient ferrule length, the clinician may consider crown lengthening procedures (Figs 6.19a and b) or orthodontic extrusion (Fig. 6.20). This will allow the distance between crown margin and alveolar crest to be widened and increase the potential ferrule length. However, these methods may result in reducing the root length and making the crown-to-root ratio unfavourable. In such cases, composite resin posts and core are preferred where ferrule effect may not be required. Thus, balance is mandatory between the ferrule length achieved and the remaining root length. These considerations determine the choice of post and core material.

Certain indirect factors do affect ferrule functioning. The fiber reinforced posts, indicated where thin dentin remains, provide ferrule effect without any collar covering. Similarly, composite/bonded cores also provide ferrule effect because they act as 'monobloc' with the resin post.

III. Fiber Reinforced Posts

The metal post and core provides optimum strength; however, need for color masking and discoloration of crown/gingiva with time, are the significant drawbacks. Furthermore, metal shines through all ceramic restorations and negates the transmission of light.

In an effort to overcome the disadvantages of metal posts, fiber reinforced posts have been developed and are being used as posts. The commonly used posts, their properties and technique of use is described.

a. Carbon Fiber Posts

Carbon fiber posts (Mirafit carbon, Endopost, etc.) are considered viable alternatives to metals when properties like strength, stiffness, lightness and resistance to corrosion and fatigue are concerned. The carbon fiber posts bond to tooth structure; the modulus of elasticity (rigidity) being similar to dentin are significantly more flexible than metal posts. The carbon fiber posts are black in color and are radiolucent, which makes it difficult to detect radiographically. Replacing carbon with quartz fiber results in a tooth colored post (Figs 6.21a and b).

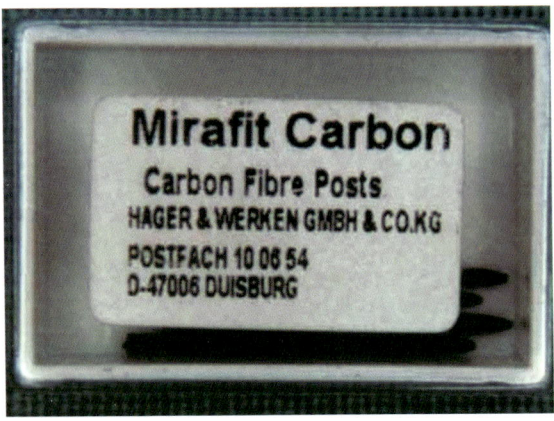

Fig. 6.21a: Carbon fiber post

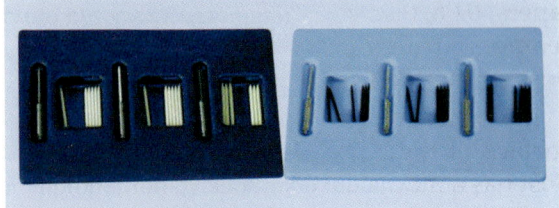

Fig. 6.21b: Carbon fiber post

Technique: The suitable sized post is selected according to the configuration of the post space prepared.

The inside of the canal is etched with 37% phosphoric acid for 10–15 seconds. The canals are washed thoroughly with water and dried with paper points. The primer is applied inside the canal and light cured. Similarly, primer is applied to the post and light cured. The dual cure cement is applied inside the root canal and the post is inserted with pressure. The exposed area of the post is coated with bonding agent and composite, creating initial shape of the core. The core portion is cured for 40 seconds. Finally, trim and contour the core according to the anatomy of the crown.

Advantages
- Superior mechanical properties.
- Modulus of elasticity is similar to that of dentin.
- Sufficient bonding to tooth structure and core composite.

Disadvantages
- Unesthetic (black color)
- Radiolucent

b. Silica Fibers

a. *Quartz fiber post:* The quartz fiber posts are the modified and improved version of the carbon fiber posts.

i. ***Light post/DT light post:*** These are available in different tapered designs for better adaptation to the prepared root canal. They are 20.0 mm long, available in three diameters (0.9, 1.0 and 1.2 mm at the apex) and three tapers, 0.06, 0.08 and 0.10. The matched set of reamers/drills are available to prepare the post space (Fig. 6.22).

Micro-mechanical tags are provided on the surface of the posts for better retention. The post has a modulus of elasticity similar to that of dentin, allowing functional stresses to be dissipated rather than concentrated in the root, thereby reducing the potential for root fracture. The translucent posts transmit light to the apical end and therefore may be used with light or dual cure cements.

A retrieval kit for post removal is available separately.

ii. *Aesthetic/aesthetic plus post:* The post uses white quartz fibers surrounding carbon fibers (Aesthetic post) and all white quartz fibers (Aesthetic plus). These posts have high flexure strength and low modulus of elasticity as good as carbon fiber posts.

Technique: The technique for placement of quartz fiber post is similar to that of carbon fiber posts.

Advantages
- Radiopaque (allow post-operative evaluation).
- Modulus of elasticity is similar to that of dentin; reduces the risk of tooth fracture.
- Complete and non-traumatic removal is possible.

- High tensile strength and superior fatigue resistance.
- Bonds well to the tooth and core material.

b. *Glass fiber post:* The glass fiber posts are improved version of the quartz fiber posts. The improved versions are esthetically pleasing along with maintaining properties of fiber posts (glass fibers have lower modulus of elasticity than carbon/quartz fibers) (Figs 6.23a and b).

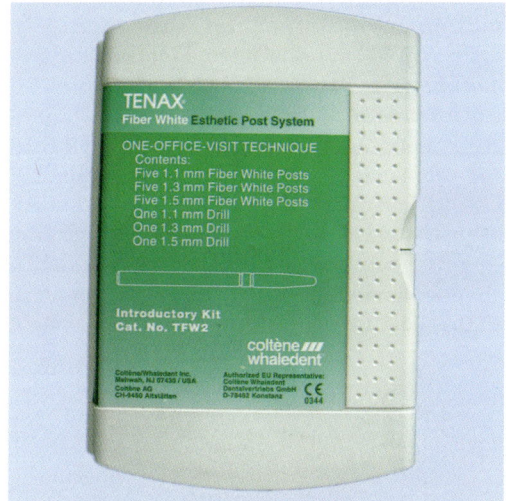

Fig. 6.23a: Tenax fiber glass post (outer)

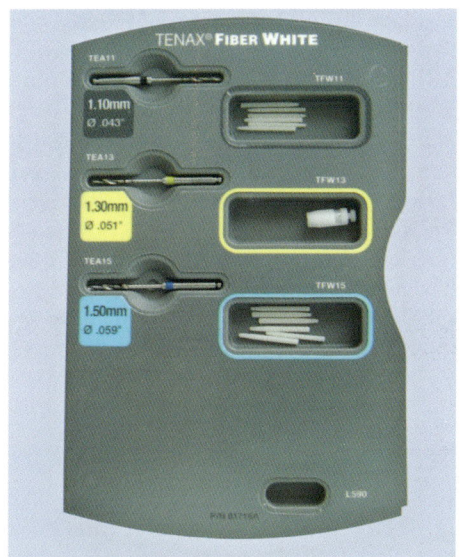

Fig. 6.23b: Tenax fiber glass post (inner)

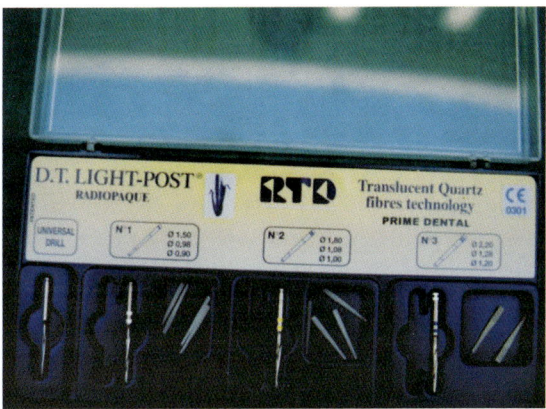

Fig. 6.22: DT light post

i. *Luscent anchor post:* The Luscent anchor post is designed to transmit natural tooth color for esthetic purposes. It is available in three diameters with 300 tapers. The luscent anchor post can be easily removed in case of retreatment.

ii. *Fiberkov post:* The bundles of glass fibers impregnated in resin provide the requisite white color to the post. The post is available in four diameters and three degree tapered along with matching drills (diameter 1, 1.2, 1.4 and 1.6 mm).

iii. *Fiber white para post:* Post is parallel and has color coded ring around the head for identification. Available in 4 sizes (diameter 1.14, 1.25, 1.4 and 1.5 mm).

Technique: After the post space preparation, an appropriate size of the post is chosen and tried in for a fit. The canal can be refined with the color coded drills, if need be. The canal is conditioned with self-curing primer and adhesive. The light cured/dual cured cement is backfilled into the canal space with a syringe tip. Thin film of cement is then applied to the post and seated immediately. The post is immediately light cured and a composite core is built on the post.

c. Polyethylene Fiber Reinforced Post

It is available as Ribbond and Ribbond-THM (Thinner Higher Modulus). It is used both as post and core material. Ribbond-THM is made of thinner fibers with a higher thread count and is almost half as thick as original Ribbond. Fibers are composed of woven polyethylene (Fig. 6.24). The modulus of elasticity of these fibers is similar to that of radicular dentin; suitable for fabrication of post and core as one unit.

Technique
The steps involved are:
- The obturated material is removed up to predetermined length (leaving gutta-percha at the apical end) as described

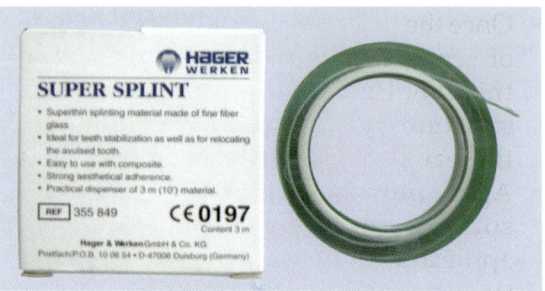

Fig. 6.24: Splint fiber

earlier. The natural internal form of the pulp space is maintained. The final depth of the post portion depends on the shape and diameter of the root canal. For single rooted teeth, the greater the irregularities and undercuts in the canal, the less depth of the post is required. For multi-rooted teeth, the greater the divergence of the canals, the less depth of the post is required.

- Verify the removal of gutta-percha and cement, etc. by evaluating radiograph of the prepared canal.
- Make a countersink having rounded angles at the opening of the canal. This will eliminate sharp angles between the post and core and thereby minimizes stress concentration and cracking at the post and core junction.
- Measure the depth of the prepared canal with a periodontal probe. Different thicknesses of Ribbond are available depending upon the need (for narrow canals, thin Ribbond preferred). Cut a piece of Ribbond measuring twice the depth of the prepared canal and three to four times the height of the anticipated core. Most canals require the use of at least a second piece of Ribbond. The second piece will usually be shorter than the first. Use the widest Ribbond that will fit in the canal in a double thickness. The rigidity and fracture resistance of the post and core is also dependent on the properties of the composite used along with the post. The greater mass of Ribbond fibers is preferred.

- Once the canal is clean and dry, use a liquid or semi-gel etchant from a syringe to etch the canal walls and all exposed tooth structures for 15 seconds. Thoroughly, rinse the canal and remove excess moisture. Apply primer and adhesive to the internal surface of the root canal using a micro applicator.
- Wet the Ribbond with unfilled adhesive resin.
- Mix the dual or self-cure luting composite. Using a small syringe such as Endo-Eze or a Centrix syringe with a needle tube, place the syringe tip at the apical end of the canal before injecting the luting composite. Start injecting the composite slowly while withdrawing the syringe. Apply composite over the wet Ribbond also.
- Hold the Ribbond with cotton pliers and center it over the canal opening. Use the instrument to push it to the apical part of the canal. If space permits, insert an additional piece of wet Ribbond into the canal, even if second piece could be inserted half the depth of the canal preparation. The first piece is sufficient for retention of the post. The purpose of the second piece is to produce a greater density of Ribbond at the post-core junction. The free ends emerging from the canal will be used to form the core. Do not cure till now.
- After placement of the Ribbond in the canal, remove the excess flowing composite with a disposable brush or instrument. Complete the core build up using a filled and/or flowable composite and cure with light. Finish and shape the core using diamond rotary instruments. If the Ribbond becomes exposed and has fuzzy appearance, place a layer of unfilled bonding adhesive over the exposed fibers and cure it.

Advantages
- A Ribbond post like a natural tooth is translucent and esthetically pleasing as opposed to a metal post that is opaque.

- The Ribbond post along with resin adapts to the irregularities and undercuts within the root canal and becomes retentive and anti-rotational after curing.
- Since, the Ribbond post adapts to the irregularities and is bonded to the tooth, it acts to cross-splint the tooth. The wedging effect, subsequently leading to root fracture, is avoided.
- The Ribbond post and core does not require additional preparation after root canal treatment, which eliminates the possibility of root perforation.

Advantages of fiber posts
- Bonding with the substrate: Fiber posts are placed using bonding agent along with dual cure resin cement such bonding provides monobloc effect.
- Micro retention achieved with fiber posts is far superior to other posts.
- Fiber posts are minimally invasive; one-half the length of root is sufficient as compared to metal posts where 'length' provides retention.
- Parallel posts or half-parallel-half-taper posts, as envisaged in metals, provide retention and stress distribution. Small taper posts provide good retention and good potential for distribution of stress.
- Metal posts exhibit corrosion potential, which may contribute to de-cementation and even root fracture. Fiber posts overcome the problem of corrosion (Titanium and ceramic also do not corrode).
- Removal of fiber post is easy, without disturbing the dentin substrate.
- Fiber posts are more fatigue resistant. Fiber posts may flex slightly, when necessary; some fiber posts have greater flexure strength than stainless steel and titanium.
- Most of the fiber posts are radiopaque, as required.
- Fiber posts (except carbon fiber black) are esthetically pleasing; overcome the need of applying masking over the post.

Disadvantages of fiber posts: The fiber posts can undergo degradation because of repeated mechanical loading and under conditions of moisture. This degradation may lead to a reduction in the modulus of elasticity and flexural strength with an increased risk in debonding.

The chemical composition and shape of routinely used fiber posts are described in Table 6.2.

IV. All-ceramic Post

The major advantage of an all-ceramic post and core is its dentin like shade. The dentin like shade of ceramic post-core is related to the deeper diffusion and absorption of the transmitted light in the ceramic mass. All-ceramic restorations transmit a certain percentage of the incident light to the underlying core and post on which it has been placed. Thus, with all-ceramic posts and cores, the colour of the final restoration will be derived from an internal shade of the ceramic post, similar to the optical behaviour of the natural teeth. In addition, a ceramic post does not reflect intensively through thin gingival tissues, and provides translucency in the cervical root areas. All-ceramic posts and cores provide an excellent biocompatibility and do not exhibit galvanic corrosion.

The main obstacles for using dental ceramics, as post and core materials are their low fracture strength and toughness. High toughness ceramics, such as the glass infiltrated alumina ceramic, In-ceram, and the dense sintered alumina ceramic, show three

Table 6.2: Chemical composition and shape of routinely used fiber posts

Post	Fibers	Resin matrix	Shape
Rely X fiber post (3M ESPE)	Glass	Resin	Double tapered
FRC post-plus (Ivoclar-Vivadent)	Glass	UDMA, TEGDEMA, Ytterbium trifluoride, high dispersed silicon dioxide	Tapered
GC fiber post	Glass	Methacrylate	Double tapered
DT light post illusion	Quartz	Epoxy	Double tapered
D1 light post	Quartz	Epoxy	Double tapered
Macrolock illusion post	Quartz	Epoxy	Tapered, circumferential head grooves, spiral head serrations
Radix fiber post (dentsply)	Zirconium enriched glass	Epoxy	Double tapered
DT light safety lock	Pre-conditioned quartz	Epoxy	Double tapered
Dentin post-X	Glass	Epoxy	Tapered with a retentive hand
Snowpost (abrasive technology)	Zirconia-rich glass	Epoxy	Cylindrical with long apical bone
Refor-post	Glass	Bis-GMA	Serrated
Fiber-Kleer (serrated post)	Glass	Bis-GMA, UDMA, HDDMA	Serrated
Composi-post	Carbon	Epoxy	Two-stage parallel

to six times higher flexural strength and toughness than do conventional feldspathic and glass ceramics. Contemporary zirconia powder technology contributes to the fabrication of new biocompatible ceramic materials with improved mechanical properties, i.e. further increase in flexural strength and toughness. The zirconium oxide ceramic have shown promising results for the fabrication of all-ceramic posts and cores.

Zirconium has several advantages over other ceramics owing to fundamental differences in their physical properties (ZiReal post is Zirconia ceramic with a small titanium insert at the apical part).

The ceramic posts are inherently brittle. It is difficult to remove a fractured ceramic post. The modulus of elasticity of these posts is equal to metals, which make the post stiffer. The stiffer post produces more stresses.

Constructing All-ceramic Posts

Different techniques used for constructing all-ceramic posts are:
  i. Slip-casting technique
  ii. Copy milling technique
  iii. Two piece technique
  iv. Heat Press technique

i. Slip-casting Technique

With this technique, the core and the post are made in one piece from the aluminium oxide ceramic material, In-ceram. However, because of the limited fracture strength, this method was initially used only in wide root canals.

Procedure
- The preparation of the root canal is similar to the preparation for a metal post and core. The minor undercuts, if any, are eliminated using conventional techniques.
- At the coronal end of the root canal, a small keyhole is created to prevent rotation of the post and core.
- A prefabricated plastic or metal post is placed in the root canal and a high precision impression is taken.

- The die is prepared and the impression is cast with the special In-ceram material. The duplicate die is used for formation of post using slip casting technique.
- The bottom of the second die is ground with a carbide bur until a tiny opening appears. During the slip casting, this hole serves as an external relief that prevents air impaction in the slip mass.
- Finally, horizontal and vertical sections are created on the die with diamond disks, which must not reach the root canal. This procedure is necessary to prevent a post fracture, which might occur through the shrinkage of the In-ceram plaster during the sintering process.
- A wax-up of the core is then fabricated on the master die. A 5.0 mm diameter wax sprue is attached to the incisal edge of the core, providing the entrance for the slip injection.
- Two putty silicon molds of the wax-up and the master casts are fitted together with internal retentive undercuts. After the removal of the wax-up, the die of the special In-ceram material is adapted in between. Finally, the two silicon molds are joined with rubber rings. With this procedure, a void space, previously occupied by the core wax up and the sprue, is provided for the slip injection.
- The alumina slip is mixed and ultrasonically vibrated to a homogenous consistency according to the manufacturer's instructions and injected through the injection spine of the silicon mold. After the slip has dried, the core is carefully carved to its final shape with a scalpel. One coat of stabilizer is applied to the finished core. The sintering is done for the In-ceram ceramic.
- After sintering, the all-ceramic post and core is filled to the master cast.
- For the subsequent glass infiltration firing, the post and core is placed on a platinum foil covered with a mixture of lanthanum glass powder and the special liquid

supplied with the In-ceram system. The excess glass is removed using coarse grit diamond and 50 µm air abrasions.

- The fit of all-ceramic post and core is checked in the patient's tooth. Rubber dam is applied for moisture control. The root canal is roughened with a diamond-coated reamer and rinsed with 70% alcohol. A self-curing dentin adhesive agent is used prior to cementation with self-cure resin cement. If a phosphate monomer containing resin composite is used for the cementation, the In-ceram post and core needs only be sandblasted, and ultrasonically cleaned with 90% alcohol. The post is finally cemented.
- After the resin cement has set, the tooth preparation is finalized with appropriate instruments.

ii. Copy Milling Technique

The glass infiltrated alumina ceramic and its fabrication process have been adapted to the celay copy milling method, as an alternative to the slip-casting technique. The celay system involves a manually guided copy-milling process in which a pre-designed resin pattern is surface traced and copied in ceramic. The ceramic substructures are prefabricated blanks made of pre-sintered aluminium oxide ceramic. In-ceram ceramic restorations made with celay method presents a 10% higher flexural strength (about 500 MPa) than do conventional In-ceram restorations.

The clinical indications and procedures are similar to those of the conventionally slip cast post and cores already described.

For the copy-milling technique, the resin 'pre-post and core' pattern can be made by a direct or indirect method.

- *Direct method:* The resin analog of the post and core is molded on the patient's tooth, similar to the conventional technique for cast metal posts and cores. This method is simplified by using prefabricated plastic or metal posts along with resin composite as core.

- *Indirect method:* An impression of the prepared tooth is taken and a working cast is prepared using stone plaster. The resin pre-post and core is molded as in the indirect fabrication method for metal posts and cores. For molding of the internal inlay of the post and core, a light curing resin with increased viscosity can be used.

The resin pre-post is mounted to the tracing chamber of the celay machine. The pre-post is mounted vertically, so that the incisal edge of the core is attached to a jig of the retentive device and the end of the post is connected to a pin on the top of the cup holder. Then, the resin pattern is surface traced and copied in ceramic by synchronized grinding in the milling chamber. After completion of the copy-milling process, the ceramic post and core is cut off with a diamond disk, fitted to the master die, glass-infiltrated and finished.

iii. Two-piece Technique

The fracture strength of In-ceram posts and cores is less than that of metal posts and cores. Usually, these are recommended for wider root canals. In case of regular root canals, In-ceram ceramic does not seem to provide a sufficient strength.

After the development of Zirconia ceramic posts, it became possible to combine both materials. For a two-piece post and core construction, a post made of Yttrium oxide (Partially stabilized zirconia is used in conjunction with an all-ceramic core made of alumina or alumina magnesia ceramics), fabricated either by the copy milling or the slip casting technique.

The zirconia ceramic posts are commercially available in three ISO sizes (050, 090, 110).

These can be fabricated by both direct and indirect methods.

- *Direct method:* The selected zirconia ceramic post is tried in the prepared root canal. A core is formed intraorally by adapting the light curing resin composite to the inserted post. After the removal of the resin core from the post, the core is copied in ceramic in the celay machine.

- *Indirect method:* An impression of the inserted post is taken and a cast is prepared. The core is then formed with the light curing resin composite celay technique on the master cast. Finally, it is also copied in ceramic.

As an alternative to the copy-milling core fabrication, the slip casting technique can be used as described earlier, with a minor modification. A plastic post is inserted in the root canal of the special In-ceram plaster die. This plastic post provides accurate space for the zirconia ceramic post and does not cause any problem because it is burnt out during the sintering firing. After the core wax-up and the two silicone molds are made, the slip is injected as described for slip casting technique.

After glass infiltration firing, the infiltrated alumina core and the zirconia post are sand blasted and ultrasonically cleaned in 90% alcohol.

For cementation, adhesive resin is applied to the bonding surface of the post and core, and luted to the tooth. Primarily, the ceramic core is placed on the prepared tooth and immediately afterward, the post is inserted in the root canal through the canal of the core. After setting of the luting agent, the post is shortened at its protruding occlusal end, and the tooth preparation is completed with appropriate instruments.

iv. *Heat Press Technique*

The heat press technique has recently found application in all ceramic post and core fabrication. It is based on the IPS Empress system. In this system, a castable, pre-cerammed leucite reinforced glass ceramic material is heated and processed in an investment mold after the burn out of the wax analog (lost wax technique). In the heat press technique, a glass ceramic core is heat pressed over a prefabricated zirconium dioxide post and both materials are fused into a solid post and core restoration.

For the root canal preparation, special reamers are used so that the canal can receive a zirconia post with the appropriate diameter (1.4 or 1.7 mm). After the impression is taken and the master cast is constructed, the core wax pattern can be molded in the laboratory.

An intra-oral direct method can also be employed with the use of a self-curing resin after insertion of the post in the root canal. Then the heat press procedure, which is identical for both methods, is followed.

A 3.0 mm diameter and 6.0 to 8.0 mm long wax sprue is attached to the core with an inclination that allows a uniform flow and expansion of the glass ceramic. At that time, the post and core is invested in a phosphate bonded refractory die material. The heat press procedure is performed in a specially designed furnace. The ceramic ingot is first heated at 1,180°C and is pressed with 0.3–0.4 MPa pressure under vacuum. After cooling and divesting the post and core, all ceramic construction is fitted to the master cast. It is tried in the patient's mouth and adhesively cemented as previously described.

V. Dentin Posts (Biological Posts)

The dentin post is a newer concept in which the post is fabricated from the root dentin of the stored extracted teeth. The extracted teeth, preferably incisors or single rooted, are stored in Hank's solution or artificial saliva. The root canal of the tooth to be restored is prepared in routine. The cementum of the stored tooth is grinded by copy milling technique preferably to have two dentin posts; alternatively, the canal of the extracted tooth is filled with composite and the cementum is grinded to have single post. The shape of the post is fabricated according to the configuration of the prepared canal. The silicone impression of the prepared canal guides the fabrication of the dentin post. The post is finally luted into the root canal using adhesive luting agents. The core portion can be fabricated with composites and finally restored with full veneer crowns (Figs 6.25a–d).

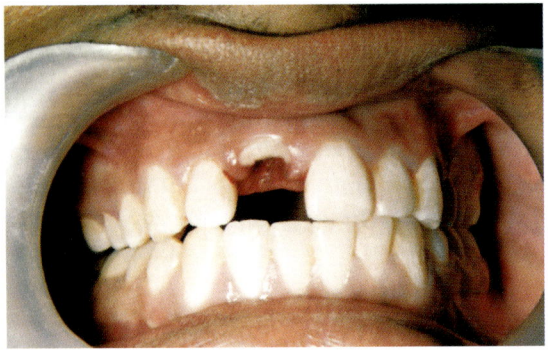

Fig. 6.25a: Preoperative

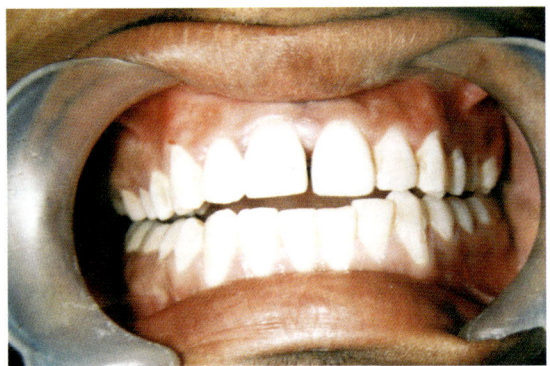

Fig. 6.25d: Postoperative

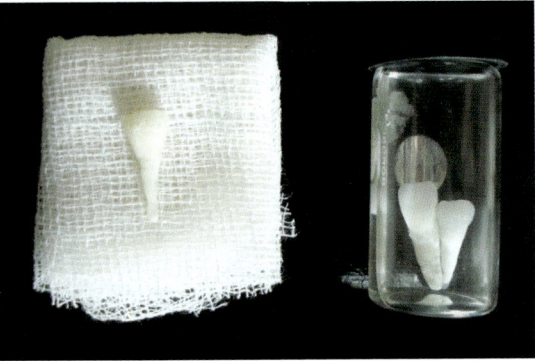

Fig. 6.25b: Tooth stored in solution

VI. Miscellaneous Post Systems

a. *Integrapost System*

The integrapost system is an esthetic post reinforced over the titanium alloy. It is biocompatible and corrosion resistant along with being stiff (Figs 6.26a–b).

b. *Fiberfill Post System*

The fiberfill system implies simultaneous obturation of the prepared root canal with the insertion of fiber reinforced post system. The system consists of an adhesive bonding agent, a light-curable calcium hydroxide based resin sealer and a fiber post with an apical terminus of gutta-percha. The primer in the system is a

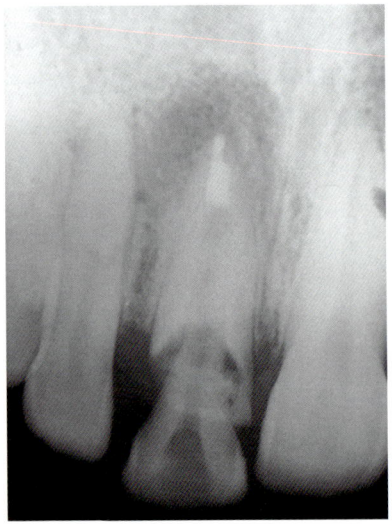

Fig. 6.25c: Radiograph showing dentin post

The dentin posts have successfully been tried in deciduous teeth and are also showing promising results in permanent teeth.

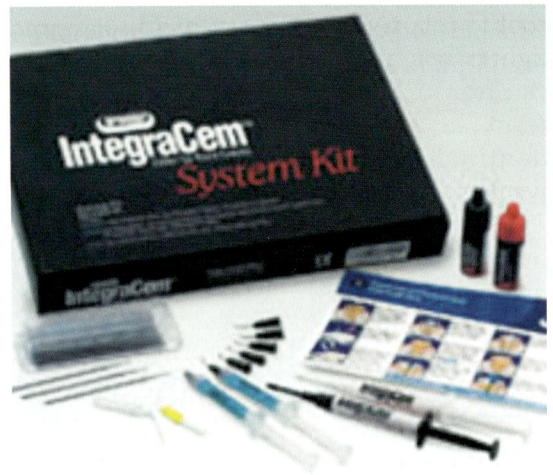

Fig. 6.26a: Integracem

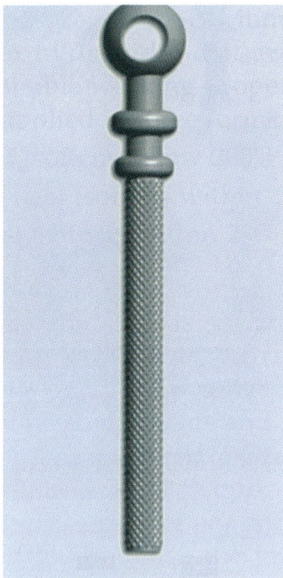

Fig. 6.26b: Integrapost

two-fold self-etching and priming liquid that allows the sealer to chemically bond to the root dentin. This system is time and cost effective.

VII. Light Transmitting Plastic Post

Occasionally, the post space presents a problem in routine post-core protocol, viz. flared canals, wider canals, internal resorption, and/or caries inside the root dentin. In such cases, the tooth is internally rebuilt with composite resin to structurally reinforce the root to retain a post and core. A clear plastic light transmitting post was introduced, which can transmit light to polymerize composite resin placed deeply. The composite acts as a dentinal substitute and rehabilitate the weakened roots.

The light transmitting posts are also indicated in case of caries in the coronal portion of the root canal or trauma to the immature incisors. The internal resorption and inadequate access cavity preparation or any other misadventure may also lead to such type of canal configuration warranting the use of light transmitting posts.

Technique: The light transmitting plastic post (Luminex light transmitting post) is selected

according to the internal configuration of the root canal. The post is tried and adjusted in length. The internal root dentin is acid etched, rinsed and dried. A dual cured bonding agent is applied inside the root, air blown to make it uniform and cured. A micro-hybrid composite is injected into the canal and the light transmitted post is pushed into the uncured composite resin to its full depth. The light transmitting post allows the passage of light through its body but does not bond to the composite material. A hemostat is used to rotate and remove the light transmitting post, leaving an ideal shape for post placement. Luscent anchor post of same matching size can then be inserted and cured in routine. Plastic post can be fabricated in clinics (Figs 6.27a–g).

CORES

It is established that every endodontically treated tooth may not require a post. Most of the teeth, especially the molars can be successfully restored without a post. The remaining tooth structure usually supports the core, which is sufficient to withstand the occlusal forces.

The post is considered only in case the remaining tooth structure is not sufficient to support the core. Many a times, the cusps are destroyed and/or undermining of cusps warrants the use of posts along with core.

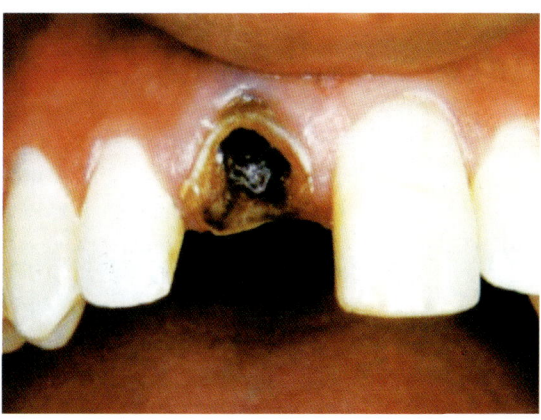

Fig. 6.27a: Preoperative

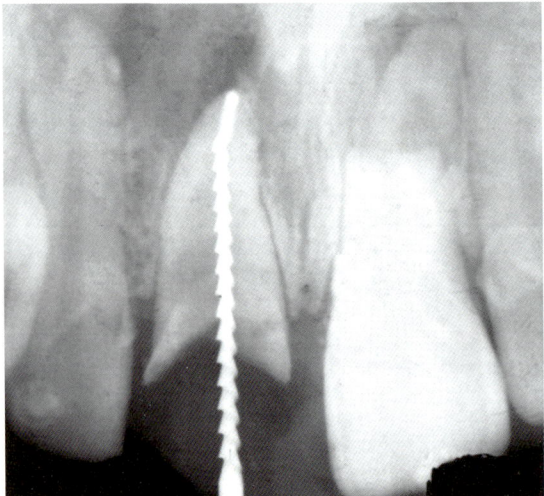

Fig. 6.27b: Evaluating root canal

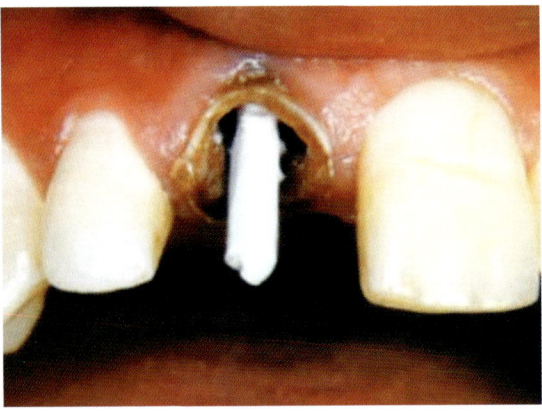

Fig. 6.27c: Evaluating plastic pin

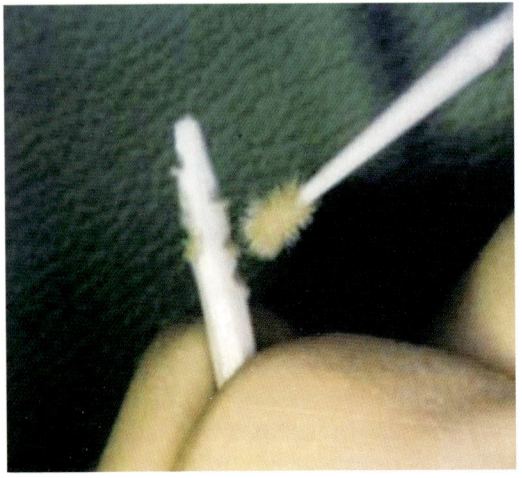

Fig. 6.27d: Applying bonding agent

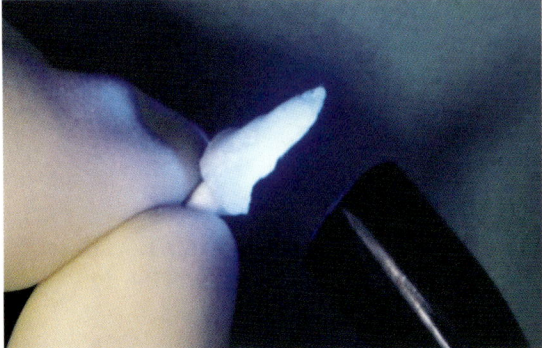

Fig. 6.27e: Final pattern

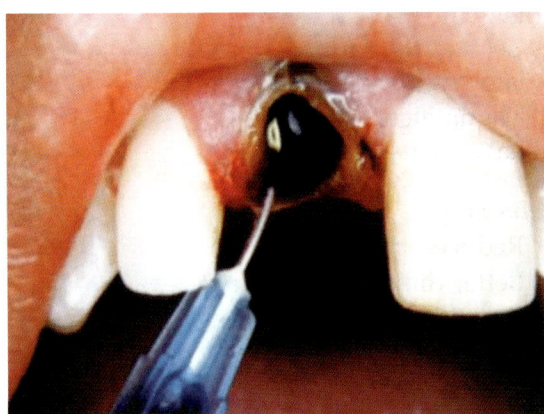

Fig. 6.27f: Applying acid etch on the inner wall

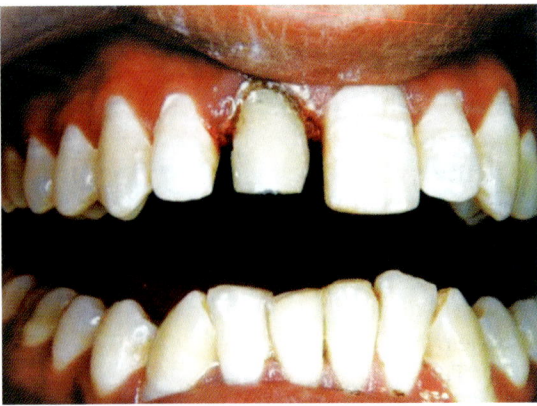

Fig. 6.27g: Core preparation

Various materials have been used and are being used as core without a post or along with the post. The commonly used materials are:

a. Amalgam

Amalgam was the most preferred core material; however, over the years, especially with the increasing popularity of all-ceramic crowns, it is no longer preferred. Pins are indicated for anchoring amalgam in teeth with extensive coronal damage. Amalgam pin cores are usually not employed for teeth where the appropriate dentin is not available (premolars and anteriors).

A coronal radicular amalgam post core has been employed; the pulp chamber along with 2.0–4.0 mm of each canal is filled with amalgam. The concept is of amalgapin used as secondary retentive device. The bulk of amalgam is utilized for strength and retention.

The amalgam cores are usually given under metal crowns or metal ceramic crowns.

Advantages
- Reduced marginal leakage
- Better dimensional stability
- Good compressive strength
- Good modulus of elasticity

Disadvantages
- Low tensile strength
- Corrosion with base metals

b. Composite Resin

Composite resin cores can be used along with pins and posts as well. They are quite strong and easy to manipulate. The resin adapts well to retentive pins and possesses as much tensile strength as amalgam cores. Composites cores are recommended in teeth with minimum tooth structure loss (Figs 6.28a and b).

The disadvantage with composite core is that the microleakage is greater than amalgam cores. Tensile bond strength for cast crowns is less during cementation. However, the retentive capacity increases with time. The crown margins should extend well past core margins.

Lumiglass composite has been tried as core material. Lumiglass core build-up composite

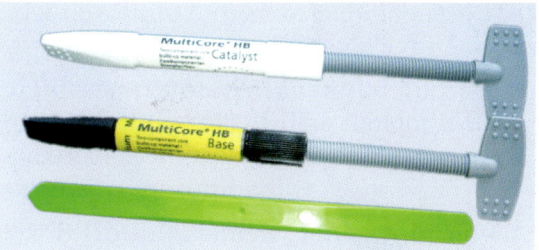

Fig. 6.28a: Composite core material

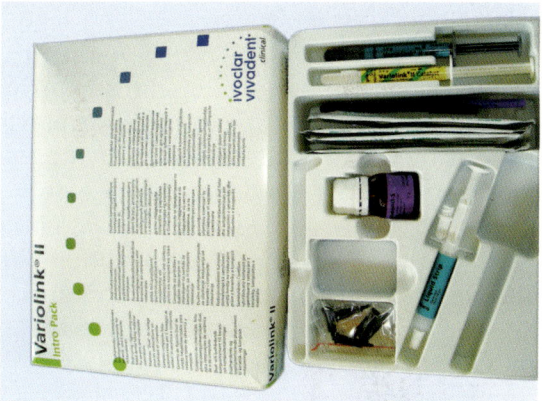

Fig. 6.28b: Composite core material

is formulated to optimize with fiber posts. Light cure Lumiglass is translucent, and can be easily cured in thickness of up to 8.0 mm thickness.

Lumiglass exhibits good handling characteristic for easy manipulation. It is radiopaque, and has better physical properties. The esthetic neutral shade is ideal for use with all-ceramic crowns.

Advantages
- Easy manipulation
- Good compressive strength
- Rapid/deep polymerization

Disadvantages
- Poor dimensional stability
- Polymerization shrinkage

c. Glass-ionomer Cement

Glass-ionomer cement has also been used as core material. It is preferred in cases where caries susceptibility is high and also in teeth with minimal tooth structure left. However, it is avoided in teeth under lateral loads.

Advantages
- Adhesive
- Anticariogenic
- Easy manipulation

Disadvantages
- Low resistance to fracture
- Sensitive to moisture

d. Glass-cermet Core

A combination of glass-ionomer cement and silver alloy in the ratio of 7:1 has been used as a core material. The glass-cermet cement possesses all the mechanical properties required for core and additionally helps in caries reduction by releasing fluorides. However, the black color of the glass-cermet limits its use only under metal crown or metal-ceramic crowns.

e. Prefabricated Post and Cast Core

The prefabricated post is tried in the root canal as usual. A core of resin or wax is fabricated over the post by either direct or indirect technique. The post and its attached core pattern are invested and one-unit metal cast is prepared. Such a system is no longer used, since it does not provide any additional advantage.

f. Prefabricated Post and Composite Resin Core

A composite resin core over the prefabricated post is considered as a simple and effective method. The entire procedure can be accomplished in a single appointment. The prefabricated post is fitted in routine and over the coronal end, composite core is build following manufacturer's instructions.

Care is taken to extend the finish lines for the final restoration well below the composite core. Auxiliary pins can be used to resist the rotational forces. A few authors have reported that the prefabricated post/composite resin core did not adequately resist torque without auxiliary pins. The auxiliary pins embedded in core material across a tooth may have a 'buttressing effect' and resist splitting forces on the root.

Restoration of Teeth after Root Amputation

In hemisection and radisectomy procedures, one root is extracted and the other root(s) along with the trunk (mostly) is utilized for restoration purposes (Figs 6.29a–e). Indications for root removal include:
- Severe periodontal involvement of the single root (may be mesio-buccal and disto-buccal in maxillary molars)
- Severe furcation involvement
- Severe root caries/resorption inside the root, which cannot be treated
- Endodontically unmanaged root, for example, instrument fracture, perforation, etc.

Restoring Mandibular Molar

In mandibular molars, either mesial or distal root is retained.
a. *Retaining distal root:* In case, the distal root is retained, it is advantageous being straight, has the widest canal and can accommodate the deepest post. It is more posterior and gives a greater arch length. It is wider in a bucco-lingual than mesio-

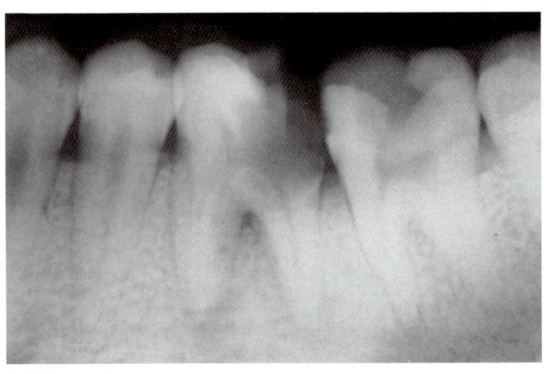

Fig. 6.29a: Badly mutilated mandibular first molar

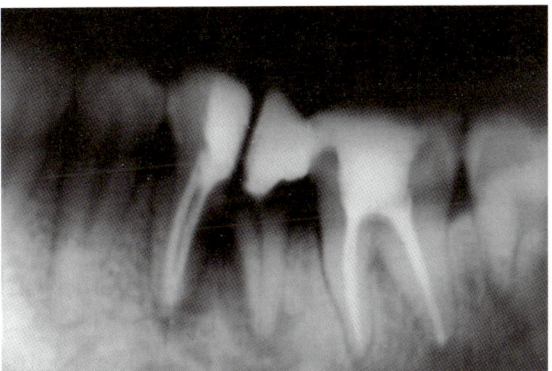

Fig. 6.29b: Hemisection of molar

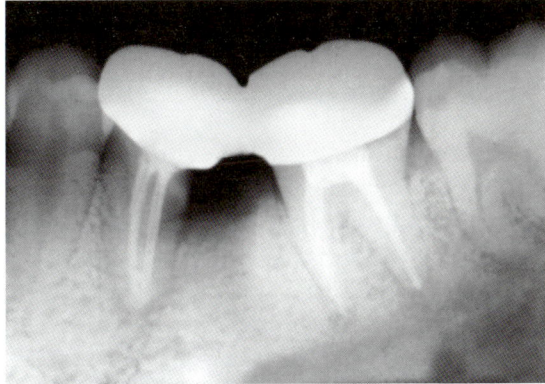

Fig. 6.29e: Radiograph showing final restoration

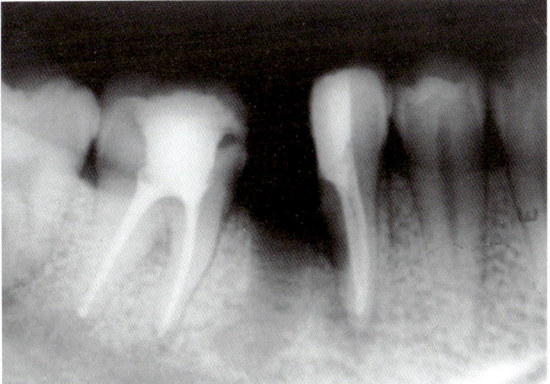

Fig. 6.29c: Extraction of distal root

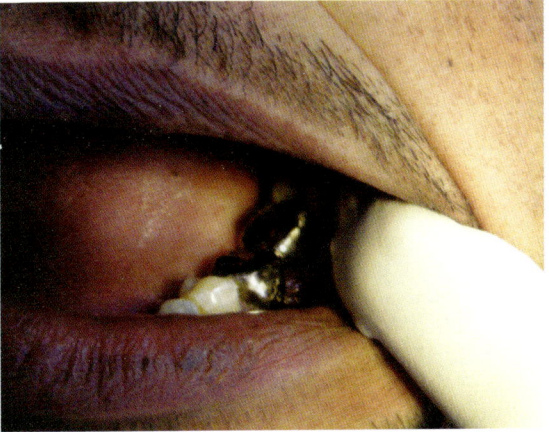

Fig. 6.29d: Restoration with cast crowns

distal direction and is handled like a bicuspid in its preparation for post and core. When the distal root has two canals,

the disto-buccal canal is usually the larger and should receive the post. The orifice is widened bucco-lingually to avoid perforation.

b. *Retaining mesial root:* In case, the mesial root is retained, the straighter mesial canal (mesio-lingual canal) is prepared to hold a single post. Additional retention may be gained by using a small preparation at the orifice of the unused canal. This also provides anti-rotational device for the post and core preparation. Because of the curved nature of these canals, care must be exercised not to make the posts so long that they deviate from the prepared canal space and lead to perforation. Both mesial canals can be used for twin posts. They must be parallel in the cervical third of canal, if a cast post is used but can deviate if prefabricated plastic posts are used. Total retention is equal to the sum of post lengths. The root is treated as a bicuspid and is prepared along with the adjacent tooth to receive a restoration in a bridge form.

c. *Retaining mesial and distal roots (bisection):* In case, both the roots are retained, it is usually not possible to create a satisfactory environment for future cleaning around both the roots. The two roots are usually not divergent enough to gain a sizeable inter-proximal space where the furcation has been located. Minor orthodontic tooth movement can be helpful.

The re-contouring is usually accomplished in two phases:

  i. Initial contouring when the amputation is performed
  ii. Final contouring during tooth preparation for crown fabrication

The re-contouring is mainly completed in first phase. The line angles are blended smoothly. Sharp projections or spurs are eliminated. The inter-proximal areas between the amputated root and adjacent tooth must be kept open to allow for optimal plaque control. The furcation area should be fluted to allow for proper tissue adaptation.

In the final phase of re-contouring, the occlusal table should be narrowed and the excursive contacts should be eliminated.

Restoring Maxillary Molar

In maxillary molars, the most commonly unmanaged root is the mesio-buccal root. The other roots are usually managed clinically. However, in certain cases, disto-buccal root is also extracted along with the mesio-buccal (Palatal root is to be preserved for post and core restoration).

a. Retaining Disto-buccal and Palatal Roots

The channel for post is prepared in the palatal root. Preparation of the areas adjacent to the retained root is critical. The trifurcation formed by the missing and remaining roots, if more, may pose clinical difficulties. This is to be minimized to prevent the residual furcation from acting as a 'shelf' for plaque accumulation.

The preparation at the gingival margin resembles a figure eight shape as the preparation is bevelled between the remaining two roots. The shape of the final restoration at the gingival margin will depend on the horizontal depth of the concavity created between the two roots. Flatter contours with mild concavities are preferred. The final coronal restoration for this preparation has an occlusal configuration similar to that of a molar but with the mesio-buccal or disto-buccal portion reduced to lessen the occlusal stress where no root is present. At the gingival margin, there is a large embrasure where the amputated root was formerly present.

b. Retaining Palatal Root Only

Sometimes, both the buccal roots are extracted and only palatal is retained. The palatal root is the widest of the maxillary roots and circumferential concavities on palatal roots are far more subtle than concavities on the other maxillary roots. The single remaining root must be used in conjunction with another tooth/teeth since it is not strong enough to function alone. The natural buccal curvature of the palatal root creates a severe undercut on its straight buccal surface. A bevelled shoulder preparation of the buccal surface of the palatal root is required to parallel it with adjacent teeth and allow preparation of the undercut margin. The restoration must be narrow bucco-lingually, which may place the occlusal table in a cross-bite relation.

Bibliography

1. Abu Kasim NH, Madfa AA, Hamdi M and Rahbari GR. 3D-FE analysis of functionally graded structured dental posts. Dent. Mater.: 2011;30:869–80.
2. Akkayan B and Gulmez T. Resistance to fracture of endodontically treated teeth restored with different post systems. J. Prosthet. Dent.: 2002;87: 431–7.
3. Asmussen E, Peutzfeldt A and Heitman T. Stiffness, elastic limit and strength of newer types of endodontic posts. J. Dent.: 1999;27:275–8.
4. Bandeca M, El-Mowafy O, Shebl A and Poro-Neto S. Non-metallic post endodontic restoration: a systematic review. Int. J. Dent.: 2010;9:57–62.
5. Bateman G, Ricketts DN and Saunders WP. Fiber-based post systems: a review. Br. Dent. J.: 2003; 195:43–8.
6. Bitter K and Kilebassa M. Post-endodontic restorations with adhesively luted fiber-reinforced composite post systems: A review. Am. J. Dent.: 2007;20:353–60.
7. Brodbeck U. The Zi Real post: A new ceramic implant abutment. J. Esthet. Rest. Dent.: 2003;15: 10–23.

8. Brown PL and Hicks NL. Rehabilitation of endodontically treated teeth using the radiopaque fiber post. Compendium.: 2003;24:75–8.

9. Cagidiaco MC, Goracci C, Garcia-Godoy F and Ferrari M. Clinical studies of fiber posts: a literature review. Int. J. Prosthodont.: 2008;21:328–36.

10. Dallari A, Rovatti L, Dallari B, Mason PN and Suh B. Translucent Quartz-fiber post luted in vivo with self-curing composite cement: Case report and microscopic examination at two year clinical follow up. J. Adhes. Dent.: 2006;8:189–95.

11. Demirel F, Saygili G and Sahmali S. Microleakage of endodontically treated teeth restored with prefabricated posts and tooth colored restorative material. Int. J. Periodontics Rest. Dent.: 2005;25:73–9.

12. Deutsch AS, Musikant BL, Cavallari J and Lepley JB. Prefabricated posts: A literature review. J. Prost.Dent.: 1983;49:498–503.

13. Dietschi D, Duc O, Krejci I and Sadan A. Biomechanical considerations for the restoration of endodontically treated teeth: a systematic review of the literature - part 1: composition and micro- and macrostructure alterations. Quint. Int.: 2007;38:733–43.

14. Erkut S, Gulsahi G, Caglar A, Imirzalioglu P, Karbhari VM and Ozmen I. Microleakage in overflared root canals restored with different fiber reinforced dowels. Oper. Dent.: 2008;1:96–105.

15. Fernandes AS and Desai GS. Factors affecting the fracture resistance of post-core reconstructed teeth: A review. Int. J. Prosthod.: 2001;14:355–63.

16. Ferrari M, Mannocci F, Vichi A, Cagidiaco MC and Mjor IA. Bonding to root canal: structural characteristics of the substrate. Am. J. Dent.: 2000;13:255–60.

17. Ferrari M, Mason PN, Goracci C, Pashley DH and Tay FR. Collagen degradation in endodontically treated teeth after clinical function. J. Dent. Res.: 2004;83:419–29.

18. Ferrari M, Vichi A and Garcia-Godoy F. Clinical evaluation of fiber reinforced epoxy resin posts and cast post and cores. Am. J. Dent.: 2000;13:15B–18B.

19. Fishelberg G. Clinical response to a vacant post space. Int. Endod. J.: 2004;37;199–204.

20. Freedman GA. Esthetic post-and-core treatment. Dent. Clin. N. Am.: 2001;45:103–16.

21. Gao H, Zhang ZT, Fan L, Wang DS, Zuo HJ and Sheng Y. Development of novel polyimide composite core materials reinforced with carbon fibers. Chinese J. Prosthodont.: 2007;3:210–2.

22. Gegauff AG. Effect of crown lengthening and ferrule placement on static load failure of cemented cast post cores and crowns. J. Prosth. Dent.: 2000;84:169–79.

23. Glazer B. Restoration of endodontically treated teeth with carbon fiber posts-a prospective study. J. Can. Dent. Assoc.: 2000;66:613–8.

24. Goodacre CJ and Spolnic KJ. The prosthodontic management of endodontically treated teeth: a literature review. Part I: Success and failure data, treatment concepts. JPD 3, 243, 1994, Part II: Managing the apical seal, Part III: Tooth preparation considerations. JPD: 1995;4:122–8.

25. Goracci C and Ferrari M. Current prospective on post systems: a literature review. Aust. Dent. J.: 2011;56:77–83.

26. Grande N, Butti A, Plotino G and Somma F. Adapting fiber-reinforced composite root canal post for use in non-circular shaped canals. Pract. Proced. Aesthet. Dent.: 2006;18:593–9.

27. Grecca FS, Rosa ARG, Gomes MS, Parolo CF, Bemfica JRD and Frasca LCF. Effect of timing and method of post space preparation on sealing ability of remaining tooth filling material: In vitro microbiological study. JCDA: 2009;75:583–583e.

28. Grossmann Y and Sadan A. The prosthodontic concept of crown-to- root ratio: A review of literature. J.Prosth.Dent.: 2005;93:559–62.

29. Gutman J. The dentin-root complex: anatomic and biological considerations in restoring endo-dontically treated teeth. J. Prosth.Dent.: 1992;67:458–67.

30. Hashim NS, Moaleem MM and Al-attas H. Tooth colored post system: review of literature. IJCD: 2013;4:50–6.

31. Hayashi M and Ebisu S. Key factors in achieving firm adhesion in post-core restorations. Jap. Dent. Sci. Review: 2008;44:22–8.

32. Heffernan MJ, Aquilino SA, Diaz-Arnold AM, Haselton DR, Stanford MJ and Vargas MA. Relative translucency of six all-ceramic systems. Part I: core materials. J. Prosthet. Dent.: 2002;88:4–10.

33. Hew YS, Purton DG and Love RM. Evaluation of pre-fabricated root canal posts. J. Oral Rehab.: 2001;28:207–11.

34. Heydecke G and Peters MC. The restoration of endodontically treated, single-rooted teeth with cast or direct posts and cores: a systematic review. J. Prosthet. Dent.: 2002;87:380–6.

35. Hyashi M. Fracture resistance of pulpless teeth restored with post-cores and crowns. Dent. Mater.: 2006;22:477–85.

36. Jhavar N, Bhondwe S, Mahajan V and Dhoot R. Recent advances in post systems: a review. J. Appl. Dent. Med. Sci.: 2015;1:128–36.

37. JOE Editorial Board. Post space preparation: an online study guide. J. Endod.: 2008;34;e139–41.

38. Kakehashi Y, Luthy H, Naef R, Wohlwend A and Scharer P. A new all ceramic post and core system: Clinical, technical and in vitro results. Int. J. Periodontics Rest. Dent.: 1998;18:587–93.

39. King PA, Setchell DJ and Rees JS. Clinical evaluation of a carbon fibre reinforced endodontic post. J. Oral Rehab.: 2003;30:785–89.

40. Koutayas S and Matthias K. All ceramic post and cores: The state of the art. Quint. Int.: 1999;30:383–92.

41. Kumar M, Chauhan A, Olepu S and Sharma A. Advances in post systems- Pit and falls to avoid. Asian J. Sci. Tech.: 2014;5:625–7.

42. Lamichhane A, Xu C and Zhang F. Dental fiber-post resin base material: a review. J. Adv. Prosthodont.: 2014;6;60–5.

43. Lanza A, Aversa R, Rengo S, Apicella D and Apicella A. 3D FEA of cemented steel, glass and carbon posts in maxillary incisors. Dent. Mater.: 2005;21:709–15.

44. Lassila LV, Tanner J, Le Bell AM, Narva K and Vallittu PK. Flexural properties of fibre reinforced root canal posts. Dent. Mater.: 2004;20:29–36.

45. Liaw DJ, Wang KL, Huang YC, Lee KR, Lai JY and Ha CS. Advanced polyimide materials: Syntheses, physical properties and applications. Prog. Polym. Sci.: 2012;37:907–74.

46. Lindblad RM, Lassila LV, Salo V, Vallittu PK and Tjaderhane L. Effect of chlorhexidine on initial adhesion of fiber-reinforced post to root canal. J. Dent.: 2010;38:796–801.

47. Lopes GC, Baratieri LN, Caldeira de Andrada MA and Maia HP. All-ceramic post, core, and crown: technique and case report. J. Esthet. Restor. Dent.: 2001;13:285–95.

48. Malferrari S, Monaco C and Scotti R. Clinical evaluation of teeth restored with quartz fiber reinforced epoxy resin posts. Int. J. Prosthodont.: 2003;16:39–44.

49. Manning KE, Yu DC, Yu HC and Kwan EW. Factors to consider for predictable post and core build ups of endodontically treated teeth Part II. Clinical application of basic concepts. J. Can. Dent. Assoc.: 1995;61:696–701.

50. Mannocci F, Bertelli E, Sheriff M, Watson TF and Ford TRP. Three year clinical comparison of survival of endodontically treated teeth restored with either full cast coverage or with direct composite restoration. JPD: 2002;88:297–301.

51. Mannocci F, Sherriff M,Watson TF and Vallittu PK. Penetration of bonding resins into fibre-reinforced posts: A confocal microscopic study. Int. J. Endodont.: 2005;38:46–51.

52. Michalakis K, Hirayama H, Sfolkos J and Sfolkos K. Light transmission of posts and cores used for anterior esthetic region. Int. J. Periodontics and Rest. Dent.: 2004;24:462–9.

53. Morgano SM, Rodrigues AHC and Sabrosa CE. Restoration of endodontically treated teeth. Dent. Clin. N. Am.: 2004;48:397–416.

54. Naumann M, Preuss A and Frankenberger R. Reinforcement effect of adhesively luted fiber reinforced composite versus titanium posts. Dent. Mater.: 2007;23:138–44.

55. Newman MP. Fracture resistance of endodontically treated teeth restored with composite posts. J. Prosthet. Dent.: 2003;89:360–7.

56. Northdurft FP and Pospiech PR. Clinical evaluation of pulpless teeth restored with conventionally cemented zirconia posts: a pilot study. J. Prosthet. Dent.: 2006;95:311–4.

57. Ozkurt Z and Kazazoglu IU. Zirconia ceramic post systems: a literature review and a case report. Dent. Mater.: 2010;29;233–45.

58. Peroz I. Restoring endodontically treated teeth with posts and cores: A review. Quint. Int.: 2005; 36:737–46.

59. Pitel ML and Hicks NL. Evolving technology in endodontic posts. Compendium: 2003;24:13–6.

60. Plotino G, Grande NM, Pameijer CH and Somma F. Influence of surface remodeling using burs on the macro and micro surface morphology of anatomically formed fiber posts. Int. Endod. J.: 2008;41:345–55.

61. Poggio C, Chiesa M, Lombardini M and Dagna A. Influence of ethanol dying on the bond between fiber posts and root canals: SEM analysis. Qunit. Int.: 2011;42:e15–21.

62. Purton DG and Pay Ne JA. Tooth-colored post systems: A Review. Oper. Dent.: 2003;28:86–91.

63. Purton DG, Love RM and Chandler MP. Rigidity and retention of ceramic root canal posts. Oper. Dent.: 2000;25:223–37.

64. Qualtrough AJE and Mannoci F. Tooth-colored post systems: a review. Oper. Dent.: 2003;28:86–91.

65. Rickets DNJ, Tait CME and Higgins AJ. Post and core systems: refinements to tooth preparation and cementation.Br. Dent. J.: 2005;198:533–41.

66. Rosentritt M, Furer C, Behr M, Lang R and Handel G. Comparison of in-vitro fracture strength of metallic and tooth colored posts and cores. J. Oral Rehab.: 2000;27:595–601.

67. Sadak FT, Monticelli F, Goracci C, Tay FR, Cardoso PE and Ferrari M. Bond strength performance of different resin composites used as core material around fiber posts. Dent. Mater.: 2007;23:95–9.

68. Sahafi A, Pentzfeldt A, Asmussen E and Gotfredson K. Effect of surface treatment of prefabricated posts on bonding of resin cement. Oper. Dent.: 2004;29:60–8.

69. Sahafi A, Peutzfeldt A, Asmussen E and Gotfredsen K. Retention and failure morphology of prefabricated posts. Int. J. Prosthodont.: 2004; 17:307–12.

70. Schwartz RS and Robbins JW. Post placement and restoration of endodontically treated teeth: a literature review. J. Endod.: 2004;30:289–301.

71. Sedgley CM and Messer HH. Are endodontically treated teeth more brittle? J. Endod.: 1992;18:332–5.

72. Slutzky-Goldberg I, Slutzky H, Gorfil C and Smidt A. Restoration of endodontically treated teeth: review and treatment recommendations. Int. J. Dent.: 2009;1–9, Art.ID 150251.

73. Soares CJ, Mitsui FH, Neto FH, Marchi GM and Martins LR. Radiodensity evaluation of seven root post systems. Am. J. Dent.: 2005;18:57–60.

74. Sorrentino R, Salameh Z, Zarone N, Tay FR and Ferrari M. Effect of post-retained composite restoration of MOD preparations on the fracture resistance of endodontically treated teeth. J. Adhes. Dent.: 2007;9:49–56.

75. Stankiewicz NR and Wilson PR. The ferrule effect: a literature review. Int. J. Endod.: 2002;35:575–81.

76. Sterzenbach G, Franke A and Naumann M. Rigid versus flexible dentine like endodontic posts—Clinical testing of a biomechanical concept: Seven-year results of a randomized controlled clinical pilot trial on endodontically treated abutment teeth with severe hard tissue loss. J. Endod.: 2012;38:1557–63.

77. Stewardson DA. Non-metal post systems. Dent. Update: 2001;28:326–32, 334–6.

78. Streacker AB and Geissberger M. The milled ceramic post and core: A functional and esthetic alternative. J. Prosthet. Dent.: 2007;98:486–7.

79. Tang W, Wu Y and Smales RJ. Identifying and reducing risks for potential fractures in endodontically treated teeth. J. Endod.: 2010;36: 609–17.

80. Theodosopoulou JN and Chochlidakis KM. A systematic review of dowel (post) and core materials and systems. J. Prothodont.: 2009;18: 464–72.

81. Ton PLB, Aquilino SA, Gratton DG, Stanford CM, Tan SC, Johnson WT and Dawson D. In vitro fracture resistance of endodontically treated central incisors with varying ferrule heights and configurations. JPD: 2005;93:331.

82. Torbjorner A and Fransson B. A literature review on the prosthetic treatment of structurally compromised teeth. Int. J. Prosthod.: 2004;17:369–76.

83. Torbjorner A and Fransson B. Biomechanical aspects of prosthetic treatment of structurally compromised teeth. Int. J. Prosthodont.: 2004;17: 135–41.

84. Tronstad L, Asbjornsen K, Doving L, Pedersen I and Eriksen HM. Influence of coronal restorations on the periapical health of endodontically treated teeth. Int. Endo. J.: 2000;167:218–21.

85. Vichi A, Grandini S and Ferrari M. Comparison between two clinical procedures for bonding fiber posts into a root canal: a microscopic investigation. J. Endo.: 2002;28:355–60.

86. Vlahova A, Kissovy C, Kazukova R and Popova E. Masking the metal color of cast post-and-core restorations by metal ceramic caps: a clinical report. JSM Dent.: 2014;2:1024.

87. Yalcin E, Cehrili MC and Canay S. Fracture resistances of cast metal and ceramic post and core restorations: a pilot study. J. Prosth. Dent.: 2005;14:84–90.

88. Zhu Z, Dong XY, He S, Pan X and Tang L. Effect of post placement on the restoration of endodontically treated teeth: a systematic review. Int. J. Prosthodont.: 2015;28:475–83.

7

Shade Matching

The main goal of restorative dentistry is to achieve esthetics and functions. The restoration should not be conspicuous and must stimulate the natural dentition under all conditions. Four basic determinants are required to achieve esthetics, viz. position, contour, texture and color. The parameters of color need special attention, since color perception involves scientific determinants along with aesthetic abilities of the operator. The knowledge of underlying scientific principles of color is essential to achieve desired esthetic results. Color combination not only improves esthetics, but also makes the restoration appear natural and attractive. Continued research on the human visual system has given us greater insight into how color discrimination is affected by environment and other features like disease, drugs and aging. Besides the clinical applications of color, the color-measuring instruments and systems are also used in research, viz. comparing visual and instrumental findings, color compatibility and color stability during tooth whitening procedures, etc. The basic fundamentals of color and light, the radiation spectrum and the optical characteristics of the object is to be understood before evaluating and selecting proper color shade for the restoration.

Basic Color Schemes

The color wheel or color circle (Fig. 7.1) is the basic tool for combining colors. Sir Isaac Newton (1666) designed the first circular color diagram. Over the years, many variations of the basic design have been made, but the most common version is a wheel of 12 colors; the primary colors being red, yellow and blue. Three secondary colors (green, orange and purple) are created by mixing two primary colors. Six tertiary colors are created by mixing primary and secondary colors.

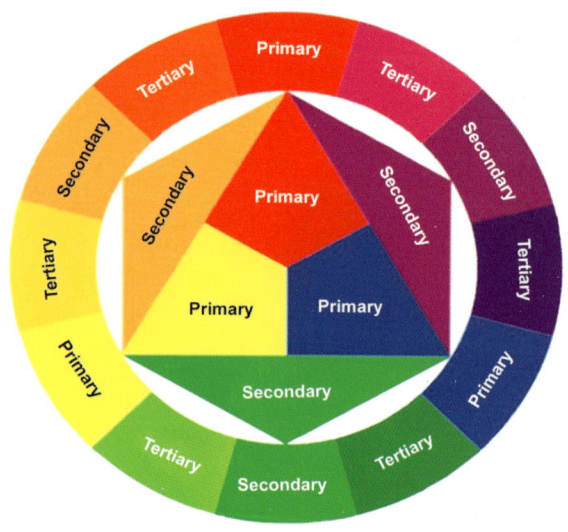

Fig. 7.1: Color wheel

The color circle can be divided into warm and cool colors.

'Warm colors' are vivid and energetic, and tend to advance in space; whereas 'Cool colors' give an impression of calm, and create a soothing impression (white, black and gray are considered to be neutral colors).

Color Harmonies (Color Chords)

The color combinations that are considered pleasing are called color harmonies or color chords. They consist of two or more colors having fixed relation in the color wheel. The combinations are described as:

- Complementary color scheme (colors that are opposite to each other on the color wheel are considered to be complementary colors; for example, red and green).
- Analogous color scheme (colors that are next to each other on the color wheel).
- Triadic color scheme (three colors that are evenly spaced around the color wheel).
- Tetradic or rectangular color scheme (four colors arranged into two complementary pairs).
- Split complementary color scheme (in addition to the base color, it uses two colors adjacent to its complement).
- Square color scheme (similar to rectangle, but all four colors spaced evenly around the color circle).

Additive Color Theory

The additive primary colors are red, green and blue. Combining one of these additive primary colors with equal amounts of another one results in the additive secondary colors of cyan, magenta and yellow (Fig. 7.2). Combining all three additive primary colors in equal amounts will produce the color white. Remember, combining additive colors creates lighter colors; so adding all three primary colors results in a color so 'light', actually seen as 'white'.

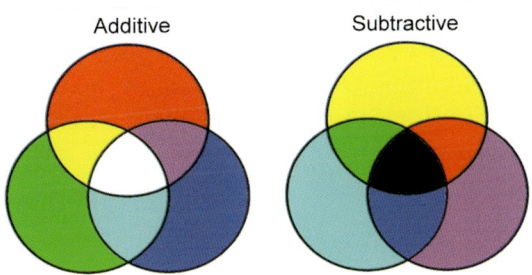

Fig. 7.2: Additive and subtractive colors

Additive Colors

Combined in equal parts:
- Blue + Green = Cyan
- Red + Blue = Magenta
- Green + Red = Yellow
- Red + Green + Blue = White

By changing the brightness of each of the three primary colors by varying degrees, one can make a wide range of colors.

Additive Colors

Combined in unequal parts:
- 1 Green + 2 Red = Orange
- 1 Red + 2 Green = Lime
- 1 Green + 1 Blue + 4 Red = Brown

Subtractive Color Theory

The subtractive primary colors are cyan, magenta and yellow (Fig. 7.2). Subtractive color mixing occurs when light is reflected off a surface or is filtered through a translucent object. For example, a red surface only appears red because it absorbs (subtracts) all of the light that is not red and only reflects or allows the red light.

Subtractive Colors Mixing

Combine	Absorbs	Leaves
Cyan + Magenta	Red + Green	Blue
Cyan + Yellow	Red + Blue	Green
Magenta + Yellow	Green + Blue	Red
Cyan + Magenta + Yellow	Red + Green + Blue	Black

Mixing of two subtractive primary colors results in a color, which is complimentary to the remaining primary. For example, if cyan and magenta is mixed it will form blue which is complimentary to the yellow (third subtractive primary color).

Perception of Color

The color perception involves various physical, psychological and physiological aspects. The perception is influenced by the light and its source, object and the observer.

Light and Light Source

The light source, the color of emitted light is described in color temperature ($^\circ$Kelvin). The lighting environment is important while perceiving color of an object (tooth). Light is defined as an electromagnetic radiation that can be detected by human eye. Natural white light falls between 380 and 770 nm along the electromagnetic spectrum. The component bands along with electromagnetic spectrum produce six different sensations, i.e. red, orange, yellow, green, blue and violet. The bands also produce infinite number of gradations with ill-defined boundaries. The color of any object is dependent on the illumination in which it is viewed. If incident light does not contain a particular wavelength segment, the object cannot reflect it. Colorants (pigments or dyes) are responsible for chromatic reflection of light. The chemical composition of a colorant selectively absorbs one part of the visible spectrum more than another. When a particular wavelength segment of light is reflected and enters the eye, the sensation of color is produced.

The quality of light source is important in determining the tooth shade. The natural light, say around mid-day (noon light) is considered ideal light source for accurate color comparison. The time of day, date, and weather conditions affect the color of sunlight. With the change in light source, the light reflected from an object changes; subsequently the color perceived can be different. The usual absence of ideal conditions in clinics has led to the use of artificial lighting (source simulating standard daylight) for color matching. Color temperature, spectral reflectance curves and color rendering index (CRI) are all used to measure the capacity to reproduce standard daylight. CRI value varies from 1 to 100 (CRI over 90 is recommended for color matching). The CRI (light) is affected by time of the day, humidity, clouds and pollution. Dental unit lights are usually incandescent lights that emit light high in the red-yellow spectrum and are low at the blue end. Regular cool white fluorescent lights are high in the green-yellow spectrum. Color-corrected fluorescent lights are also available, which can accurately perceive the color. Full spectrum light emitting diodes (LEDs) are now replacing incandescent bulbs. Shade matching ability is considered better with a light-correcting source than under natural light. A new device which eliminates the variability of different light sources, 'The Optilume Trueshade', uses full spectrum light emitting diodes and shows a color spectrum similar to mid-day light. Diffusion lenses over the LEDs mix the three colors of light (red, blue and green) emitted by the individual color diodes to create optimum, diffuse daylight. With the LEDs set at a 45-degree angle to minimize spectral reflectance or glare, the clinician can more accurately assess the true color. A unique feature of Optilume Trueshade is the ability to reduce the intensity of the light source while maintaining the color temperature. A lower intensity light allows for better perception of surface details, such as topography, ridges and enamel striations.

The recommended illuminating light source in shade matching is as follows (Fig. 7.3):
- 5500°K
- Replicate natural mid-day
- Balance all Hues in the spectral curve
- Working distance should be 12 inches
- Neutral color of the surroundings

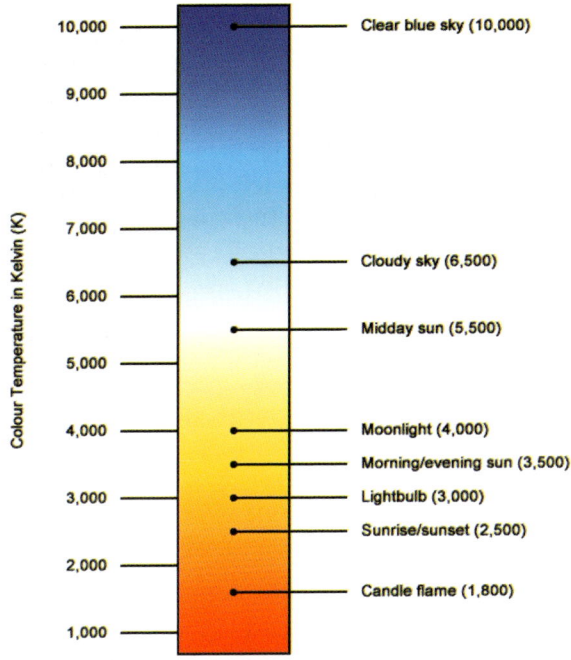

Fig. 7.3: Color temperature chart

The predominance of color (purity) influences the perception of color. It is necessary to provide similar lighting environment in the dental clinics as well as in the laboratory so as to achieve constant color purity. The ratio between the task light (which falls directly on the working area) and the ambient light (derived from the surroundings), known as the contrast ratio should be higher than 3:1, but lower than 10:1.

The Observer

The light reflected from an object stimulates the neural sensors in the retina and send a signal that is intercepted in the visual cortex of the brain. As light enters the eye, an image is focused on the retina. The amount of light entering the eye is controlled by the iris, which dilates or constricts depending on the level of illumination. The retinal rods and cones can adjust the variation of light intensity. The area around fovea centralis has mixture of sensors responsible for differences in color discrimination among observers with normal color vision. The accuracy of color perception depends on the area of retinal field stimulated by light. In high illumination, the pupil narrows and when light is dim, the pupil widens, stimulating sensors that are less accurate. As a regulator of pupil diameter, light intensity is a critical factor in color perception and shade matching. The shade assessment is highly subjective; different individuals make different interpretation of the same stimulus. A few individuals may show color blindness. In a rough estimate, 10% males and 1.0% females demonstrate color vision deficiency. Eye becomes less effective as one ages and subsequently more light is required to accomplish a task.

The Object

The quality of the color of an object (the tooth) depends on its ability to absorb, reflect, transmit or refract the light energy falling on it. The surrounding environment greatly influences the color. The ceiling and the walls reflect light, therefore, should not be painted in bright colors. Neutral colors like grey or white should be selected. Jahangiri et al (2002) evaluated the relationship between tooth shade and skin color and observed that the tooth shade was inversely related to the skin color.

Persons with medium to dark skin tone more likely to have teeth with higher value (lighter); whereas individual with lighter skin tone tended to have teeth with lower values (darker) regardless of gender and age.

Contrast Effects

Background colors considerably affect the perception of color in shade matching. Contrast effects which influence the color vision are:

i. *Simultaneous contrast* is visualized when two objects are viewed at the same time. The light or dark contrast can be correlated to the surrounding environment like skin tone, hair color and brightness of adjacent soft tissues and teeth. Hence, brighter shades should be chosen for light toned patients and darker shades for pigment-toned patients.

Color matching in a background of a rubber dam sheet is often misleading and should be avoided. Similarly, color is perceived differently with the gingival contrast; in cases of inflamed gingiva, complementary colored background is preferred. Since, tooth shades fall in orange Hue family, blue or neutral grey background should be selected to precondition the eye for better perception of color.

Actual contrast is influenced by the size and the Chroma of tooth. A brighter tooth looks larger while a darker tooth of the same dimension looks smaller.

ii. *Spatial contrast* implies the tooth when observed in different positional relationships. Recessed teeth look darker while overlapping teeth appear brighter and larger.

iii. *Successive contrast* is a phenomenon, which occurs when one color is observed after viewing another; the image of original color affects the color perception of the second object.

Effect of Surroundings

Color perception is affected by the reflection or interference from surrounding colors. The effects of clothing, make-up, especially lipstick should be neutralized. One should stare at a tooth for less than five seconds because our eyes become accommodated to the red and yellow color. The after-image which occurs when looking continuously at an object of one color can be minimized by looking at a blue object between assessing different shade tabs. Blue backgrounds, however, are not appropriate because they also cause after-images and may bias your perception to its complementary color 'orange'. The eyes should be given a break with a neutral grey background; a Pensler Shield (Kulzer) is designed to minimize background glaze.

Three Dimensions of Color

Color is usually described according to the Munsell color space in terms of Hue, Value, and Chroma. 'Hue' is the attribute of a color that enables the clinician to distinguish between different families of color; whereas 'Value' indicates the lightness of a color. 'Chroma' is the degree of color saturation. When color is determined using the Munsell system, Value is determined first followed by Chroma. Hue is determined last by matching with shade tabs of the Value and Chroma already determined.

Hue

'Hue' is the quality that distinguishes one family of colors from another. It is specified as the dominant range of wavelengths in the visible spectrum that yields the perceived color, even though the exact wavelength of the perceived color may not be present (Fig. 7.4a). Hue is a physiologic and psychologic interpretation of the sum of wavelengths. Generally, there are six Hue families, viz. violet, blue, green, yellow, orange and red; however, Hue is represented by A, B, C, or D denoting reddish-brown, reddish-yellow, grey and reddish-grey respectively on the commonly used VITA Classic shade guide.

Value

Value is the lightness/darkness of any object. 'Value' or brightness, is the amount of light returned from an object (Figs 7.4b and c). Munsell described Value as a white-to-black grey scale. Bright objects have lower amounts of grey, and low-value objects have larger amounts of grey and will appear darker. The brightness of a crown is usually increased in two ways: by lowering Chroma, or by increasing the Value (reflectivity of the surface). Lower Value means less light returns from the illuminated object and the rest is being absorbed or scattered elsewhere. Value differences are more noticeable and are more significant in restorations. In Hue A of VITA

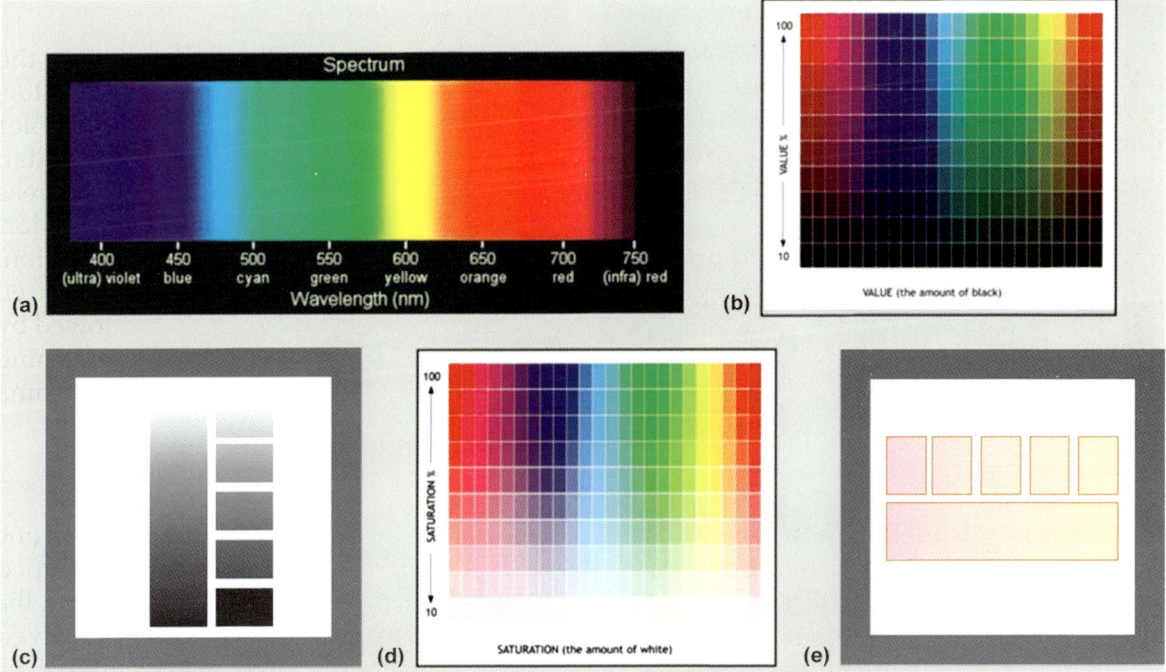

Figs 7.4a–e: Three dimensions of color. a. Hue; b and c. Value; d and e. Chroma

shade guide, A1 is the brightest while A4 is the darkest. Value relates to a color brightness specific to the black and white area. Value relates to the quality and not the quantity of the color's greyness. Hasegawa (2000) observed negative correlation between age and Value. It has been established that the amount of luster directly affects the Value. The luster control is difficult; especially in glazing porcelain. Hand polishing can achieve better luster. A 'matte-finish' luster provides greater scattering of light and is more appropriate for younger age groups; whereas 'semigloss' is preferred in middle age and 'gloss' finish luster for older age groups.

Chroma

'Chroma' is the saturation, intensity, or strength of the Hue (Figs 7.4d and e). If any dye (say red) is added into a glass of water and the same dye is added again and again the intensity increases, but the color remains the same (Hue). As more dye is added, the mixture appears darker; so the increase in

Chroma has a corresponding change in Value. As Chroma is increased, the Value is decreased (Chroma and Value are inversely related). Higher numbers on the VITA classic shade guide represent increased Chroma. Chroma cannot exist by itself but is always associated with Hue and Value. Hasegawa (2000) observed that color (reddish-yellow) of natural teeth had a tendency to increase from incisal to cervical; whereas translucency decreases. In VITA shade guide, A1 has lowest Chroma and A4 has the highest Chroma.

Opacity and Translucency

As light strikes a surface, it is either totally reflected, totally absorbed or partially absorbed and rest reflected. The objects, if reflect all/most of the light incident on them are opaque; whereas transparent objects transmit the light in totality (when part of light incident on an object is transmitted and the rest is scattered, the property is known as translucency) (Figs 7.5a and b). Human teeth are characterized by varying degrees of

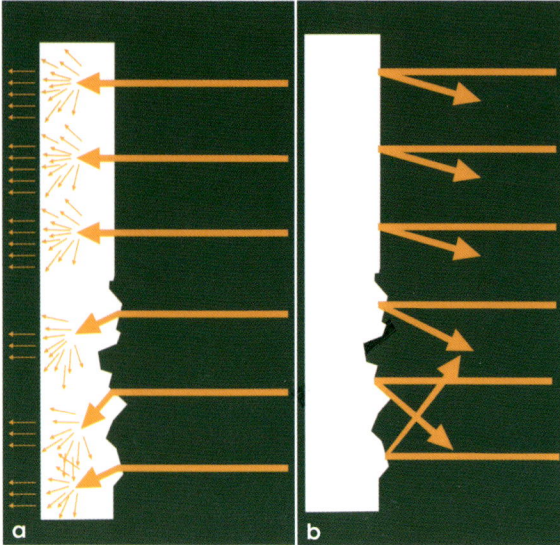

Figs 7.5a and b: Transmitted and scattered light

translucency; designated as the gradient between transparent and opaque. Generally, increasing the translucency of the object (say crown) lowers its Value, because less light returns to the eye. With increased translucency, light is able to pass the surface and is scattered within the restoration. The translucency of enamel varies with the angle of incidence, surface texture/luster, wavelength and level of dehydration. Highly translucent teeth tend to be lower in Value, since they allow light to transmit through teeth; whereas, opaque teeth have higher Values. There might be inter-tooth as well as intra-tooth differences in the translucency. The extent varies depending upon the age of the individual (reparative and degenerative changes in enamel and dentin due to age). Thus, operator is the final authority to decide upon the level of translucency.

Fluorescence

Fluorescence is the absorption of light by an object and its spontaneous emission in a longer wavelength (emission of light at a different wavelength from that of incident light). In a natural tooth, it primarily occurs in the dentin because of the higher amount of organic material. The near-UV light is absorbed and fluoresced back, primarily in the blue end of the spectrum; however, it may occur at all wavelengths (teeth fluoresce in the range of 340–410 nm). The more the dentin fluoresces, the lower the Chroma. Fluorescent powders are added to crown and other preparation to increase the quantity of light returning back to the viewer, blocking out discolorations, and decreasing the Chroma. This is especially beneficial in high-value shades, as it can raise the Value without negatively affecting the translucency when placed within the dentin porcelain layers.

Gloss

Gloss is an optical property associated with a smooth surface that produces lustrous surface appearance and thus reduces the effect of color difference. It also lightens the color appearance; associated with a smooth surface which can be created on a restoration by finishing and polishing procedures that increases the 'Value' of the final results.

Opalescence

Opalescence is the phenomenon in which a material appears to be of one color when light is reflected from it and of another color when light is transmitted through it. A natural opal is an aqueous disilicate that fragments transilluminated light into different spectrum by refraction. Opals act like prisms and refract different wavelengths to varying degrees. The shorter wavelengths refract more and also require higher critical angle to escape an optically dense material. The hydroxyapatite crystals of enamel also act as prisms. Wavelengths of light have different degrees of translucency through teeth and the restorative materials. When illuminated, opals and enamel will transilluminate the 'reds' and scatter the 'blues' within its body; thus, enamel appears bluish even though it is colorless. The opalescent effects brighten the tooth enamel and give it optical depth and vitality.

Metamerism

The colors (usually two) that match under a given lighting condition but have different spectral reflectance are called 'metamers' and the phenomenon is known as 'metamerism' (pairs of objects having the same appearance in a given environment but having different spectral curves). The metamerism impact is important. Shade guides, teeth and the restorative materials are all composed of different materials and have different spectral curves. Since, the lighting environment during shade selection is different, the chain of metamerism of tooth-guide restorative material should be recognized. The patients should be informed of the effect of metamerism on the final shade selection. The problem of metamerism can be avoided by selecting a shade and confirming it under different lighting conditions such as natural daylight and fluorescent light.

Color Determination/Measurement

The determination/measurement of color is carried out using techniques as:
a. Visual technique
b. Instrumental technique (Commission Internationale deL'Eclairage-CIE)

A. Visual Technique

A popular system for visual determination of color is the Munsell color system, the parameters of which are represented in three dimensions (Fig. 7.6). Value (lightness) is determined first by the selection of a tab that most nearly corresponds with the lightness or darkness of the color. Value ranges from white (10/) to black (0/). Chroma is determined next with tabs that are close to the measured Value but are of increasing saturation of color. Chroma ranges from achromatic or grey (/0) to a highly saturated color (/18). Hue is determined last by matching with color tabs of the 'Value' and 'Chroma' already determined. Hue is measured on a scale from 2.5 to 10 in increments of 2.5 for each of the

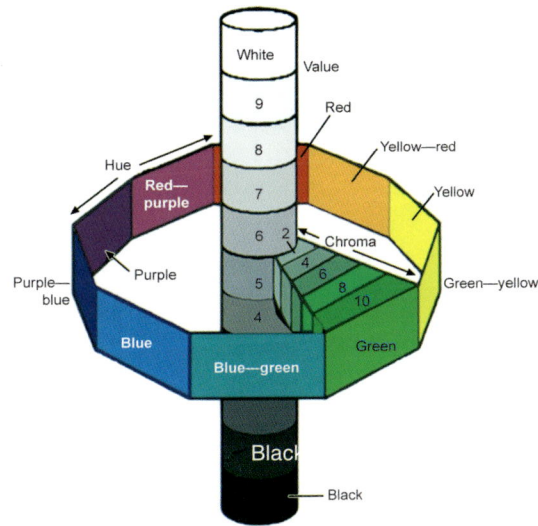

Fig. 7.6: Munsell color system

10 color families (red, R; yellow–red, YR; yellow, Y; green–yellow, GY; green, G; blue–green, BG; blue, B; purple–blue, PB; purple, P; red–purple, RP).

Visual color determination of shade selection has been found to be unreliable and inconsistent. Visual color assessment is dependent on the observer's physiologic and psychologic responses. Inconsistencies may also result from uncontrolled factors such as fatigue, aging, emotions, lighting conditions, previous eye exposure, object and illuminant position, and metamerism. A few authors, after evaluating various shade guides, observed inconsistencies and opined that there was a need for more scientific and consistent means of shade matching in restorative dentistry.

B. Instrumental Technique

An organization called CIE (Commission Internationale de L' Eclairage) determine color values that are accepted worldwide to measure color. The values used by CIE are called L*, a* and b* and the color measurement method is called CIELAB.

In this system, the color space consists of three coordinates; L* (defines lightness), a* (red–green chromacity) and b* (yellow–blue chromacity) (Fig. 7.7). The L* refers to the

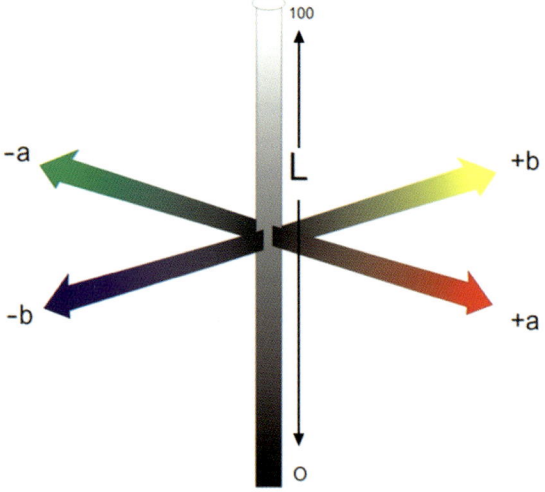

Fig. 7.7: L*a*b* system

illuminating light emitted from the device may be scattered, absorbed, transmitted, reflected and displaced as a result of translucent optical nature of teeth and dental ceramics. Colorimeters are preferred for flat surfaces, rather than the curved translucent surfaces usually observed on teeth.

The non-uniform color properties of teeth involve a complex layering of tooth structure coupled with subtle color changes that challenge even the best instruments. Additionally, high cost and technical difficulties of these instruments limit their use in routine practice.

Shade-taking Devices

These devices have been designed to aid clinicians and technicians in specifying/ measurement of tooth color. The initial color-measuring device designed for clinical use was a filter colorimeter, chromascan; however, it had limited success due to its inadequate design and accuracy. Since, esthetics is a major focus in restorative dentistry, newer devices were planned to overcome the challenges of shade matching. Color-measuring devices usually consist of a detector, signal conditioner, and software that process the signal in a manner that makes the data usable in the dental operatory or laboratory. The early shade taking instruments, viz. dental color analyzer, digital shade guide, Ikam, Shadescan, etc. are out of market or undergoing upgradation. The shade-taking devices are:

i. *Colorimeters*

The colorimeters generally use three or four silicon photodiodes that have spectral correction filters. These filters act as analog function generators that limit the spectral characteristics of the light striking the detector surface. Colorimeter measures and filters light in red, green and blue areas of visible spectrum. The filter colorimeters are considered inferior to spectrophotometers and spectro-

lightness coordinate, and its value ranges from 0 for perfect black to 100 for perfect white. The a* represents the difference between green (Δa*) and red (+a*). Positive a* values reflect the red color range and negative values indicate green color range. Similarly, b* represents the difference between yellow (+b*) and blue (Δb*). Positive b* values indicate yellow color range while negative values indicate the blue color range. The differences in the lightness and chromaticity coordinates (ΔL*, Δa*, Δb*) as a result of UV light exposure are determined first, and the total color change (ΔE*ab) can be calculated using the relationship

$$\Delta E^*ab = (\Delta L^{*2} + \Delta a^{*2} + \Delta b^{*2})^{1/2}$$

Instrumental color analysis, offers a potential advantage over visual color determination, because instrumental readings are objective and can be quantified. Spectro-photometers and colorimeters have been used with modifications in an attempt to overcome problems with visual shade matching in dentistry. Photoelectric tristimulus colorime-ters have the potential to overcome some of the shortcomings of the visual method; however, they also exhibit certain limitations. In dentistry, the results of a colorimetric device can be altered because the standardized

radiometers (aging of filter affects accuracy). However, because of their consistent and rapid sensing nature, these devices can be used for quality control. Complete tooth image is provided through the use of three databases, viz. gingival, middle and incisal third. ShadeEye and ShadeVision are examples of colorimeter (Figs 7.8b and d).

Fiber optic colorimeter (VITA Easy shade-Fig. 7.8 a) has also been introduced. As established, tooth color is caused by volume reflection, i.e. passage of incident light through the tooth followed by backward emergence. The sideways displacement of photons influence the results of usual methods of shade-matching. This problem is overcome by using large-field illumination and small-field observation. Fiber optic colorimeter works on this principle.

ii. Digital Cameras

Digital cameras, an improved version, is also being used for shade matching. Instead of focusing light upon film to create a chemical reaction, digital cameras capture images using Charged Couple Devices (CCD), which contain millions of microscopically small light-sensitive elements. Like photodiodes, each photosite responds only to the total light intensity that strikes its surface. To achieve color image, the sensors use filters to look at the light in its three primary colors in a manner similar to the filtered colorimeter. There are several ways of recording the three colors in a digital camera. The highest-quality cameras use three separate sensors, each with a different filter over it. Light is directed to the different filter/sensor combinations by placing a beam splitter in the camera. The beam splitter allows each detector to see the image simultaneously. The advantage of this method is that the camera records each of the three colors at each pixel location. ShadeRite Dental Vision System (Fig. 7.8d) and ShadeScan (Fig. 7.8c) combines digital color analysis with colorimetric analysis; whereas SpectroShade (Fig. 7.8e) combines digital color imaging with spectrophotometric analysis. Clear Match is a software that uses high resolution images comparing shades over the VITA Easyshade, version 4.0 and 5.0, are recently introduced for correct shade matching (Fig. 7.8f).

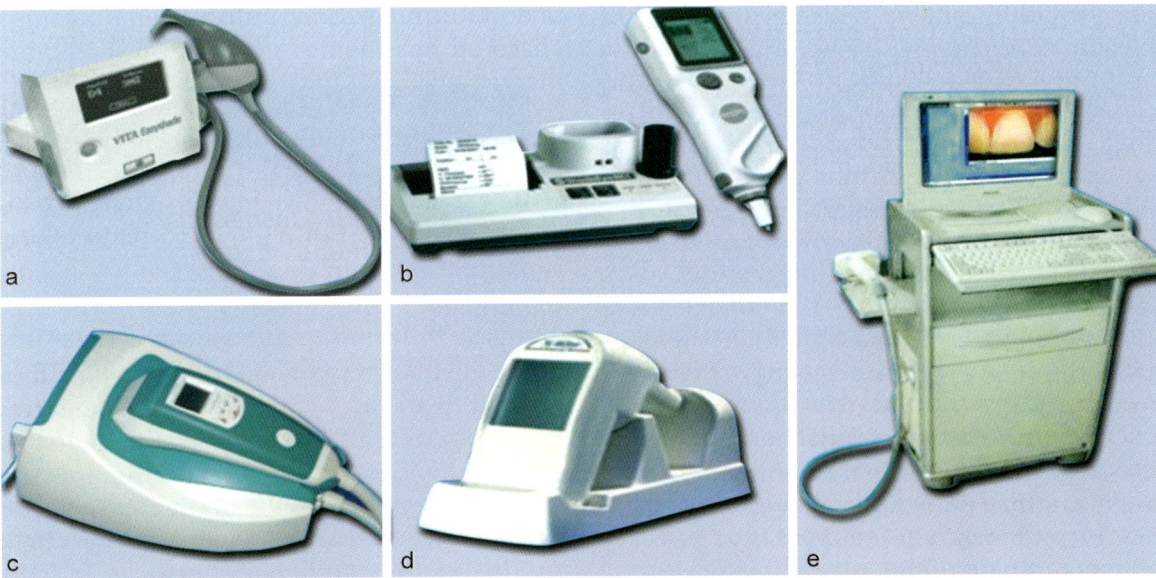

Figs 7.8a–e: Shade taking devices. a. VITA Easyshade; b. ShadeEye NCC; c. ShadeScan; d. ShadeRite dental vision system; e. SpectroShade

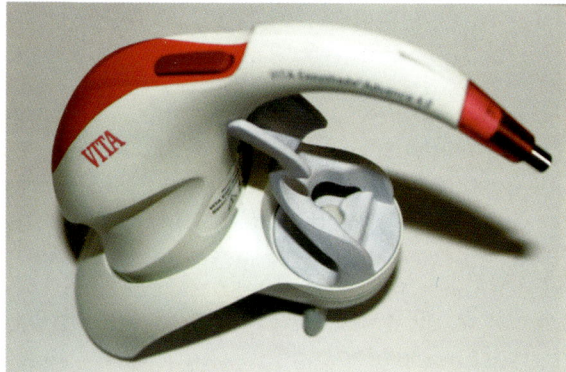

Fig. 7.8f: VITA Easyshade Advance 4.0

Dental shade matching by using digital images may be feasible when suitable color features are properly manipulated. Separating the color features into feature spaces facilitates favourable matching. A study was performed recently that uses support vector machines (SVM), which are outstanding classifiers, in shade classification. It provides a feasible technique for dental shade classification that uses the camera of a mobile device. The findings reveal that the proposed SVM classification might outperform the shade-matching results of previous studies that have performed similarity measurements of ÄE levels or used an S, a*, b* feature set.

iii. *Spectrophotometers and Spectroradiometers*

Spectrophotometers and spectroradiometers are designed to achieve the most accurate color measurements. Spectrophotometers differ from spectroradiometers primarily because they include a stable light source. These instruments basically utilize two types of designs. The traditional scanning instrument consists of a single photodiode detector that records the amount of light at each wavelength. The light is divided into small wavelength intervals by passing through a monochromator. The second design uses a diode array with a dedicated element for each wavelength. This design allows for the simultaneous integration of all wavelengths. Both designs are considerably slower than filter colorimeters; however, color-measuring is effective.

It is established that spectrophotometers provide 33% increase in accuracy of shade matching. Crystateye (Olympus-Japan) utilizes light photography with spectrophotometer. The system is beneficial, since the 'virtual shade tabs' in the computer database can be matched with the natural tooth image to analyze the correct shade. The shade is matched from inside the oral cavity, devoid of external light which may cause discrepancies.

Shade-X (Grandville, MI) is 3.0 mm probe diameter spectrometer. It has two databases to match the color; dentin (more opaque) and enamel (translucent). VITA Easyshade (Germany) and Spectroshade (Switzerland) also uses the principles of digital camera and LED spectrophotometer. Different measurement modes can be carried out using these devices.

Shade Guides

Initial shade guides were derived from tooth colors rather than from the distribution of shades observed in the general population. Clark (1931) introduced a custom shade guide based on visual assessment of human teeth, recorded in Munsell's Hue, Value and Chroma. Sproull (1971) suggested that an ideal shade guide should consist of shade (color) tabs that are well distributed and logically arranged in color space. He also preferred Munsell Color system. The issues regarding color mismatches of shade tab and porcelain shades from the same manufacturer; (more so the color mismatch with different manufacturers) was of concern to the operator and the technician. In the mid nineties, Miller acknowledged that the material of the shade guide should be same as that of the restoration and the thickness of the shade guides should not be more than the average porcelain veneer.

The limitations of shade guides led to dissatisfaction of clinicians, technicians, and the patients. A new generation of shade guides were developed to address these deficiencies. Shofu introduced the Natural Color Concept, while VITA proposed a 3-dimensional shade guide system (VITA 3D-Master). The Natural Color Concept system consists of 208 color blends based on 38 basic shades, arranged in L*a*b* color space according to Munsell's Hue, Chroma and Value. In addition, the shade guides and veneering material are made of the same material to avoid the effect of metamerism. The VITA 3D-Master shade guide (Fig. 7.9a) features a systematic colorimetric distribution of 26 shade tabs within the tooth color space. The manufacturer claims that this shade guide demonstrates an equidistant distribution in the color space. The shade guide is organized into 5 primary Value levels, with a secondary distribution based on Chroma and Hue. These Value groups are arranged from lightest (Value level 1) to darkest (Value level 5), from left to right. Intermediate shades can be achieved based on mixing formulas. The manufacturer advocates a 3-step process: Value is determined first in making a shade determination, and then the Chroma and Hue are determined. The selection process is simplified because the choices decrease as one proceeds. The shade tabs arrangement in the VITA Classical (Fig. 7.9b) is by Hue; whereas in Chromascop guides (Fig. 7.9c), the tabs are arranged in five Value levels. Within each level are tabs that represent different Chromas and Hues. The lightest Value level has only two Chroma steps of single Hue and the darkest Value level has three Chroma steps of one Hue. Groups 2, 3, and 4 have three

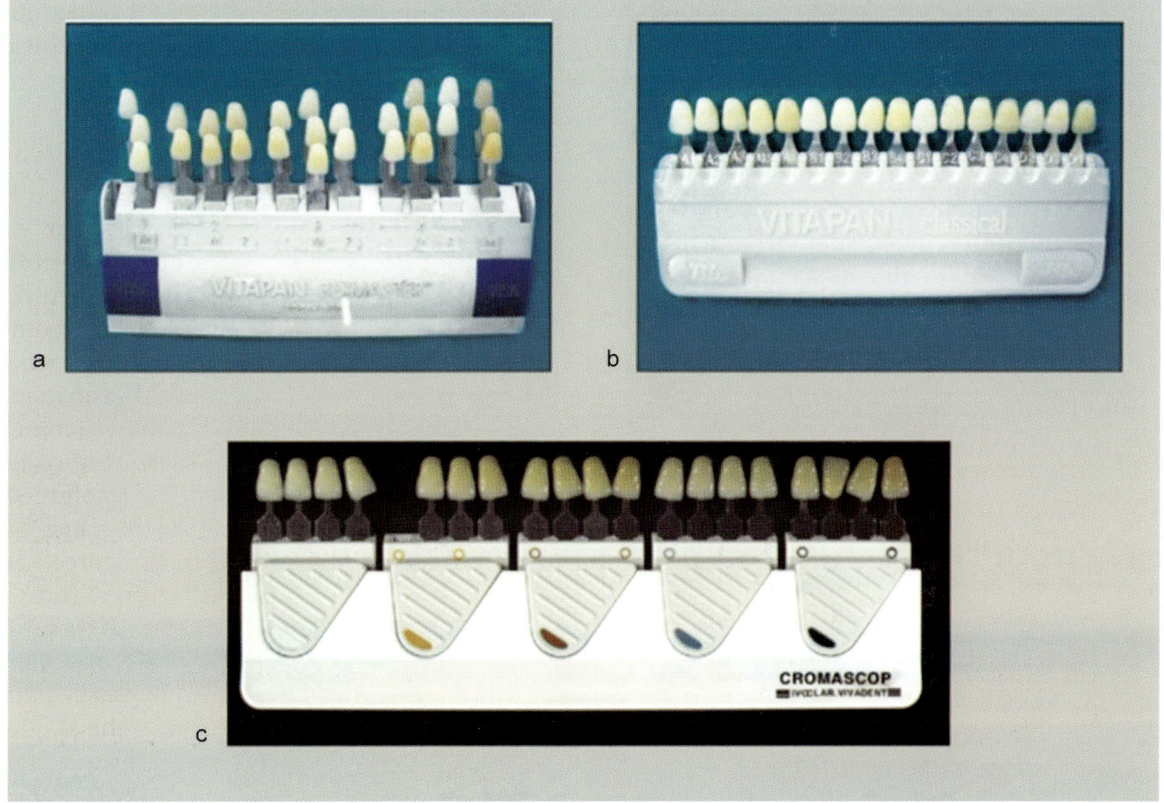

Figs 7.9a–c: Shade guides. a. VITA 3D-Master shade guide; b. VITA Classical shade guide; c. Chromascop shade guide

Chroma levels of the middle and orange Hue and two Chroma levels in each Hue shift toward yellow or red. The sequence of shade selection is Value, then Chroma, followed by Hue.

Types of Shade Guides

The different types of dental shade guides are:

i. *Hyashi shade guide:* Based on Munsell system Hue, it consists of 125 color tabs. The tabs have 5 Hues; 5 Values for each Hue and 5 Chromas for each Hue.

ii. *Clark shade guide:* It is based on analysis of color of more than 6000 teeth. It contains 60 tabs (3 basic Hue, 19 Value and 6 Chroma). Value (known as Brilliance) is considered important dimension.

iii. *Spectatone:* Spectatone is based on Hue and consists of 256 tabs. It used 12 Hues, but the shade guide represents only six Hues. The missing Hues could be selected by interpolation. Once the closest Hue was selected, the viewer had 36 Value and Chroma variations of this Hue. Since there were 6 Hues, a total of 256 selection tabs were available, and an additional 256 tabs could be created by interpolation. The system enabled the viewer to move about in the color space to every Hue, Value and Chroma needed to achieve the closest match to the tooth being replicated.

iv. *VITApan classic:* VITApan classic is based on Munsell system Hue and contains 16 tabs. The commonly available Hue shades are A (orange), B (yellow orange), C (Grey orange) and D (Brown orange). The most commonly chosen shade were in the range of reddish brown Hue, given the overall ranking of A3, A2, C2, B2, B3, C3. Shades in D are rarely selected (reddish-grey).

Limitation of VITApan classic
- Not uniformly positioned throughout tooth color space.

- No standard incremental difference between adjacent shade.
- In between shades, for example, A 2.5, is inaccurate

v. *VITApan 3D-master shade guide:* Based on CIELab system, it contains 26 tabs. The shade samples are grouped in six lightness levels each of which has Chroma variations in evenly spaced steps. The shade is spaced in steps (E) of CIELab 4 units in the lightness dimension and CIELab 2 units in the Hue and Chroma dimensions.

The manufacturer recommends selecting the lightness level first (i.e. Value first) with this system and then selecting the Chroma or saturation and finally the Hue. A form is available to facilitate the laboratory shade prescription, which can include intermediate step (since the guide is evenly spaced, intermediate shades can be formulated by combining porcelain powder of different shades). The Value levels (1–5) are arranged from left to right.

The types of VITApan 3D master shade guides are:

a. *VITApan 3D master tooth guide:* VITA 3D master tooth guide features fired porcelain shade samples built up with cervical, dentin and incisal as used in conventional shade guide.

b. *VITApan 3D master color guide:* In contrast to VITApan 3D master tooth guide, porcelain sample contains dentin color without cervical incisal distinction.

The 3D master is based on the Value system rather than grouping the shade by Hue as in VITA classic and other shade guide.

vi. *Extended shade guides:* Most commercial shade systems cover a limited range than the colors found in natural teeth, and the steps in the guide are greater than can be perceived visually. Some porcelain systems are available with extended range shade guides. Two such guides are:

a. *Visually optimal shade guide:* Analoui et al (2004) designed an optimal shade guide with the use of a hierarchical technique. The hierarchical clustering is a mathematical procedure for creating a sequence of partitions within a data set. In this approach, the similarity between all tooth samples in the population is computed. The hierarchical clustering approach facilitated a series of shade guide with varying number of tabs. The average error (e) between colors from each shade guide and the extracted teeth was also computed.

b. *Dentin shade guide:* In case of all-ceramic crowns and veneers, the shade of the prepared dentin is also to be communicated to the dental laboratory. Dentin shade guides provide specially colored die materials that match the dentin shade and enable the technician to match the color of the restoration.

vii. *Custom shade guide:* The color of certain teeth may not match the commercial shade guides; consequently, the final shade of the restoration is compromised. The extensive use of surface staining has severe drawbacks, because the stains increase surface reflection and vent light from being transmitted through porcelain. The custom shade guides overcome these problems. An infinity number of shades are created by using different combinations of porcelain powders in varying distributions.

The fabrication of a custom shade guide, especially one having an expanded shade range can be helpful. Although, fabrication of such a guide is time consuming, it provides a more realistic representation of what is achievable. Unlike most shade guides, a custom guide is made of the same material as the final restoration, thus reducing metamerism.

viii. *Modified shade guides:* Many a times, a tooth approximates a specific shade; however, the characterizations/deviations on the tooth need to be communicated to the laboratory. In such cases, the shade guides are modified adding the characterization/deviation features onto the shade guide tabs. The glare of the shade guides is removed, adding dental surface stains (colorants). Aluminum oxide abrasion is recommended to remove the glaze; alternatively, emery discs can also be used. The colorant may be applied, and modified until the proper effect is achieved. Once the guide closely resembles the tooth to be matched, it should be placed in a vial to avoid smearing, and sent to the laboratory along with a description of the colorants used and the effects desired.

Drawbacks of Shade Guides

The shade guides have certain inherent drawbacks, such as:

- The colors in a shade guide vary from guide to guide.
- The porcelain color may not match the color of the shade guide.
- The colors of the shade guide are not arranged in a manner simulating color space of the natural teeth.
- The colors of shade guide do not duplicate the manner in which porcelain is fabricated.
- Only central incisors are used as a standard for color matching.

Differences in Standard Shade Guides and Restorations

- Standard shade guide tabs are thicker than the natural teeth.
- Light is reflected and transmitted through a shade guide tab providing it translucency; whereas in restorations, light is reflected and barely transmitted making it look dense and opaque.

Shade Selection

The principles followed during shade selection are:

1. Shade selection for indirect restorations (crowns, inlays, onlays and laminates) should be carried out prior to tooth preparation (the moisture lost during preparation may change color).
2. Lipstick and/or other facial cosmetics should be removed prior to shade matching. The bright colored clothes should also be covered with grey or bluish napkins.
3. The patient should be viewed at eye level so that most color-sensitive part of the retina is utilized. The shade determination should be carried out in 5 seconds time interval (eye fatigue after that time affects the accuracy of selection). Refresh eye by observing at grey or light blue background in between the assessments.
4. The middle third of the teeth should be matched with middle third of the shade guide tabs (middle represents the body color of the restoration).
5. Shade comparison should be made under different lighting conditions. Normally, the patient is taken to a window and the color is confirmed in natural daylight after initial selection under incandescent and fluorescent light (restoration should match the natural color in all lighting conditions).
6. The teeth to be matched should be clean. Observe the teeth adjacent to the teeth to be restored and confirm initial selection by placing it between the adjacent teeth.
7. Shade matching should be undertaken at the start of the patient's visit.
8. Shade comparison should be made quickly, with the color samples placed under the lip directly next to the tooth being matched.
9. The eye should be rested by focusing on a gray–blue surface immediately before a comparison since this balances all the color sensors of the retina and resensitize eye to the yellow color of the tooth.
10. Always seek a second opinion in shade selection.
11. The patient should also be involved in shade selection process (it increases patient's confidence and minimizes dissatisfaction after placing the restoration).
12. The shade characteristics such as crack-lines, incisal translucency or opacities should be informed to the laboratory.

Clinical shade matching is shown in Figs 7.10a and b.

Problems in Shade Matching

The common problems encountered in shade matching are:

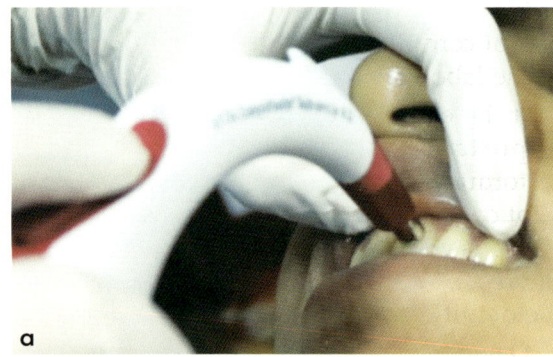

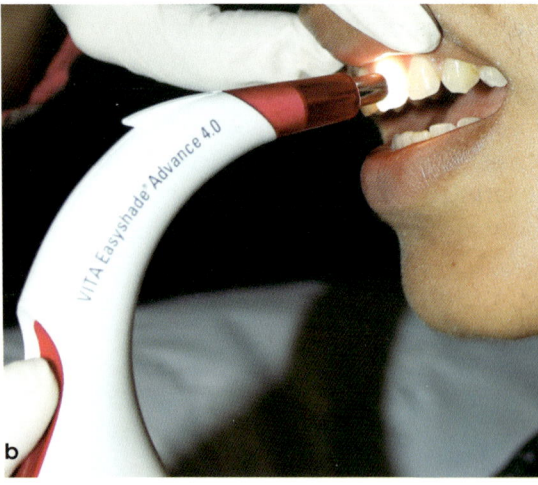

Figs 7.10a and b: Clinical shade matching with VITA Easyshade Advance 4.0

- Poor light quality
- Shade guide not properly conceived
- Taking too long to select the shade (prolong staring cause errors)
- Color matching with the material being used
- Taking shades at the end (eyes are tired by that time and the patient's teeth are dehydrated)
- Effect of background color (oversaturated background colors, say burnt orange affects shade selection)
- Disinfection of shade guides removes glazed layer (old shade guides do not present exact picture)
- Use of single modality during shade matching
- Optical illusion should also be taken care of.
- Not conveying the photographic results to the laboratory

It is established that Value is more important than base color. The Value restoration enables it to withstand dark and light color. The color can be incorrect and the Value is correct, there are more chances that the restoration will blend in with the rest of the dentition.

Dagg H et al (2004) investigated some of the factors on which accurate shade taking depends. Four main factors were investigated, namely difference between the two types of porcelain used, effect of light quality, effect of porcelain thickness and experience of the observer. These results indicate that the most influential factor on shade taking was the light quality.

Indirect restorations should be verified visually along with the instrument system in the laboratory before sending the same to the clinician. The verification and modification, if any, will save the chairside time of the operator and the patient both.

It is recommended that both instrumental and visual color matching method should be used, as they compliment each other leading to better esthetic results.

Shade Modification

Porcelain fusing is a result of time and temperature; so a restoration can be taken rapidly to higher temperature or at lower temperature and held at that given temperature for a longer period of time. The type of porcelain and the number of times it has been tried (under temperature) will determine the temperature at which the desired maturation occurs. Smoothness and gloss is evaluated for the temperature used for fabrication of porcelain (the material used in ceramic restoration is important for successive use of shade modifications).

The concept of shade modification is an art; the 'stains' are metallic oxides in a modified porcelain base. Most of the colorant hits have wider range of colors. The useful colors are orange, yellow, grey, violet and brown of different Hue and concentrations; and white with different translucencies.

Orange and yellow colorants are useful in Hue changes. Brown helps in lowering Value and increasing chrome, especially useful in cervical position. Violet is used to neutralize basic Hue; it reduces Chrome, lower Value and helps achieving translucent appearance in incisal one-third.

The surface modifications should be reserved for minor changes to improve initial results. The initial shade should be matched while the teeth are moist (dry teeth appear white and opaque).

Communicating Color

The principles of color and shade matching should be clear to the operator and the laboratory technician. The main challenge is to communicate or transfer the 'shade' to the technician. Transferring the 'shade number' is not sufficient. It should involve the detailed information related to color, texture and related shade characteristics (cracks, hypo-calcified areas, incisal translucency, halo, etc.).

The operator relies on shade guide to be communicated to the technician. Along with shade guides, various means of communicating color to the technician have been tried. The routinely used means are as follows:

i. *Color sketches:* Fine line markers are used to sketch the color zones and the translucency areas. These sketches help the technician understand areas of transition from one shade to other and also the relative translucency and transparency required at different zones. The sketches, though improve perception of the actual color component, fail to provide the exact information.

ii. *Photographs:* Colored photographs are considered fine way of communicating shade to the technician. The photograph should be clicked along with the shade guide tab, which improves the color perception by the viewer. The photographs provide a vivid description of the relative translucency, opacity, color zones and the incisal variations. Intra oral camera is also of great help for communicating shade.

iii. *Shade mapping:* Proper drawings and even photographs may not be adequate for understanding the shade. Shade characterization drawn on the cast that duplicate size, shape and contours, is the shade mapping, which is considered appropriate for shade communication. An image of the selected shade tab(s) near the tooth to be restored should accompany the cast and the writing. The visual translucency, characterization and color bleaching is superior to the paper drawings.

iv. *Digital images/data network:* Digital images can be sent electronically or on CD. Later, the same can be discussed with the technician, which enhances the shade duplication process. The network data has also facilitated transmission of shade to the laboratory.

v. *Modified shade guides:* The customized and modified shade guide, as described, are considered better method for communicating shade to the laboratory.

Bibliography

1. Ahmad I. Three-dimensional shade analysis: Perspectives of color. Part II. Practical Periodontics and Esthet. Dent.: 2000;12:557–64.
2. Aladuljabbar R and El-Masri S. Design of web content management system for dental laboratories. Int. J. Comput. Sci. Issue: 2013;10: 82–9.
3. Al-Dwairi Z, Shaweesh A, Kamkarfar S, Borzabadi-Farahani A and Lynch E. Tooth shade measurements under standard and non-standard illumination and their agreement with skin color. Int. J. Prosthodont.: 2014;27:458–60.
4. Alshiddi IF. Communication between dental office and dental laboratory: From paper-based to web-based. Pakistan Oral Dental J.: 2014:34: 555–9.
5. Analoui M, Papkosta E, Cochran M and Matis B. Designing visually optimal shade guides. J. Prosthet. Dent.: 2004;92:371–6.
6. Apratim A, Eachempati P and Kumar K. Digital shade matching: an insight. Res. J. Pharma. Biol. Chem. Sci.: 2015;6:1072–9.
7. Barrett AA, Grimaudo NJ, Anusavice KJ and Yang MC. Influence of tab and disk design on shade matching of dental porcelain. J. Prosthet. Dent.: 2002;88:591–7.
8. Bayindir F, Bayindir YZ, Gozalo-Diaz DJ and Wee AG. Coverage error of gingival shade guide systems in measuring color of attached anterior gingiva. J. Prosthet. Dent.: 2009;101:46–53.
9. Blaes J. Today's technology improves the shade-matching problems of yesterday. J. Indiana Dent. Assoc.: 2002-03;81:17–9.
10. Boksman L. Shade selection; accuracy and reproducibility. Ontario Dentist: 2007;24–27.
11. Bona AD, Barrett AA, Rosa V and Pinzetta C. Visual and instrumental agreement in dental shade selection: Three distinct observer populations and shade matching protocols. Dent. Mater.: 2009;25:276–81.
12. Brewer JD and Wee AS. Advances in color matching. Dent. Clin. N. Am.: 2004;48:341–58.
13. Cal E, Guneri P and Kose T. Comparison of digital and spectrophotometric measurements of color shade guides. J. Oral Rehabil.: 2006;33:221–8.
14. Cal E, Sonugelen M, Guneri P, Kesercioglu A and Kose T. Application of a digital technique in evaluating the reliability of shade guides. J Oral Rehabil.: 2004;31:483–91.

15. Capa N, Malkondu O, Kazazoglu E and Calikkocaoglu S. Evaluating factors that affect the shade matching ability of dentists, dental staff members and lay people. JADA: 2010;141:71–6.

16. Chang JY, Chen WC, Huang TK, Wang JC, Fu PS, Chen JH and Hung CC. Evaluation of the accuracy and limitations of three tooth-color measuring machines. J. Dent. Sci.: 2015;10:16–20.

17. Christensen GJ. Improving dentist-technician interaction and communication. J. Am. Dent. Assoc.: 2009;140:475.

18. Chu SJ, Trushkowsky RD and Paravina RD. Dental color matching instruments and systems. Review of clinical and research aspects. J. Dent.: 2010; 38s:e2–16.

19. Dagg H, O'Connell B, Claffey N, Byrne D and Gorman C. The influence of some different factors on the accuracy of shade selection. J. Oral Rehabil.: 2004;31:900–4.

20. Da Silva JD, Park SE, Weber HP and Ishikawa-Nagai S. Clinical performance of a newly developed spectrophotometer system on tooth color reproduction. J. Prosthet. Dent.: 2008; 99: 361–8.

21. Denissen H, Dozic A. Photometric assessment of tooth color using commonly available software. Eur J Esthet Dent: 2010;5:204–15.

22. Dozic A, Kleverlaan CJ, El-Zohairy A, Feilzer AJ and Khashayar G. Performance of five commercially available tooth color measuring devices. J. Prosthodont.: 2007;16:93–100.

23. Egger B. Natural color concept: A systematic approach to visual shade selection. QDT: 2003;26: 161–70.

24. Fondriest J. Shade matching in restorative dentistry: The science and strategies. Int. J. Perio. Restor. Dent.: 2003;23:467–79.

25. Haddad HJ, Jakstat HA and Arnetzi G. Does gender and experience influence shade matching quality? J. Dent.: 1991;37:40–4.

26. Hall NR. Tooth color selection: the application of color science to dental color matching. Aust. Prosthodont.: 1991;5:41–6.

27. Hassel AJ, Grossman AC, Schmitter M, Balke Z and Buzello AM. Inter-examiner reliability in clinical measurement of L*C*h* values of anterior teeth using a spectrophotometer. Int. J. Prosthodont: 2007;20:79–84.

28. Hassel AJ, Zenthofer A, Corcodel N, Hildenbrandt A, Reinelt G and Wiseberg S Determination of VITA Classical shades with the 3D-Master shade guide. Acta. Odontol. Scand.: 2013;71:721–6.

29. Ishikawa-Nagai S, Yoshida A, Da Silva JD and Miller L. Spectrophotometer analysis of tooth color reproduction on anterior all-ceramic crowns. Part 2. Color reproduction and its transfer from in-vitro to in-vivo. J. Esthet. Rest. Dent.: 2010;22:53–63.

30. Ishikawa-Nagai S, Yoshida A, Sakai M, Kristiansen J and Da Silva JD. Clinical evaluation of perceptibility of color differences between natural teeth and all-ceramic crowns. J. Dent.: 2009; 37:e57–63.

31. Jankar AS and Kale YJ. Dentist and lab communication: Key to better restorations. Ind. J. Basic and Applied Res.: 2012;1:136–42.

32. Jarad FD, Russell MD and Moss BW. The use of digital imaging for color matching and communication in restorative dentistry. Br. Dent. J.: 2005;199:43–9.

33. Johnston WM. Color measurement in dentistry. J. Dent.: 2009;37:e2–6.

34. Joiner A. Tooth color; a review of the literature. J. Dent.: 2004;32:3–12.

35. Khanshayar G, Dozic A, Kleverlaan CJ and Feilzer AJ. Data comparison between two dental spectrophotometers. Oper. Dent.: 2012;37:12–20.

36. Kuehni RG. The early development of the Munsell system. Color Res. Appl.: 2002;27:20–7.

37. Lasserre JF, Pop-Ciutrila JS and Colosi HA. A comparison between a new visual method of color matching by intraoral camera and conventional visual and spectrometric methods. J. Dent.: 2011; 39:e29–36.

38. Lehmann KM, Devigus A, Igiel C, Wentaschek S, Azar MS and Scheller H. Repeatability of color-measuring devices. Eur. J. Esthet. Dent.: 2011;6, 428–35.

39. Lindsey DT and Wee AG. Perceptibility and acceptability of CIELAB color differences in computer-simulated teeth. J. Dent.: 2007;35: 593–9.

40. Lynch CD, McConnell RJ and Allen PF. Trends in indirect dentistry:7. Communicating design features for fixed and removable prostheses. Dent. Update: 2005;32:502–10.

41. Marcucci B. A shade selection technique. J. Prosthet. Dent.: 2003;89:518–21.

42. McLaren EA and Schoenbaum T. Combine conventional and digital methods to maximize shade matching. Dentalaegis: 2012;8:1–4.

43. Oh W, Koh IW and O'Brien WJ. Estimation of visual shade matching errors with two shade guides. Quint. Int.:2009;40:833–6.

44. Oh W, Pogoncheff J and O'Brien WJ. Digital computer matching of tooth color. Materials: 2001;3:3694–9.

45. Paravina RD. Performance assessment of dental shade guides. J. Dent.: 2009;37:15–20.

46. Paravina RD. Critical appraisal. Color in dentistry: match me, match me not. J. Esthet. And Rest. Dent.: 2009;21:133–9.

47. Paravina RD, Majkic G, Imai FH and Powers JM. Optimization of tooth color and shade guide design. J. Prosthodont.: 2007;16:269–76.

48. Paravina RD, Stankovic D, Aleksov L, mladenovic D and Ristic K. Problems in standard shade matching and reproduction procedure in dentistry: A review of the state of the art. Med. And Biol. 1997;4:12–6.

49. Park JH, Lee YK and Lim BS. Influence of illuminants on the color distribution of shade guide. J. Prosthet. Dent.: 2006;96:402–11.

50. Pohjola RM, Hackman ST and Browning WD. Evaluation of a standard shade guide for color change after disinfection. Quint. Int.: 2007;38: 671–6.

51. Preston JD, Ward LC and Bobrick M. Light and lighting in dental office. Dent. Clin. North Am.: 1978;22:431–51.

52. Ristic I and Paravina RD. Color measuring instruments. Acta. Stomatologica Naissi: 2009;25: 925–32.

53. Russell MD, Gulfraz M and Moss BW. In vivo measurement of color changes in natural teeth. J. Oral Rehabil.: 2000;27:786–92.

54. Sikri V. Color: Implications in Dentistry. J. Conserv. Dent.: 2010;13:249–55.

55. Sorensen JA and Tores TJ. Improved color matching of metal-ceramic restorations. Part I: A systematic method for shade determination. J. Prosthet. Dent.: 1987;58:133–9.

56. Spencer LM. Shade selection environment and technique. Dent. Clin. North Am. J.: 1996;52:358–62.

57. Stephen J. Precision shade technology; contemporary strategies in shade selection. Prac. Proced. Aesthet. Dent.: 2002;14, 79–83.

58. Tashkandi E. Consistency in color parameters of a commonly used shade guide. Saudi Dent. J.: 2010;22:7–11.

59. Wang J, Lin J, Seliger A, Gil M, Silva JD and Ishhikawa-Nagai S. Color effects of gingiva on cervical regions of all-ceramic crowns. J. Esthet. Rest. Dent.: 2013;25:254–62.

60. Weng-Kong Tand Hsi-Jian L: Accurate shade image matching by using a smartphone camera. J Prosthodontic research: (2016) August, online version.

61. Wee AG, Lindsey DT, Kuo S and Johnston WM. Color accuracy of commercial digital cameras for use in dentistry. Dent. Mater.: 2006;22:553–9.

62. Wyble DR and Rich DC. Evaluation of methods for verifying the performance of color measuring instruments. Part I:Repeatability. Color Res. Appl.: 2007;3:166–88.

63. Yuan JCC, Brewer JD, Monaco ED and Davis EL. Defining a natural tooth color space based on a 3- dimensional shade system. J. Prosthet. Dent.: 2007; 98:110–9.

64. Zenthofer A, Wiesberg S, Reinelt G, Rammelsberg P and Hassel AJ. Selecting VTA classical shades with the vita 3D-Master Shade Guide. Int. J. Prosthodont.: 2014;27:376–82.

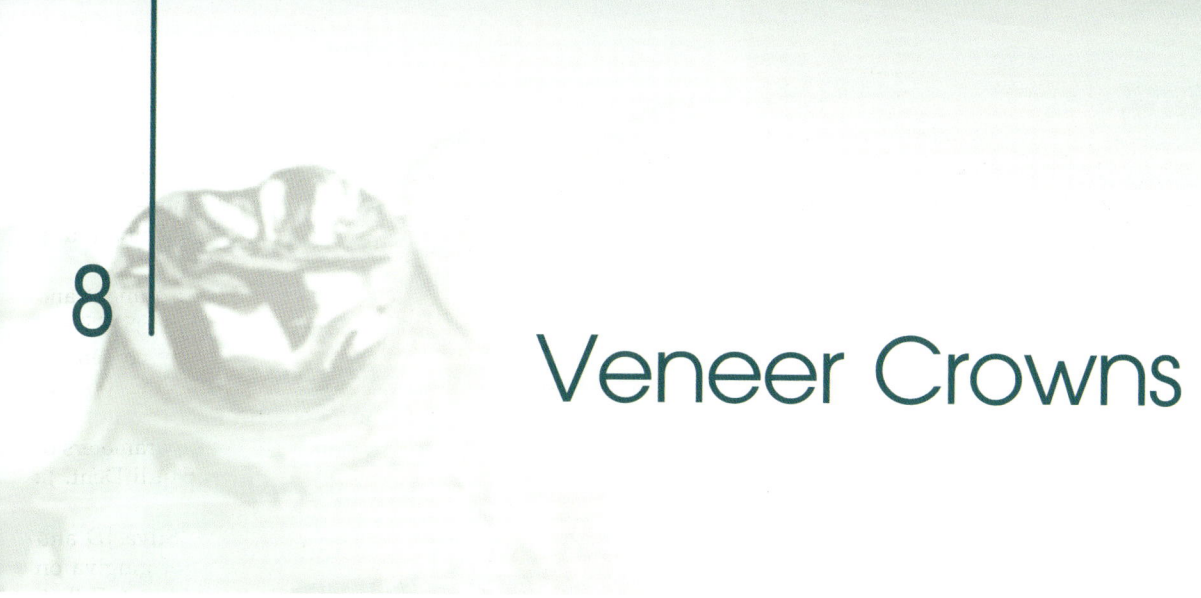

8

Veneer Crowns

Crown is an artificial replacement that restores the missing tooth structure by surrounding part or all the remaining structure with a material such as cast metal, porcelain, acrylic, composite or a combination of materials such as metal and porcelain, metal and acrylic, etc.

A full veneer crown is one, which encompasses the entire crown structure. These crowns cover all the tooth surfaces, i.e. mesial, distal, facial, lingual and occlusal.

A partial veneer crown, also termed 'partial coverage crown' is a conservative approach covering part of the total crown, i.e. may be one-half, three-quarter or seven-eighth of the coronal structure. These crowns provide better esthetics; however, the retention is compromised to some extent.

The full veneer crown has better retention and support. It also protects the remaining tooth structure. The chances of marginal leakage are less because of lesser exposed area. The mildly tilted/rotated teeth can be re-aligned by restoring with full veneers; the teeth may need to be root canal treated to achieve proper tooth preparation. The preparation is less conservative than partial veneer crown.

According to the material used for fabrication, the full veneer crown may be of following types:

i. All-Metal Crown (Cast Metal Crown)

All metal crown, also known as cast metal crown, is fabricated using noble metal alloys or base metal alloys. These are indicated where high strength is priority rather than esthetics.

ii. Porcelain Fused to Metal (PFM) Crown

The crown is fabricated using metal substructure upon which a ceramic veneer is fused. These are indicated where both strength and esthetics are required and sufficient tooth structure is available.

iii. All-ceramic Crown

All-ceramic crown is fabricated without support of the metal. High strength porcelain (Procera, All Ceram, etc.) may be used in routine. These are indicated for both anterior and posterior teeth, where esthetics is the priority. An all-ceramic crown provides better esthetics.

iv. Resin Bonded Porcelain Crown

Resin bonded porcelain crown is similar to porcelain veneer providing coverage on all surfaces along with conserving the tooth tissue. The strength of these restorations is largely reliant on the resin bond as there is no reinforcing ceramic core. Excellent esthetics can be achieved along with much less destructive preparation as compared to all-ceramic and porcelain fused to metal crowns. These crowns are preferably indicated in younger patients having large, vulnerable pulps.

Indications of Full Veneer Crowns

- For extensively decayed/decalcified/restored/fractured teeth. When the supporting tooth structure is less as in smaller abutment tooth, where crown length is not sufficient to provide retention and resistance for partial veneer crown, the full veneer crown is preferred.
- For endodontically treated tooth/severely stained/malformed tooth like peg incisors, etc.
- For tilted/rotated tooth or for gaps like mesial diastema, which cannot be treated by orthodontic means.
- For long span bridges.

Contraindications of Full Veneer Crowns

- For patients with uncontrolled caries and periodontal disease.
- Cases of bruxism and severe deep bite.

Armamentarium

The armamentarium required for preparation of full veneer crown is as follows:

- Handpiece
- Flat-end long tapered diamond bur
- Round-end long tapered diamond bur
- Flame/football/wheel diamond bur
- Thin short needle diamond
- Enamel hatchet
- Torpedo diamond
- Small inverted cone bur

Salient Features

The salient (must have) features required for any type of veneer crown are as follows:

- No undercuts
- Single path of insertion

- Minimum 3.0 mm axial preparation at gingival (cervical) half shall be parallel
- Occlusal/incisal/labial/lingual reduction depends upon the material to be used
- Short clinical crowns may need extra retentive features in the form of pins, groove, etc.
- Margin selection according to the clinical and mechanical needs

While preparing the tooth for any type of crown, diamond points should be used in decreasing grade of abrasive particle size. The diamond points are labeled with various color codes for easy identification.

The color code specifications are:

White: Superfine (15–20 µm)
Yellow: Extra-fine (28 µm)
Red: Fine (60 µm)
Blue: Regular (125 µm)
Green: Coarse (151 µm)
Black: Super coarse (181 µm)

PREPARATION FOR FULL VENEER CROWN

The amount of tooth reduction depends upon the space required to accommodate different materials as per need and choice of the patient. The basic principles of tooth preparation must be kept in mind while preparing the tooth for full crowns. There is no fixed sequence of steps for tooth reduction; however, the following sequence is preferred.

- Occlusal/incisal reduction
- Proximal reduction
- Buccal-labial/lingual reduction
- Site and configuration of the margins
- Placing extra retentive features (if required)
- Finishing and toileting

The full veneer crowns can be of all-metal, porcelain fused to metal or all-ceramic.

ALL-METAL CROWN

All-metal crown is considered more conservative than porcelain fused to metal (PFM) crown and also provides better strength. This type of crown is indicated for posterior teeth only where esthetics is not the priority.

The preparation for all-metal crown is carried out as:

i. Occlusal Reduction

A clearance of 1.5 mm on functional cusps (i.e. buccal in mandibular and palatal in maxillary teeth) and 1.0 mm on non-functional cusp is considered adequate for all-metal crowns (slightly less cutting is sufficient for type II gold alloy). Occlusal reduction is carried out in plane of the occlusal anatomy. Depth orientation grooves can also be given, facilitating reduction, especially by the beginners. The grooves of required depth are made as reference point and join them together to achieve the required reduction (Fig. 8.1). These grooves should be made on primary grooves of occlusal surface. The final

clearance should be evaluated with strip of wax sheet. The occlusal reduction is carried out using round-end pear shaped tapering diamond. The basic morphology of all cusps should be maintained. The functional cusp should be bevelled after requisite reduction to give more space for metal, so as to provide better strength to the final restoration (Figs 8.2a and b). Angle for functional cusp bevel is about 45 degrees to the long axis (the

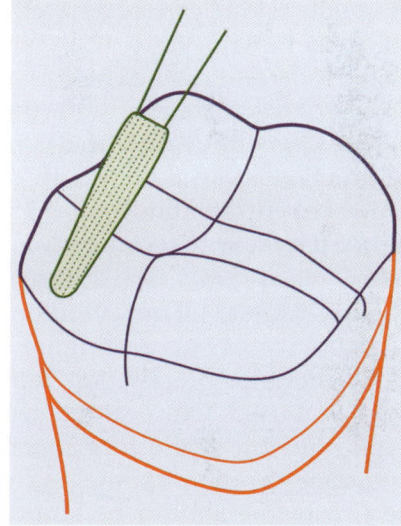

Fig. 8.2a: Maintaining cusp morphology

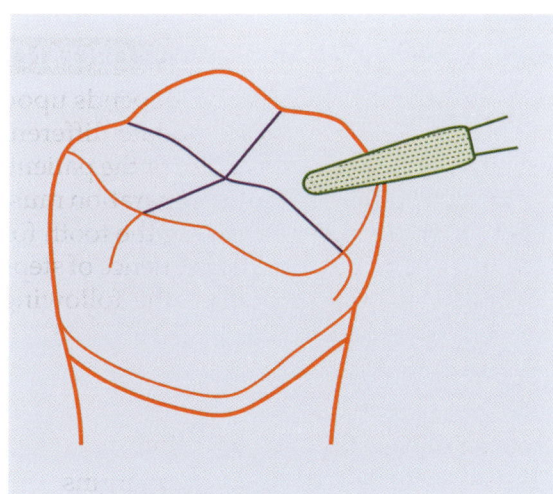

Fig. 8.1: Occlusal reduction

Occlusal Reduction

- Pear shaped tapering diamond point
- Follow original cusp configuration
- Functional cusp to be beveled after occlusal reduction
- Remove marginal ridges
- Evaluate occlusal reduction with wax or putty

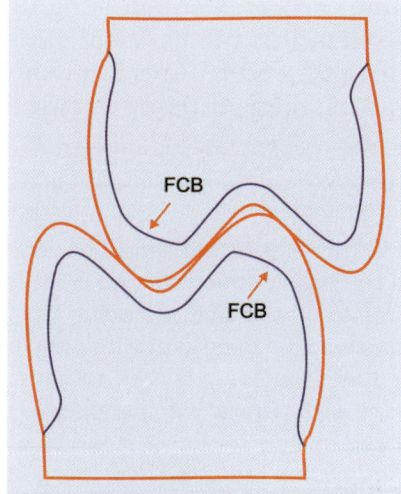

Fig. 8.2b: Beveling facial cusp

angle simulates the cuspal incline plane angle of the tooth in occlusion). A few authors are of the view that the non-functional cusp (buccal cusps of maxillary molars) should also be beveled to provide a minimum of 0.6 mm clearance so as to avoid overcontouring.

ii. Proximal Reduction

The proximal reduction should be started with short needle diamond points. This thin diamond is moved through proximal area bucco-lingually taking care of adjacent tooth. Placement of matrix strip will facilitate protection of adjacent tooth. The contact area should be broken preferably with the hand instruments. Once the contact area is free, the further reduction is carried out with the help of torpedo-shaped diamond point (Fig. 8.3). The rules of parallelism and tapering should be followed.

A 0.5 mm chamfer/1.0 mm shoulder finish line in continuity of buccal/lingual wall is made throughout the preparation depending upon the metal used. Extra care is needed in roundening the line angle from buccal and lingual surfaces to the proximal surfaces so that the finish line should be smooth and continuous (Fig. 8.4). A supragingival type of cervical finish line is usually preferred in case sufficient height is available. If not, the cervical finish line can be extended subgingivally. While extending the cervical finish line subgingivally, end-cutting burs should be preferred as gingival tissue health is to be maintained.

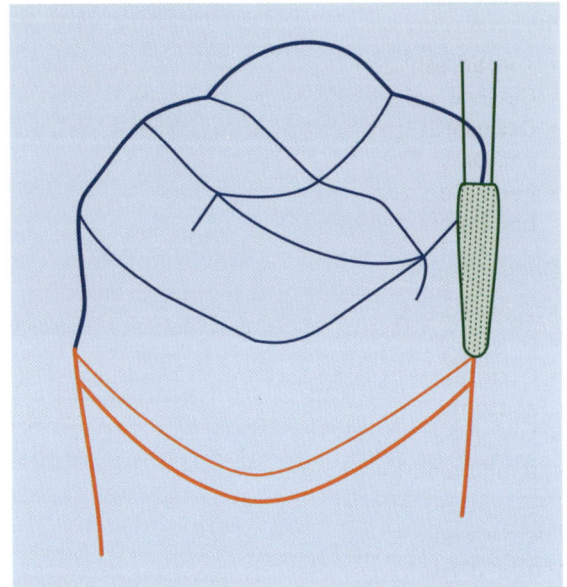

Fig. 8.3: Proximal reduction

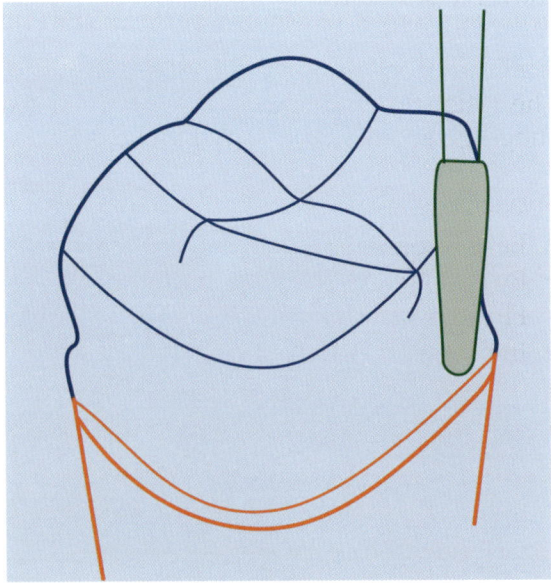

Fig. 8.4: Reshaping line angles

Proximal Reduction
- Hand instruments for breaking the contact point
- Initial cutting with thin diamond point followed by torpedo-shaped diamond point
- Reduction points to be kept within the confines of the tooth and not in between adjacent teeth
- Keep the walls parallel with permissible taper (if need be)
- 1.0 mm/0.5 mm reduction depending upon the metal

iii. Buccal/Lingual Reduction

The buccal and lingual walls are reduced with round-ended torpedo-shaped tapering diamond point. A 0.5 mm chamfer finish line is adequate in case the metal used is cast gold; whereas in base metals, the finish line should be 1.0 mm like shoulder preparation (Fig. 8.5).

Buccal Reduction

- Torpedo-shaped tapering diamond point
- Gingival 1/3rd parallel-straight
- Occlusal 2/3rd sloped inwards conforming to the anatomy
- Reduction depth (0.5 mm/1.0 mm) depending upon metal to be used

Lingual Reduction

- Torpedo-shaped tapering diamond point
- Gingival 2/3rd parallel-straight
- Occlusal 1/3rd sloped inwards conforming to the anatomy
- Reduction depth (0.5 mm/1.0 mm) depending upon metal to be used

The opposing walls should be parallel to each other and long axis of tooth for better resistance and retention form. The preparation should have 3–5° occlusal taper to achieve the convenience form.

iv. Site and Configuration of Margins

The rationale for placing supragingival and subgingival margins are as follows:

Supragingival Margins

- Easy to prepare
- By and large located on enamel
- Finishing is easy
- Impression making is simple

Subgingival Margins

- Caries/erosion/abrasion, etc.
- Proximal contact extending in gingival crest
- Need more surface area
- Esthetics

v. Placing Extra Retentive Features

It is established that a minimum of 3.0 mm occluso-gingival parallelism is mandatory to achieve the requisite retention and resistance form in full veneer crowns. If the occluso-gingival height of the preparation is short (3.0 mm or less), a groove may be created, preferably on center of the buccal side. It will provide the resistance form against rotation and facilitate retention of the crown. It should be made parallel to the long axis of tooth along the occluso-gingival height; usually 3.0 mm long, 0.5 mm wide and 0.6 mm deep (Figs 8.6a and b). The depth of groove should always be more than the width. For longer span bridges, the grooves may be created on both buccal and lingual sides.

vi. Finishing and Toileting

The line angles are slightly rounded off using carbide-finishing burs at low speed. The

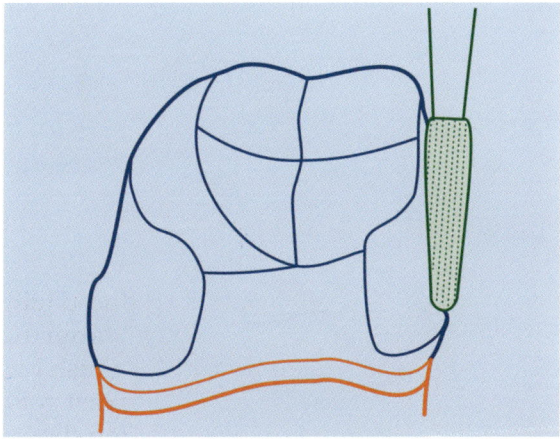

Fig 8.5: Finish lines in buccal or lingual reduction

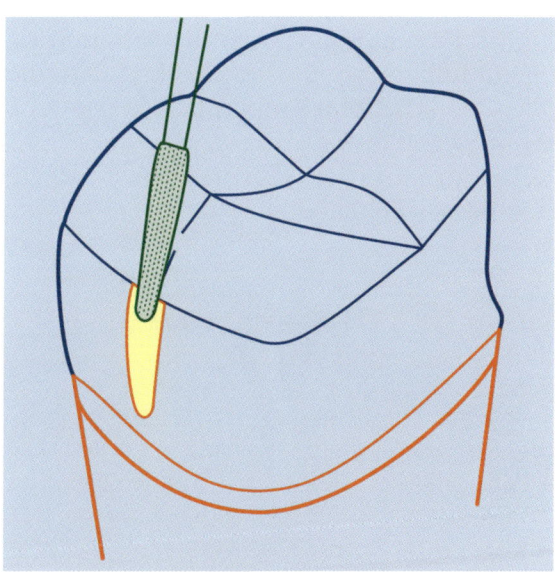

Fig. 8.6a: Making retentive grooves

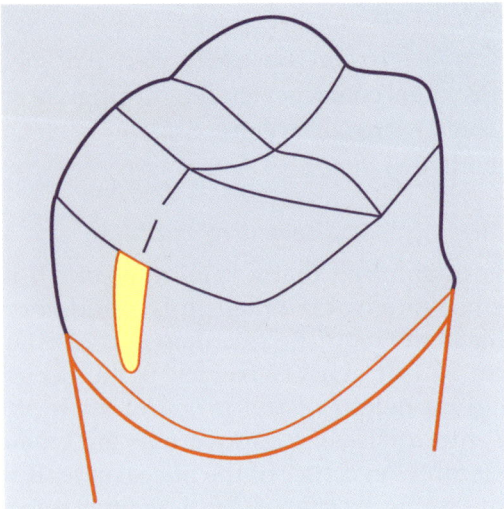

Fig. 8.6b: Final shape of the groove

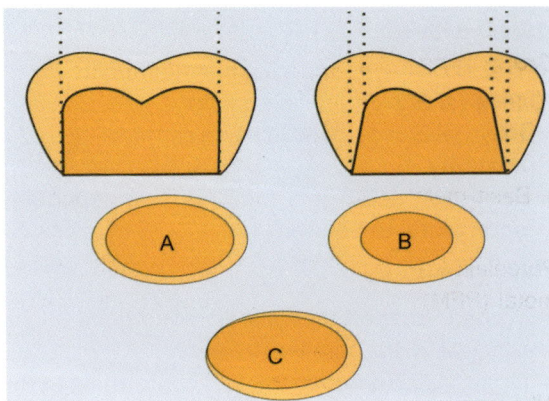

Fig. 8.8: View from occlusal side for undercuts

continuity of all finished lines should be maintained. The preparation should be cleaned off with fresh water and slow air jet (Fig. 8.7).

Once the preparation is complete, taper and the path of insertion are checked. No undercut should be detected once viewed from occlusal and buccal side. Occlusal view can be had by one eye closed because an undercut can be perceived as a near parallel when viewed with two eyes. The junction between proximal and buccal/lingual reductions, the common site for undercuts, should be checked carefully (Fig. 8.8). The final preparation is shown in Figs 8.9a and b.

The preparation features for posterior crowns are tabulated in Table 8.1.

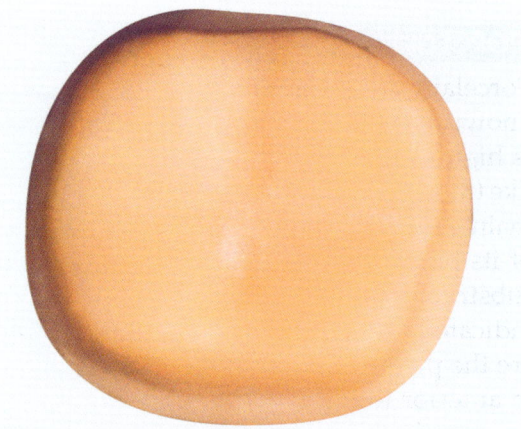

Fig. 8.9a: Final preparation

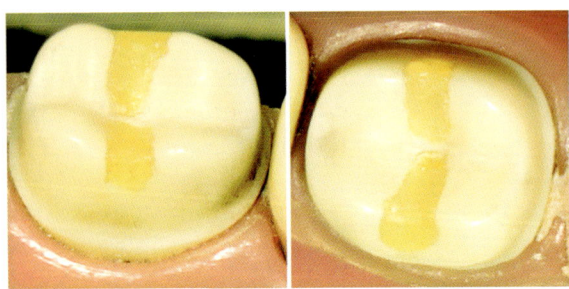

Fig. 8.7: Cleaning of final preparation

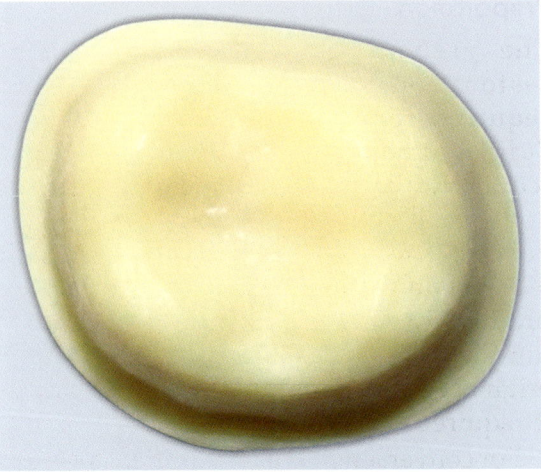

Fig. 8.9b: Final preparation

Crown type	Occlusal reduction	Finish line depth	Configuration
Table 8.1: Preparation features for posterior crowns			
All metal crown			
i. Gold	1.5 mm functional cusp 1.0 mm non-functional cusp	0.5 mm	Chamfer
ii. Base-metal	1.5 mm functional cusp 1.0 mm non-functional cusp	1.0 mm	Shoulder
Porcelain fused to metal (PFM)	2.0–2.5 mm functional cusp 2.0 mm non-functional cusp	1.5 mm buccal 0.5 mm (Gold) lingual 1.0 mm (Base-metal) lingual	Shoulder Chamfer/Shoulder
All-ceramic	2.0–2.5 mm functional cusp 2.0 mm non-functional cusp	1.5 mm	Shoulder

PORCELAIN FUSED TO METAL CROWN

Porcelain fused to metal (PFM) crown is also known as metal ceramic crown. The porcelain is highly esthetic material because of its life like translucency; however, brittle nature is the main drawback. To overcome the drawback of its brittleness, it is strengthened by metal substructure (metal coping). Metal ceramic is indicated where both esthetics and strength are the prime considerations. It may be given in anterior teeth as well as in posterior teeth ranging from single unit restoration to long span bridges.

Preparation

The preparation for a metal ceramic restoration involves tooth reduction required for both metal and porcelain. Sufficient reduction of tooth structure is required to allow for adequate thickness of both metal substructure and the porcelain veneer. The reduction should follow the biomechanical principles governing tooth preparation. The final shape of the preparation should be a miniature reproduction of original tooth form with minor modifications, if required.

For convenience, the preparation is divided into three steps:

a. Initial preparation involves gross reduction of tooth surfaces.
b. Margination involves the preparation of finish lines/margins.
c. Final finishing involves achieving a smooth, evenly reduced surface.

a. Initial Preparation

There is no definite protocol for sequencing the tooth preparation. However, following steps are preferred in routine (preparation for anterior metal-ceramic crown is described).

i. Incisal Reduction

A uniform reduction of 1.5–2.0 mm on the incisal surface is mandatory for porcelain fused to metal (PFM) crowns. The depth can be asked on the facial and lingual surfaces; alternatively flat-end tapered diamond is used to place cuts parallel to the uncut incisal edge facio-lingually at the requisite depth. Three such orientation grooves are usually made. The remaining tooth structure between the orientation grooves is removed to obtain the desired incisal reduction of 1.5–2.0 mm (Fig. 8.10). This reduction allows for adequate thickness of metal and porcelain at the incisal area. The adequate thickness reinforces the weak incisal edge and also enhances the esthetics. The plane of reduction is

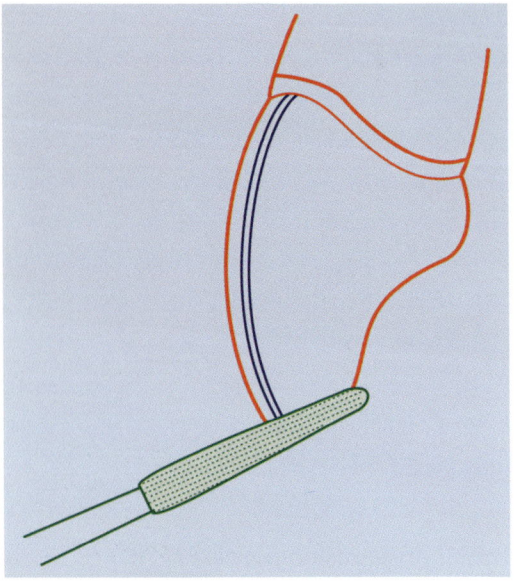

Fig. 8.10: Incisal reduction

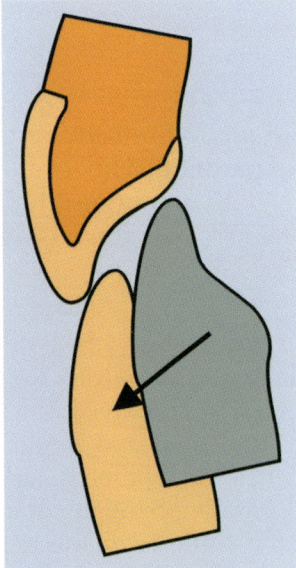

Fig. 8.11: Protrusive movement in incisal reduction

preparation allows the restoration to resist occlusal forces in a better way.

ii. *Proximal Reduction*

The proximal surface reduction should be parallel to the line of draw with an allowable 2–3° taper per wall. The diamond point is aligned parallel to the path of draw taking care not to damage the adjacent tooth. The depth of proximal surface reduction (1.5–2.0 mm) should be same as that of the facial aspect. The gingival edge from the proximal surface to the facial is to be continued. The reduction should extend lingually to a point that just clears the proximal contact with the adjacent tooth. This improves the esthetics by allowing sufficient porcelain thickness proximally to hide the metallic hue from the lingual line angle (Figs 8.12 and 8.13).

iii. *Facial Reduction*

The depth of facial reduction should be 1.5 mm or even slightly more, if other parameters allow. Any depth less than this will compromise with the esthetics because of lack of adequate porcelain thickness. The facial

perpendicular to the direction of occlusal forces and parallel to the mandibular protrusive pathway (Fig. 8.11). This implies that the incisal reduction be directed at approximately 45° to the long axis of the tooth. Such angular reduction in the incisal

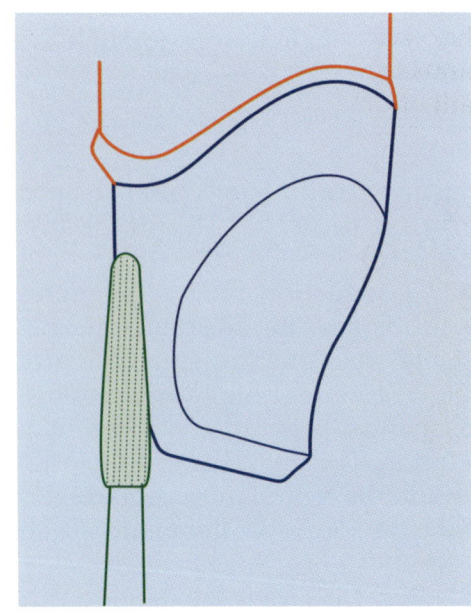

Fig. 8.12: Clearing proximal line angle

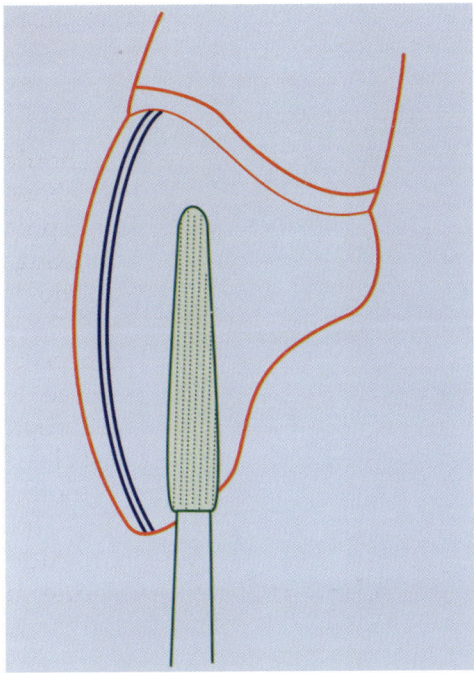

Fig. 8.13: Proximal reduction

- The incisal portion is reduced parallel to the incisal one-third of the facial surface to simulate the natural contour of that area.

The reduction in a single plane is to be avoided at all costs.

Inadequate reduction in a single straight plane results in too little space for porcelain in incisal half, while too liberal reduction in a single straight plane (produces an excessively tapered preparation) and also, may endanger the pulp in the mid-facial area (Fig. 8.15).

Facial reduction is accomplished by the use of a flat-end tapered diamond point. For convenience in achieving appropriate reduction depth, the operator may place three depth orientation grooves, one in mid-facial area and one each close to the proximal line angles. Following the placement of depth cuts, the remaining tooth structure between the depth cuts is removed and the reduction is continued around the line angles continuing along the proximal reduction (Figs 8.16 and 8.17).

In gingival third area, the diamond point is held parallel to the long axis of tooth creating shoulder at the gingival edge. Initially, the tip of the diamond is kept coronal to the gingival crest even though a subgingival extension is planned. End-cutting burs are preferred for extending the margins to subgingival areas (Fig. 8.18).

In the incisal portion, the diamond point is aligned parallel to the incisal one-third of the

surface is reduced taking into consideration morphology of the tooth form, path of insertion and relationship to the adjacent teeth. The facial reduction is carried out in two planes:

- The cervical/gingival two-thirds is reduced parallel to the long axis of the tooth [the path of draw (Fig. 8.14)].

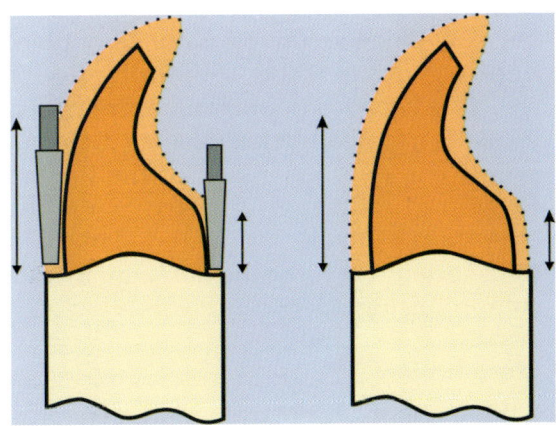

Fig. 8.14: Labial two-third and lingual one-third parallel

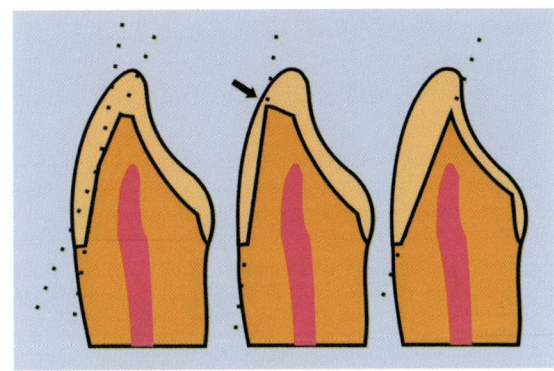

Fig. 8.15: Importance of two plane reduction

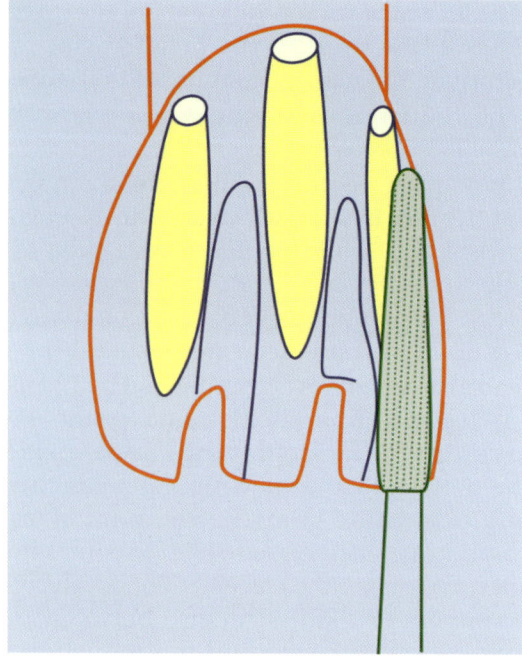

Fig. 8.16: Orientation grooves (labial)

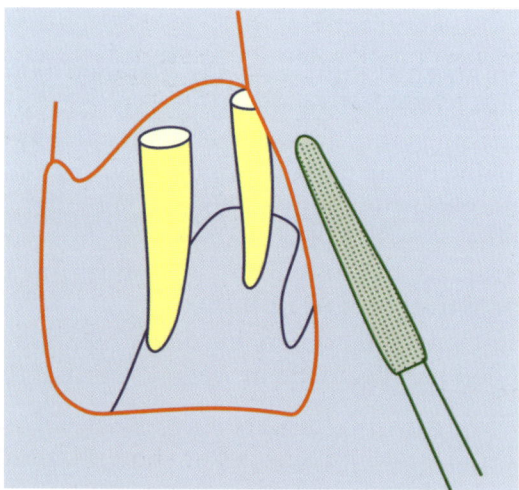

Fig. 8.17: Orientation grooves (proximal)

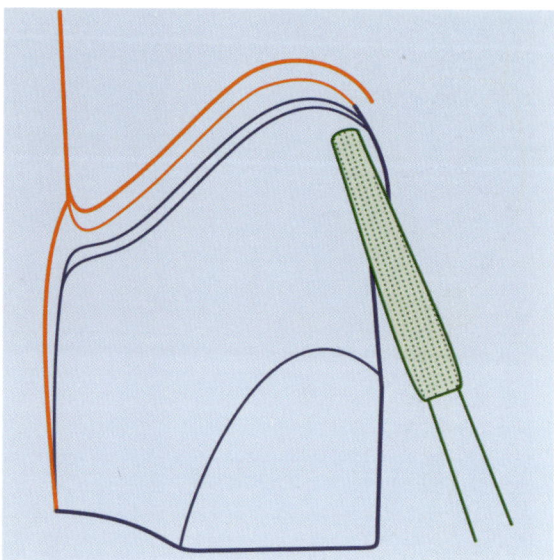

Fig. 8.18: Extending margins subgingivally

facial surface (simulating facial incisal contour).

iv. Lingual Reduction

The lingual reduction is carried out in two phases:

a. *Cingulum reduction:* This is accomplished with a torpedo diamond or round-end tapered diamond point keeping the instrument parallel with the line of draw. The lingual axial surface with a chamfer finish line is created. The depth of the chamfer should be 0.3–0.5 mm. The cingulum axial wall provides a vertical wall on the lingual surface that serves as a resisting area to help counteract the tipping forces. In case, the axial lingual wall is not prepared properly, the preparation will lack resistance form, leading to failure.

b. *Lingual fossa reduction:* The lingual fossa is reduced to a uniform depth of 1.0 mm, which provides adequate metal thickness. For convenience, the operator may place depth grooves. The remaining tooth structure between depth marks is removed by use of a football/wheel shaped diamond point. The over-extension of the lingual fossa reduction gingivally over the cingulum is to be prevented. This will foreshorten the vertical axial lingual wall, compromising retention (Fig. 8.19).

b. Margination

The three options for margin placement are:
   i. Supragingival

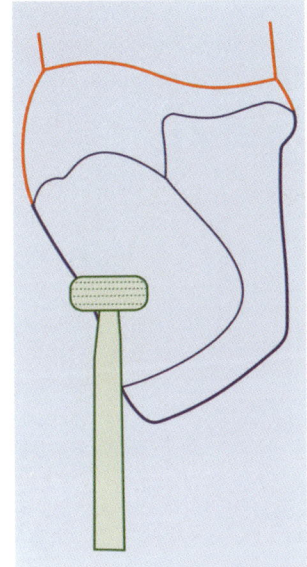

Fig. 8.19: Lingual fossa reduction

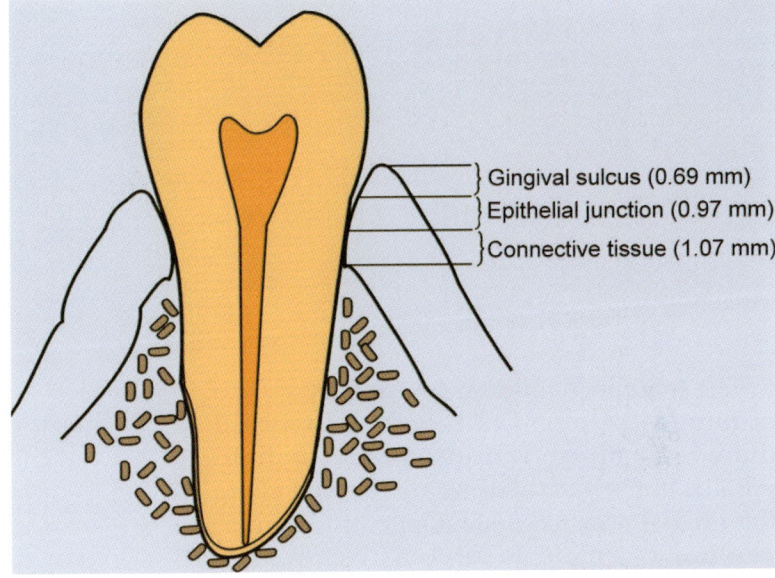

Gingival sulcus (0.69 mm)
Epithelial junction (0.97 mm)
Connective tissue (1.07 mm)

Fig. 8.20: Biological width: sum total of epithelial junction and connective tissue

ii. Equigingival (even with the tissue)

iii. Subgingival

The preparation of margins (finish lines) should preferably terminate supragingivally if sufficient height is available and the demand for esthetics is not critical. Equigingival margins provide good esthetics and are better tolerated periodontally if the restoration provides a smooth, polished cervical interface. Subgingival margins are placed 1.0 mm below the gingival crest. The depth should not exceed more than half the depth of gingival sulcus ensuring that the epithelial attachment or the biological width area is not disturbed (Fig. 8.20). A few authors prefer placing subgingival margin 4.0 mm coronal to the alveolar crest. This can be gauged by using a probe through the attachment. Tissue management techniques are recommended during preparation of finish line to protect gingival tissues, especially when a subgingival extension is planned. When the finish line is likely to be extensively subgingival, a crown lengthening procedure can often facilitate more accessible crown margins.

The general contour of the gingival tissues vis-à-vis the restoration margin is evaluated at the level of the margin. No 'lip' or 'edges' of enamel/tooth structure should remain at the finish line; such that these edges fail to reproduce when the impression is poured, resulting in an ill fitting casting. Such edges should be removed using hand instruments. The uneven shoulder is finished using end-cutting burs. Some other forms of finish lines, such as bevelled shoulder, sloped slant shoulder and heavy chamfer have also been used depending upon the clinical conditions.

The bevelled shoulder margin places a polished metal collar in the gingival sulcus. The sloped/slant shoulder can also have a metal collar or a disappearing margin. Slant shoulder with a metal collar should be used when the tooth preparation extends onto the roots and lies in the esthetically non-critical areas. However, if smile exposes the gingival margins, disappearing margins should be preferred.

An inverted bevel can be fabricated in the labial shoulder of the prepared tooth (Fig. 8.21). The metal part in the metal fused to ceramic crown is hidden under the bevel and the final restoration is esthetically pleasing.

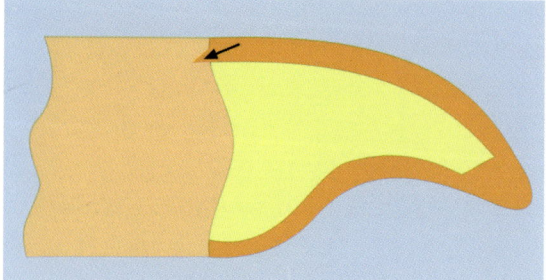

Fig. 8.21: Inverted bevel

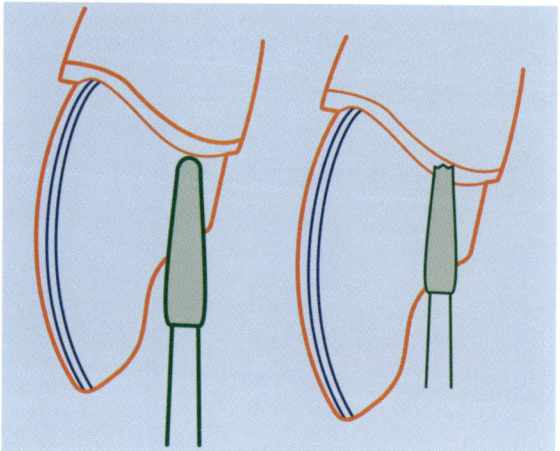

Fig. 8.22: Final finishing

The lingual chamfer is finished by means of torpedo-diamond or round-end tapered diamond points. The instrument is held parallel to the path of draw and moved along the lingual area to create a smooth chamfer. The tissue contour is carefully followed to prevent trauma to the gingival tissues. Proximally, the lingual chamfer is merged with the facial shoulder in a gradual manner to avoid sharp angles (edging) in the preparation.

The type and location of finish line may vary; however, the guiding points are:

- It should not have any unsupported 'lip' or 'edges' of tooth structure, which is liable to fracture during impression making or on the die creating problems for crown seating.
- It should be in harmony with the outline of the gingival margin. In case of subgingival margins, there should be no impingement on the biological width area.
- The finish line should be smooth and even well detected in the impression and the die.

Final Finishing

The final finishing is carried out using carbide finishing burs in descending order (say 24 fluted, 36 fluted and plain) (Fig. 8.22). The sharp angles along the edges are rounded off, prepared tooth surfaces are smoothened and the margins are redefined (Fig. 8.23). The axio-occlusal line angle, being vulnerable, should be carefully finished. The preparation should be cleaned with water and air spray. The final preparation is shown in Figs 8.24a–c.

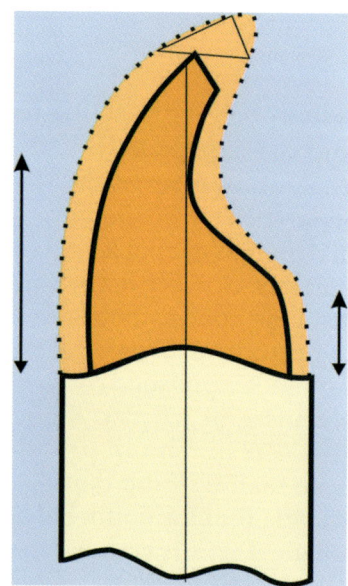

Fig. 8.23: Checking final preparation

Design for Metal Coping for PFM Crown

Various designs for metal coping have been tried and documented in literature. The gingival extension of the metal substructure relative to the shoulder margin has always been controversial (Figs 8.25a–f).

1. The thin metal collar may extend to the axio-gingival line angle. Such collar provides better esthetics, but is unesthetic.

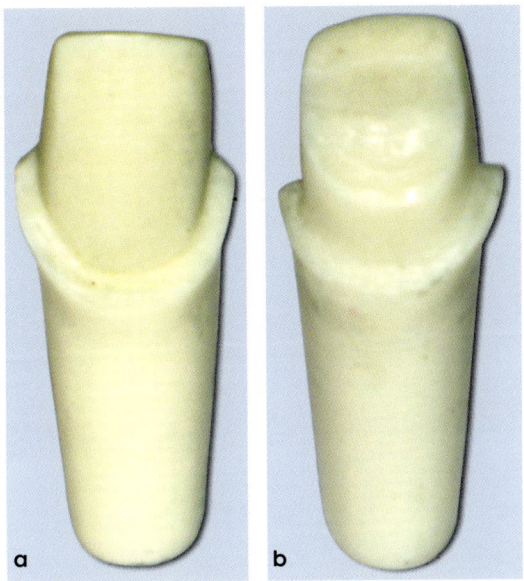

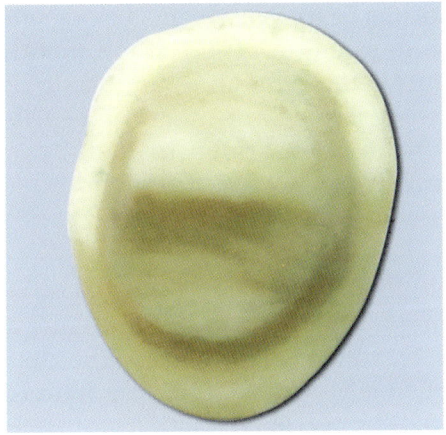

Fig. 8.24c: Incisal view

Figs 8.24a and b: (a) Labial view; (b) Lingual view

of metal improves light transmission and hence esthetics. A cutback of 1.0 mm is usually recommended to avoid weakened restoration.

2. Disappearing margin/conventional margin where metal collar is trimmed out near the margin.
3. The cervical extension of metal can be shortened to terminate 1.0–3.0 mm short of the shoulder margin. The cervical extension

ALL-CERAMIC CROWN

The all-ceramic crown, as per nomenclature, is made up of ceramic only. With the advent of pressable/castable ceramics, the all-ceramic crowns are becoming more popular as they

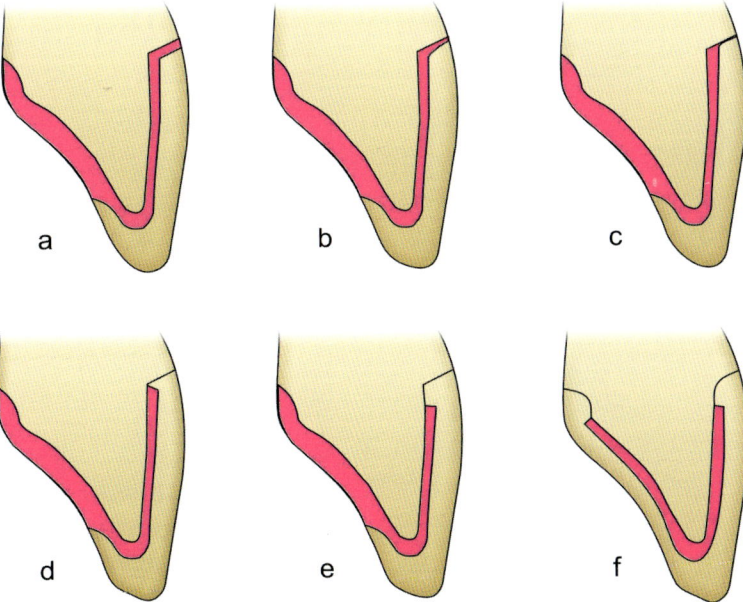

Figs 8.25(a–f): Labial margin designs for metal-ceramic restorations (Touati and Miara-J Esth Dent 1993)

provide the best cosmetic effect along with the requisite strength. There is no metal substructure beneath the all-ceramic restorations. The all-ceramics are more susceptible to fracture in comparison to metal ceramic crown. It is usually used for anterior restorations or small bridges.

Preparation

The preparation protocol is the same as for metal ceramic crowns, except the depth of reduction is less in all-ceramic crowns (depth required for porcelain only).

The preparation protocol includes:
- The labial/lingual reduction, with or without the help of orientation grooves, be kept at 1.2 to 1.5 mm (Figs 8.26a–d).
- The two plane incisal reduction is carried out to achieve 2.0 mm reduction.
- A heavy chamfer (1.0 mm) or shoulder (1.5 mm) should be provided on the proximal surfaces (proximal surfaces reduced in continuation with lingual surface taking care of the adjacent tooth) (Figs 8.27 and 8.28a and b).
- A heavy chamfer/shoulder finish line should be given on all the surfaces for better

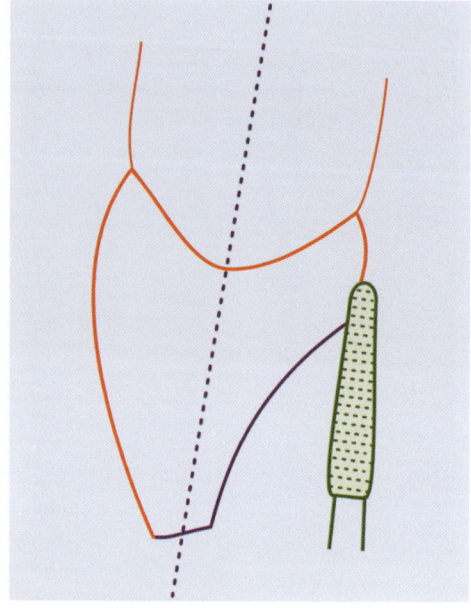

Fig. 8.26b: Proximal adjustment

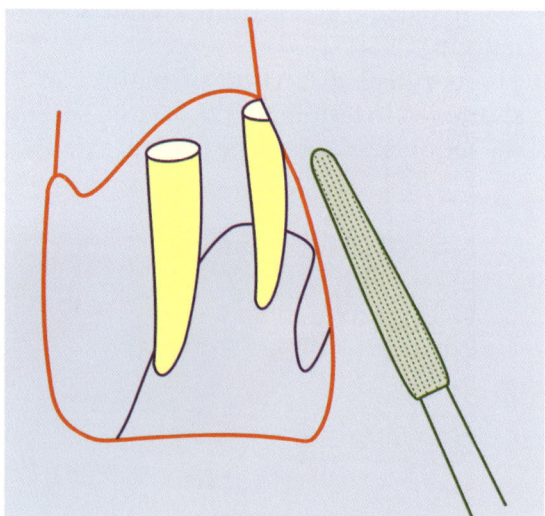

Fig. 8.26c: Proximal line angle groove

marginal integrity and structural durability. The 90° cavosurface angle provides the necessary bulk for ceramic at the margins (Fig. 8.29). All surfaces should be smooth and continuous without having any unsupported enamel.

The preparation features for anterior crowns are tabulated in Table 8.2.

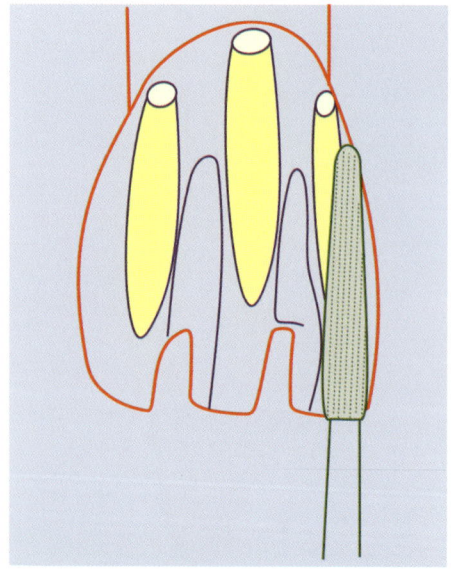

Fig. 8.26a: Labial orientation groove

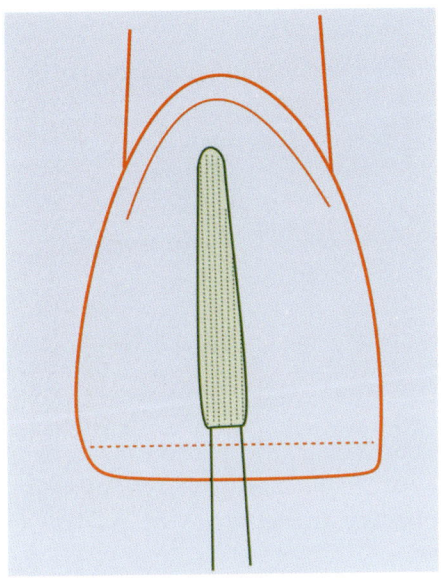

Fig. 8.26d: Final finishing

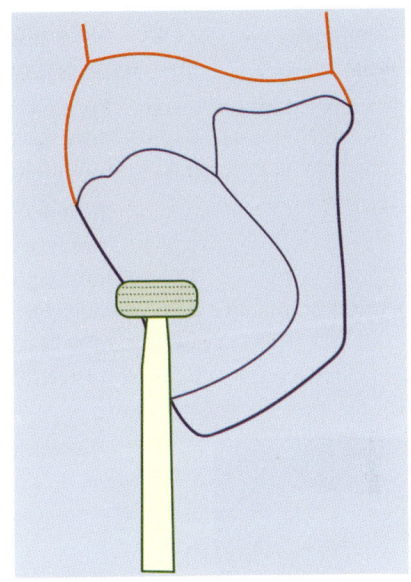

Fig. 8.27: Lingual fossa reduction

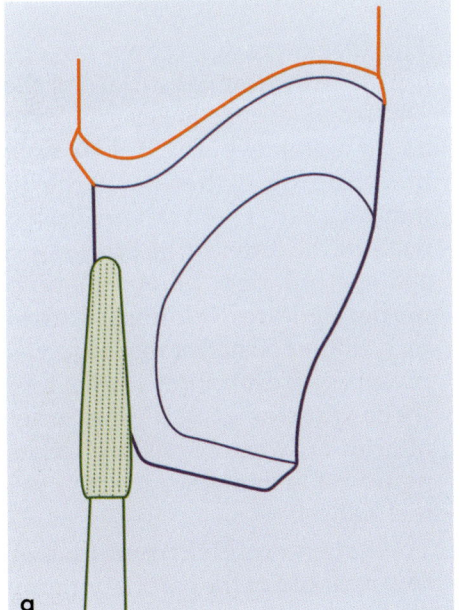

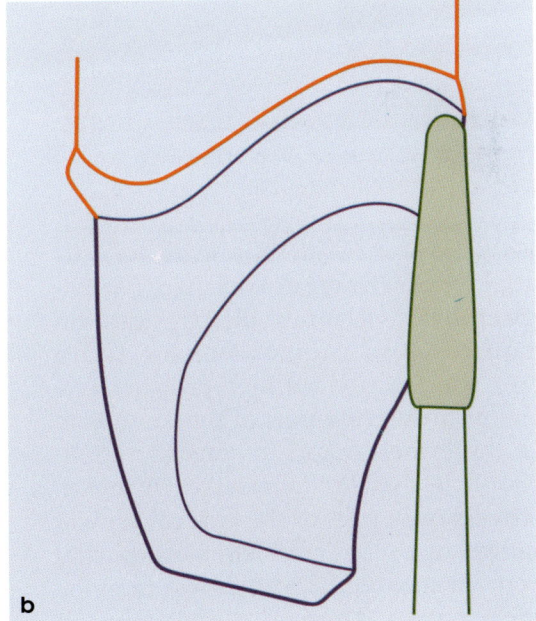

Figs 8.28a and b: (a) Proximal reduction; (b) Finish line preparation

Table 8.2: Preparation features for anterior crowns

Crown type	Incisal/Labial/Lingual reduction	Finish line depth	Configuration of finish line
Porcelain fused to metal	2.0 mm incisally 1.5 mm labially 0.5–1.0 mm lingually	1.5 mm labial 0.5 mm lingual	Shoulder Chamfer
All-ceramic	2.0 mm incisally 1.0–1.5 mm labially 1.0–1.5 mm lingually	1.0–1.5 mm both	Heavy chamfer/shoulder
Resin bonded porcelain	2.0 mm incisally 1.0 mm labially 0.5–1.0 mm lingually	1.0 mm both	Shoulder/heavy chamfer

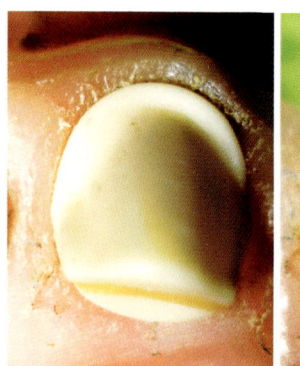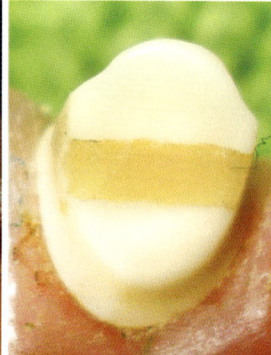

Fig. 8.29: Finished preparation

PREPARATION FOR PARTIAL VENEER CROWN

The partial veneer crown, also termed 'partial-coverage crown', is a conservative restoration that requires less preparation of tooth structure than a full veneer crown. The rationale for preserving part of the tooth is to enhance the esthetics and to conserve tooth structure. It is usually fabricated in metal, which covers only part of the clinical crown. The chances of pulpal problem with partial veneer crown are about 2.5 times less than the full veneer crown. Thermal pulp testing, if required, can be carried out even after insertion of the restoration because part of the tooth structure remains intact. Since it does not cover the entire coronal surface, it tends to be less retentive than a complete crown. It provides less resistance to displacement so may be used for intact/minimally-decayed tooth and that too having sufficient crown length; however, the procedure is technique sensitive.

There are three types of partial veneer crowns.

    i. Three-quarter crown
   ii. Seven-eighth crown
  iii. Half (proximal half/mesial-half) crown

    i. The three-quarter crown covers three-fourth of the lingual surface of the tooth. The facial surface is kept unprepared so as to conserve the tooth structure, maintaining esthetics of the original natural tooth. Three-quarter crown can be used in the anterior or posterior teeth as a single unit or as an abutment for fixed partial denture. The lingual surface of a mandibular posterior tooth is occasionally preserved; restoration known as 'reverse three-quarter crown'. Reverse three-quarter crowns are mainly indicated on mandibular molars with severe lingual inclination.

   ii. The seven-eighth crown encompasses seven-eighth of the coronal circumference of the tooth (mesio-buccal cusp of maxillary first molar not covered). It is generally indicated for maxillary molars and premolars, which are sound mesially, but may have extensive carious involvement on the distal surface.

  iii. The half (mesial-half) crown covers the mesial cusps (mesio-buccal and mesio-lingual) usually preserving the distal half.

In certain cases, the distal surface can be covered and the mesial is conserved. This preparation design is primarily indicated for the distal retainer of the mandibular fixed partial denture with tilted molar abutment. The restoration is also used as a single retainer where there has been drifting and tipping of the mandibular molar. Mesial-half crowns are contra-indicated if there are blemishes on the distal surface of the tooth.

Indications of Partial Veneer Crown

- Tooth having sufficient crown length.
- Tooth to be used as abutment should be intact or minimally restored without any attrition/cervical erosion. It should be in good alignment.
- The labio-lingual thickness of tooth should be sufficient to provide additional/auxiliary retentive features.

Contraindications of Partial Veneer Crown

- Tooth with short clinical height.
- Teeth having extensive caries/restoration.
- Tooth with extensive attrition/erosion.
- Malformed teeth.

Armamentarium

The armamentarium required for preparation of partial veneer crown is as follows:

- Handpiece
- Flat-end long tapered diamond bur
- Round-end long tapered diamond bur
- Flame/football/wheel diamond bur
- Thin short needle diamond
- Enamel hatchet
- Torpedo diamond
- Small inverted cone bur

Preparation

The partial veneer crown is not as retentive as a full veneer crown but it has adequate retention for single restoration and retainer for short span fixed partial denture. The retentive features are mandatory to compensate for the lack of retention and resistance form due to less surface area covered. The most commonly used retentive feature is groove followed by pinledge. Though, there are no hard and fast protocols for preparation of partial veneer crown, however', tooth preparation involves following steps:

   i. Occlusal/incisal preparation
   ii. Lingual reduction
   iii. Proximal preparation
   iv. Placing extra-retentive features
   v. Lingual-incisal/occlusal bevel
   vi. Finishing and toileting the preparation

ANTERIOR THREE-QUARTER CROWN

The anterior partial veneer (three-quarter) crown is prepared following the steps as:

i. Incisal Preparation

The incisal preparation is carried out using a tapered round-ended diamond point. The incisal edge is reduced lingually by 1.0 mm by keeping the instrument 45-degree to the long axis of the tooth. During incisal area preparation, facial contour of the tooth is to be maintained (Fig. 8.30).

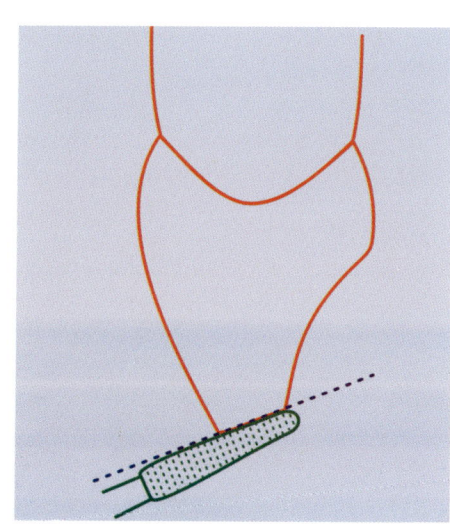

Fig. 8.30: Incisal reduction

ii. *Lingual Reduction*

The lingual reduction is carried out in two stages.

The lingual supra-cingulum preparation is carried out by flame/football/ wheel shaped diamond point. It is accomplished in two planes. A ridge should be left in the center inciso-gingivally as a guideline. A clearance of 1.0 mm should be achieved. The height of cingulum should not be over reduced as it will result in shortening of the lingual seat (Fig. 8.31).

The gingival one-third reduction is achieved parallel to the long axis of tooth using a round-ended tapered diamond point.

A chamfer cervical finish line of 0.5 mm width should be achieved which includes lingual line angles (Fig. 8.32).

iii. *Proximal Preparation*

Proximal preparation is initiated by using a thin long tapering diamond point. Proximal reduction is carried out from lingual to facial surface, protecting the facial line angle (must remain intact for better esthetics, Fig. 8.33).

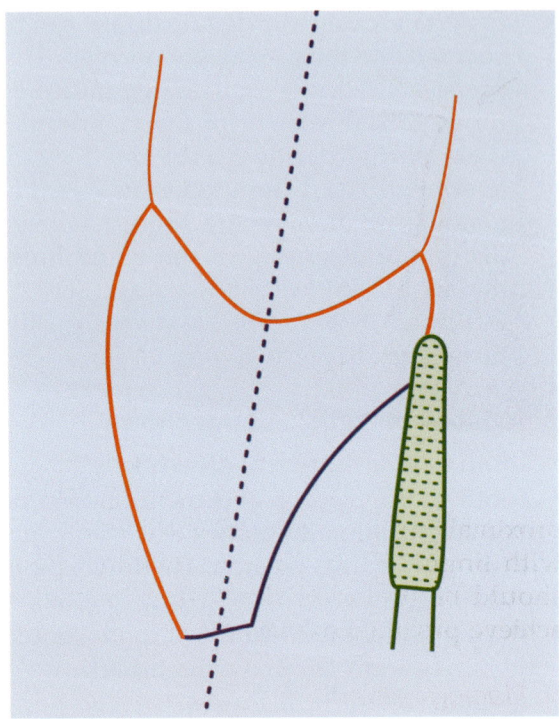

Fig. 8.32: Gingival one-third reduction lingually

A light chamfer finish line is prepared on proximal surface with the help of a long narrow round-ended bur (Fig. 8.34). The

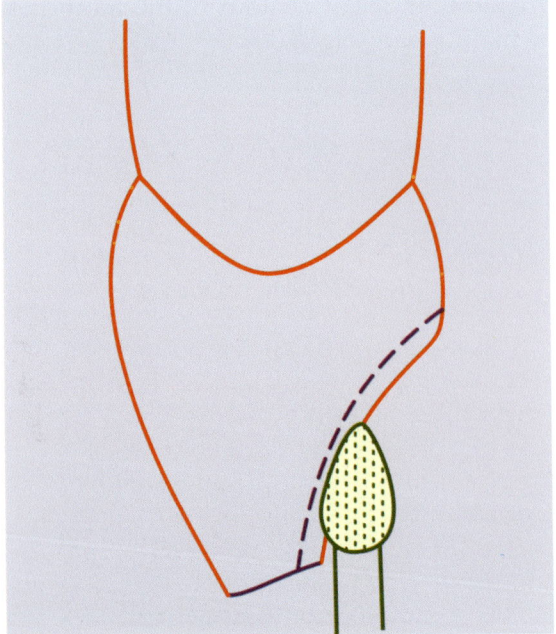

Fig. 8.31: Lingual fossa reduction

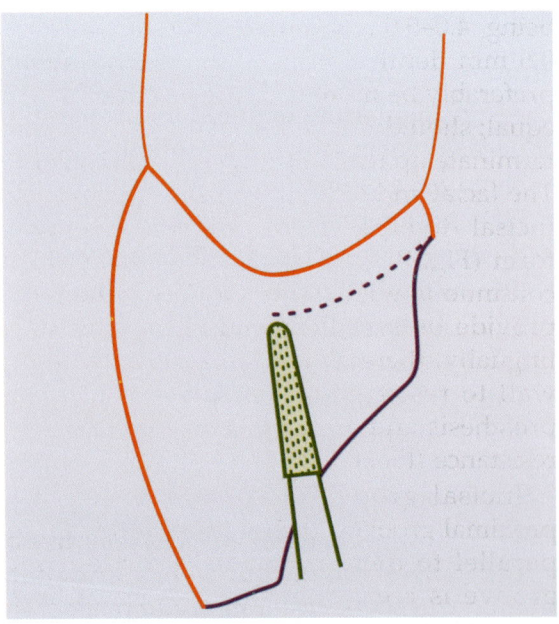

Fig. 8.33: Proximal reduction

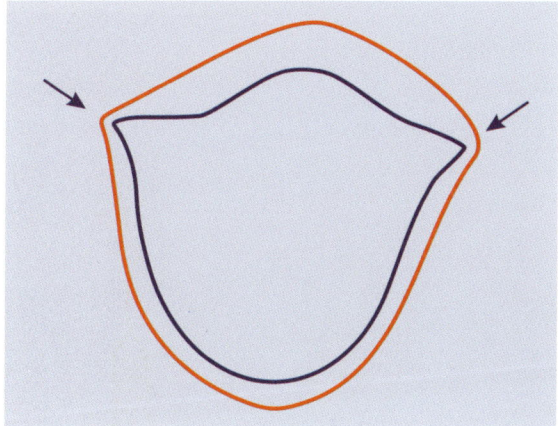

Fig. 8.34: Proximal finish lines

proximal finish line should be in continuation with lingual finish line. The contact point should be broken gently using hatchet to achieve proximal extension.

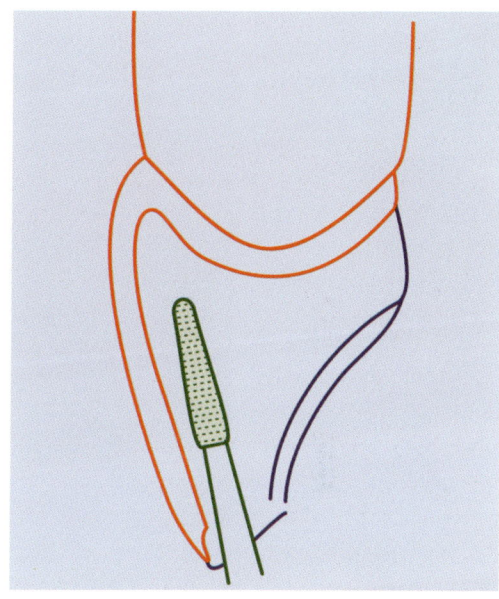

Fig. 8.35: Preparing proximal groove

iv. Placing Extra-retentive Features

The proximal grooves are the most commonly used retentive feature in three-quarter crown. The grooves are created to obtain better retention and resistance form in the preparation. The grooves should be along the lingual-proximal area; the routine dimensions being, 4.0–5.0 mm length, 0.5 mm width and 0.6 mm depth. Depth of the groove should preferably be more than the width or at least equal; should not be less in any case. It must terminate up to 0.5 mm of cervical finish line. The facial and lingual wall should have 2–5° incisal divergence to achieve convenience form (Fig. 8.35). The facial wall should be continuous with proximal flare, which will provide bulk to the facial margin; whereas lingually, there should be a definite lingual wall to resist lingual displacement of the prosthesis and also for better retention and resistance (Fig. 8.36).

Incisal groove is created to join two proximal grooves. It should be in dentin and parallel to dentino-enamel junction. This groove is created with the help of small inverted cone bur (Figs 8.37a and b).

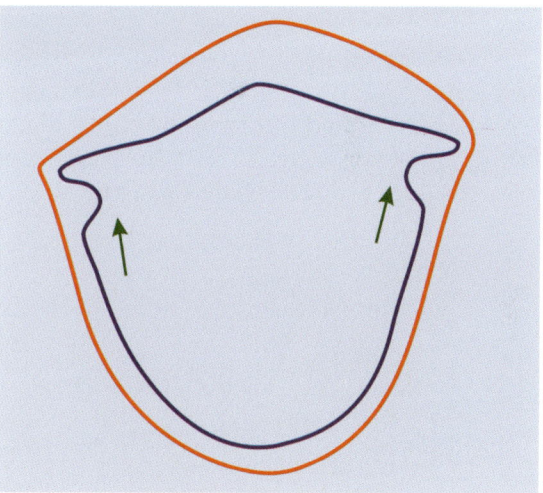

Fig. 8.36: Proximal groove

Pin ledges are also used where routine retention is not sufficient. Pin ledge is prepared in cingulum area parallel to the long axis of proximal groove. It is created by using long tapering diamond point at slow speed (Figs 8.39a–c).

A pilot hole may be made with the help of small round bur. This pinhole may be drilled 1.5 to 2.0 mm deep with twist drill, parallel to the path of insertion.

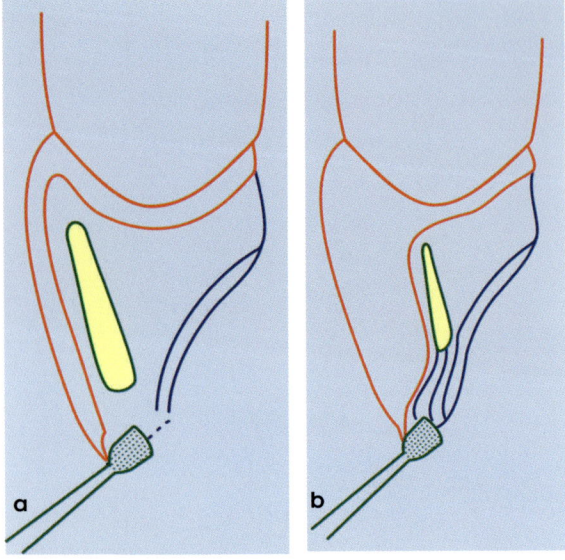

Figs 8.37a and b: (a) Incisal groove; (b) Joining proximal and incisal grooves

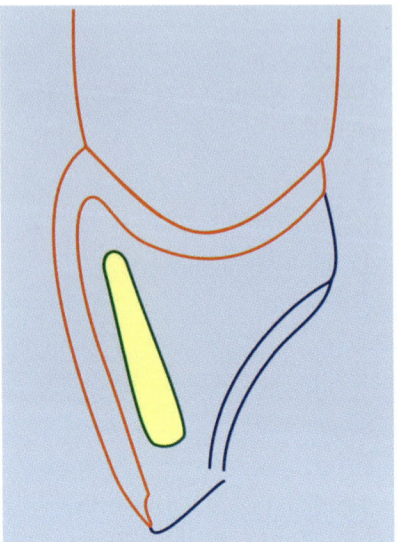

Fig. 8.38b: Facial bevel

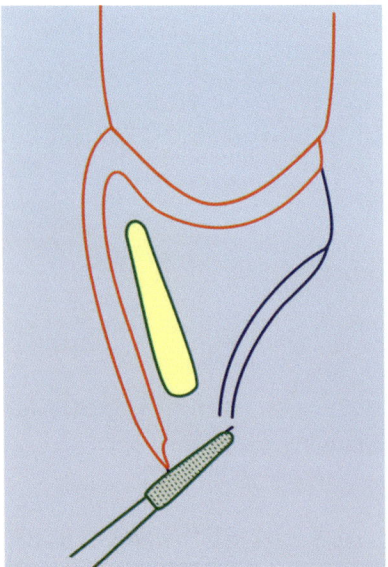

Fig. 8.38a: Facial bevel preparation

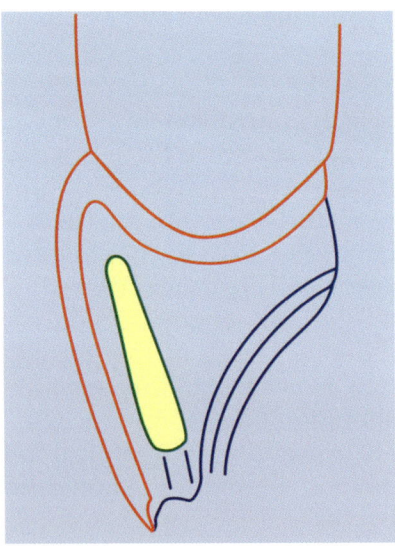

Fig. 8.38c: Final preparation

v. *Lingual-incisal bevel*

A narrow facial bevel less than 0.5 mm is given on labio-incisal finish line (lingually) using flame-shaped diamond points. This should be at right angle to incisal one-third of incisal edges (Figs 8.38a–c).

vi. *Finishing and Toileting the Preparation*

Finishing and toileting the prepared tooth is carried out using carbide-finishing burs at lower speed. All line angles should be rounded off to provide continuity of all finish lines. The preparation should be cleaned thoroughly with water and air jet before impression making (Figs 8.40a and b).

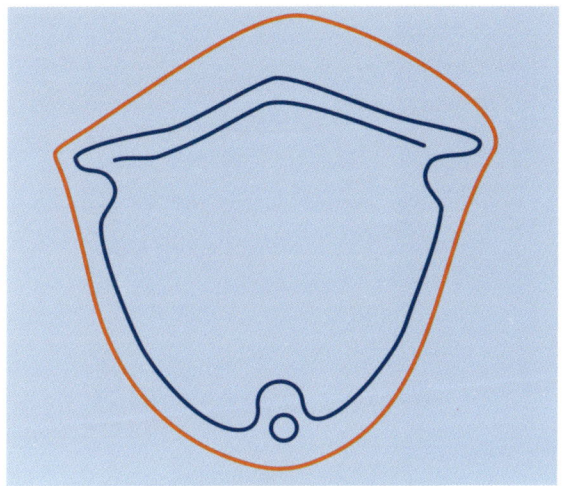

Fig. 8.39a: Pin-hole (incisal view)

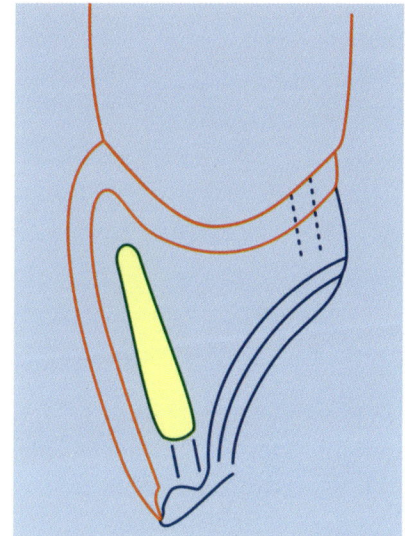

Fig. 8.39c: Final preparation

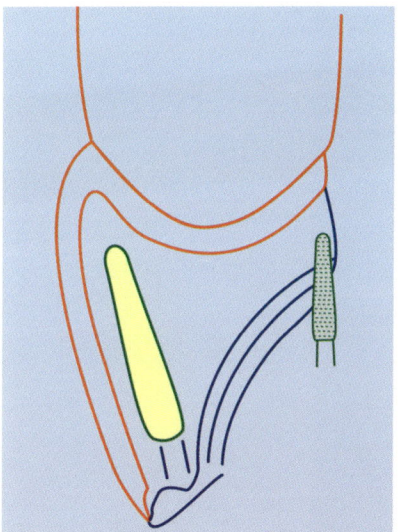

Fig. 8.39b: Preparing pin-hole

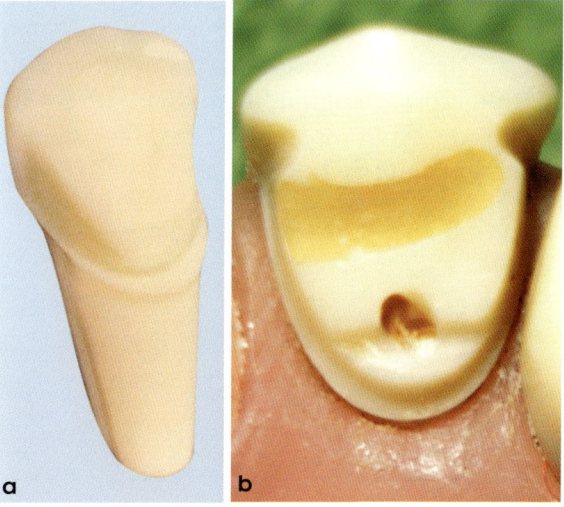

Figs 8.40a and b: (a) Finished preparation; (b) showing pin-hole

THREE-QUARTER CROWN FOR MAXILLARY PREMOLAR

The three-quarter crown for maxillary premolars is prepared following the steps as:

i. *Occlusal Reduction*

The lingual cusp is reduced to get a clearance of 1.5 to 2.0 mm followed by buccal cusp inclines to achieve 1.5 mm occlusal clearance at central groove and 1.0 mm clearance at the cusp tip. The reduction is carried out with the help of long tapering round-ended diamond point. The basic morphology of the cusps should be maintained in both outer and inner inclines (Fig. 8.41).

ii. *Lingual Reduction*

The lingual reduction is carried out using tapering round and diamond points keeping it parallel to the long axis of tooth.

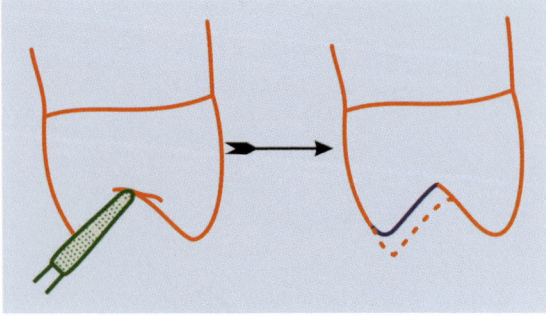

Fig. 8.41: Occlusal reduction

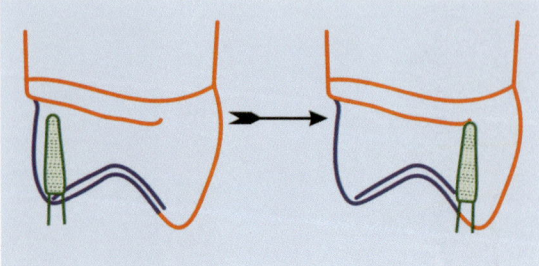

Fig. 8.43: Proximal reduction

A 0.5 mm deep cervical finish line (chamfer) is prepared all along the surface involving the proximal line angles (Fig. 8.42).

iii. Proximal Reduction

The proximal reduction is carried out from lingual to facial surface with the help of long thin carbide/diamond point. A chamfer finish line (0.5 mm deep) should be achieved in continuation of lingual finish line (Fig. 8.43).

The contact point should be broken gently with the help of hatchet and the area be finished off using round-ended carbide bur (Fig. 8.44).

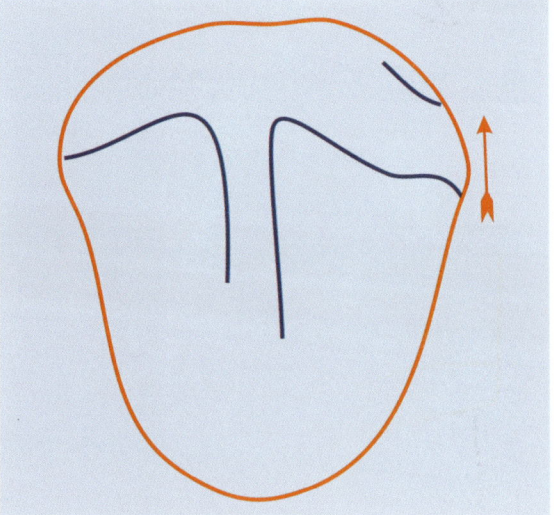

Fig. 8.44: Breaking contact point

iv. Placement of Extra-retentive Features

The proximal groove is the most common extra retentive feature used in three-quarter crown of premolars (Fig. 8.45). The groove is created from facial to the central groove. It should be approximately 0.5 mm away from the gingival finish line. The dimensions of the grooves should be the same as for anterior teeth.

The two proximal grooves are joined by making a groove of 0.5–0.75 mm depth on inner incline of the facial cusp. Facial cusp tip should be conserved and the groove should be in dentin. Inverted cone bur is used to make this groove (Fig. 8.46).

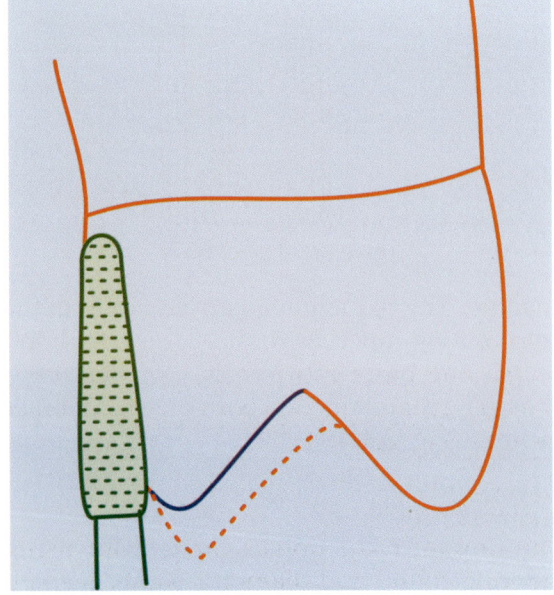

Fig. 8.42: Lingual reduction

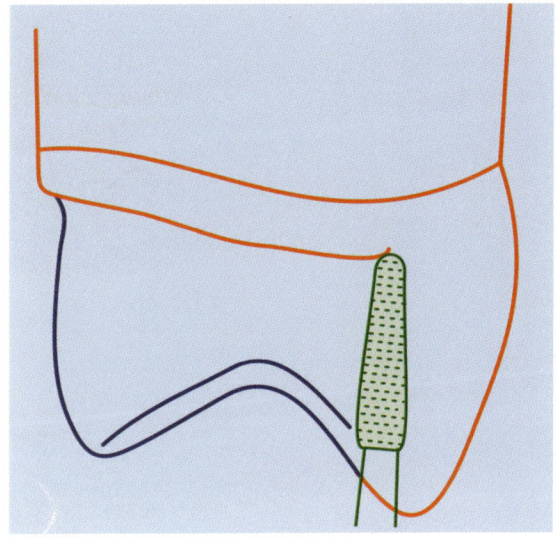

Fig. 8.45: Proximal groove

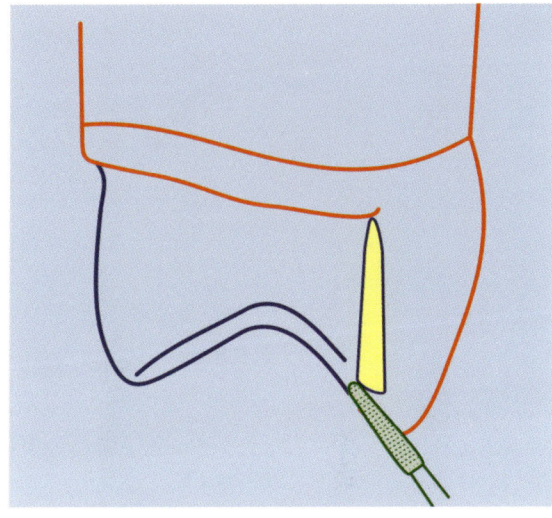

Fig. 8.47a: Preparing facial bevel

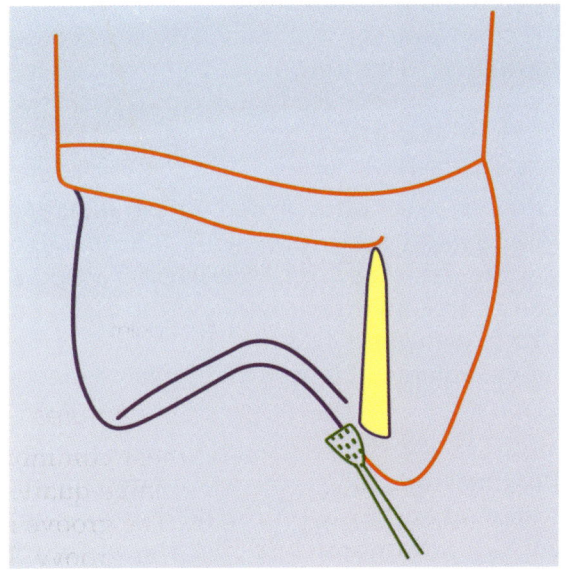

Fig. 8.46: Occlusal groove

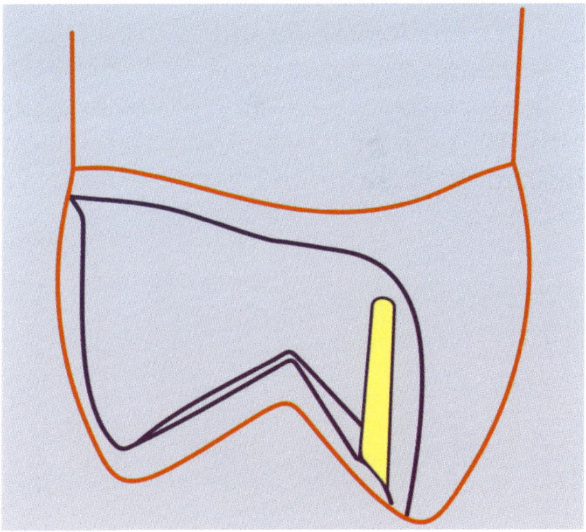

Fig. 8.47b: Facial bevel

v. Lingual-occlusal Bevel

A narrow bevel of less than 0.5 mm is given at the lingual-occlusal margin (lingually) at right angle to long axis of the tooth. A fine long flame shaped bur is used to create this bevel (Figs 8.47a and b).

vi. Finishing and Toileting the Preparation

All line angles are slightly rounded off with the help of carbide finishing bur at low speed. The continuity of all finished line angles are maintained (Fig. 8.48).

The preparation should be wiped off with water and air jet. The final preparation is shown in Fig. 8.49.

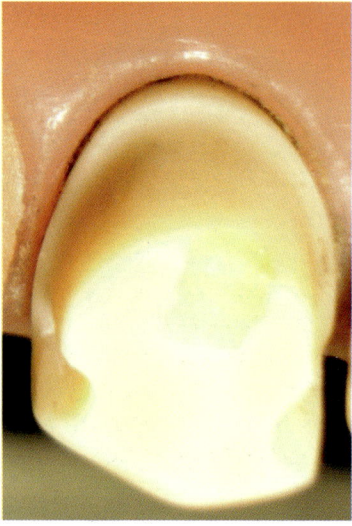

Fig. 8.48: Finished preparation

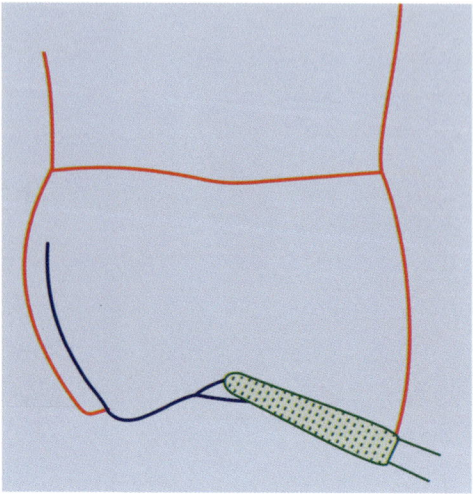

Fig. 8.50: Occlusal reduction

groove and 1.0 mm at cusp tip. The remaining cusps are reduced to achieve 2.0 mm occlusal clearance (Fig. 8.50). The basic anatomy of all the cusps must be maintained during occlusal reduction. The long round-ended tapered diamond point is used for occlusal reduction.

ii. Lingual Reduction

Lingual reduction is carried out parallel to the long axis of tooth preparing 0.5 mm deep chamfer line (Fig. 8.51). Mesial half is prepared like a three-quarter crown and the distal half like a complete crown. The round-ended tapered diamond is used for lingual reduction.

iii. Proximal Reduction

Proximal reduction is carried out from lingual to buccal surface with the help of long thin carbide/diamond bur like three-quarter preparation. A chamfer finish line (0.5 mm) should be achieved in continuation of lingual finish line (Fig. 8.52).

If sufficient tooth structure is lacking, the preparation simulates anterior three quarter crown.

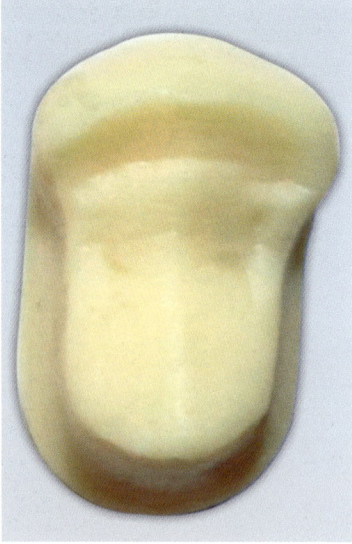

Fig. 8.49: Final preparation

SEVEN-EIGHTH CROWN FOR MAXILLARY MOLAR

The steps followed for preparation of seven-eighth crown for maxillary molars are:

i. Occlusal Reduction

Occlusal reduction is carried out in two steps. First, reduce the inner incline of mesio-buccal cusp to create 1.5 mm clearance at central

iv. Distobuccal Reduction

The distobuccal reduction is initiated along the buccal surface and extending it distally around

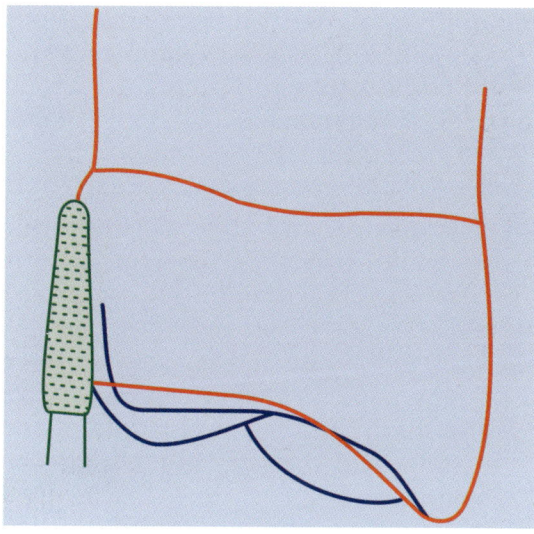

Fig. 8.51: Lingual reduction

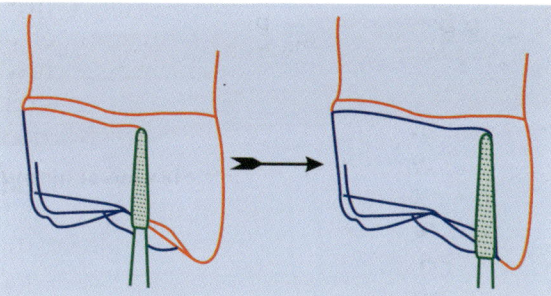

Fig. 8.52: Proximal reduction

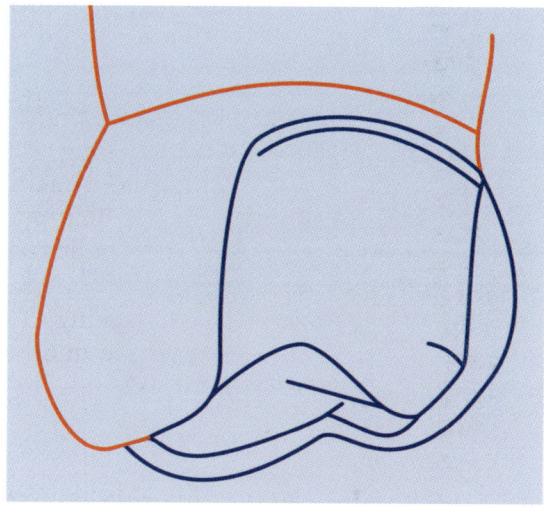

Fig. 8.53: Distobuccal reduction

the distobuccal line angle (Fig. 8.53). The finish line (0.5 mm) should be prepared in continuation with distal chamfer line. The finishing line is prepared using round-ended long tapered diamond points.

v. Placement of Extra-retentive Devices

Grooves are the most commonly used retentive features in seven-eight crown.

A 3.0 mm long buccal groove is created in the area of mid-buccal surface. It should be 0.5 mm away from the cervical finish line and the distobuccal finish line. The axial wall should converge occlusally while mesial and distal walls of the buccal groove should diverge occlusally (Fig. 8.54).

Lingual groove is prepared on the lingual surface which should be 0.5 mm away from the gingival finish line. The groove should be 3.0 mm long and converge occlusally (Fig. 8.55).

The buccal and the lingual grooves are joined together by making an occlusal groove on the inclines of the mesial cusps. It is carried

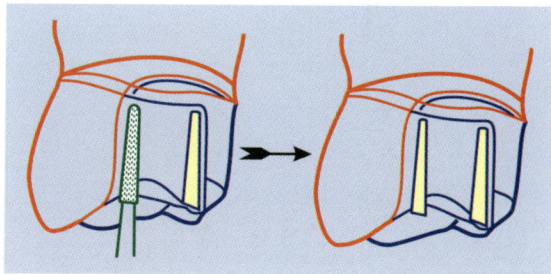

Fig. 8.54: Buccal groove preparation

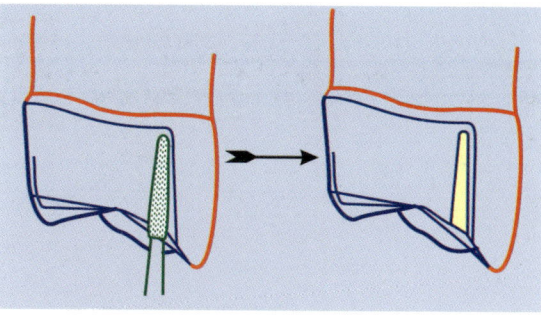

Fig. 8.55: Preparing lingual groove

out with the help of small inverted cone bur (Fig. 8.56).

vi. *Beveling incline Planes of Mesio-buccal Cusp*

A narrow bevel of less than 0.5 mm is given on the mesio-buccal cusp on the incline planes at approximately right angle to the long axis of tooth using fine long tapering diamond bur (Fig. 8.57).

vii. *Finishing and Toileting the Preparation*

All line angles are slightly rounded off using carbide-finishing burs at low speed. The

continuity of all finished line angles should be maintained (Fig. 8.58). The preparation should be cleaned with water and air spray. The final preparation is shown in Fig. 8.59.

Errors in Tooth Preparation

The impression and the cast should be evaluated for any type of error in tooth preparation. The commonly encountered errors are:

1. *Sharp line angles:* The axial line angles of the preparation should be evaluated for any sharp angles, which lead to poor fit castings and subsequently failure of the restoration.

2. *Incomplete and/or non-uniform shoulder:* Incomplete and/or non-uniform shoulder

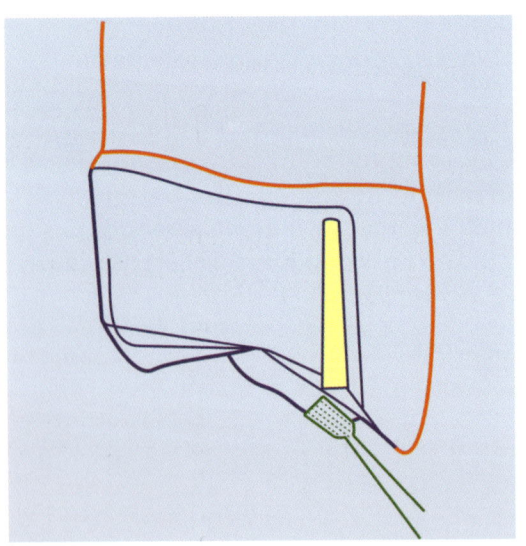

Fig. 8.56: Joining of buccal and lingual grooves (occlusal groove)

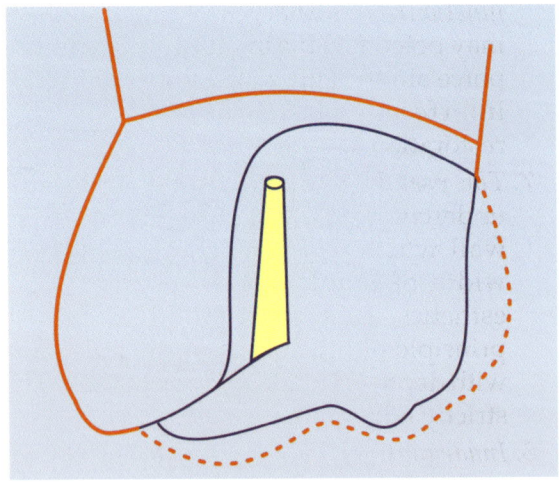

Fig. 8.58: Finished preparation

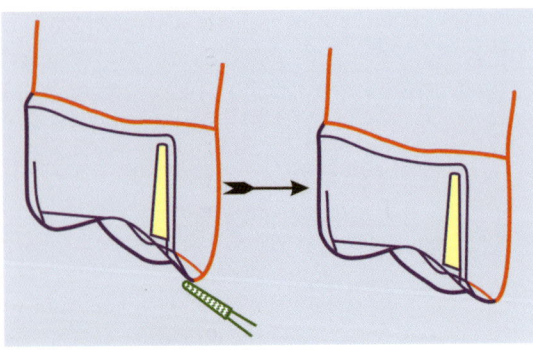

Fig. 8.57: Facial bevel

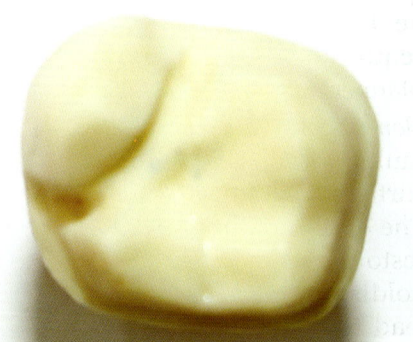

Fig. 8.59: Final preparation

can lead to premature fracture during fabrication of all-ceram restorations and esthetic problems.

3. *Rough shoulder:* Rough shoulder will compromise fit, cement line and esthetics and can result in stress fractures during seating or delayed fracture of restoration in function.

4. *Beveled or feather margin:* It is difficult to fabricate and finish porcelain over these beveled margins. Hence, these should be avoided.

5. *The J Margin:* It is incomplete chamfer providing a little room for adequate porcelain thickness for optimum esthetics. In turn, restorations become over-contoured.

6. *Sharp internal line angle (axial wall-shoulder junction):* This sharp internal line angle may potentiate the internal stresses in the porcelain and subsequent fractures. It also interferes with proper fit of the restoration.

7. *The pseudo-shoulder:* It results due to undercut near the shoulder on the axial wall which leads to reduced effective width of shoulder. It can compromise esthetics. To avoid a pseudo shoulder, principle of orientation of the bur along with depth orientation grooves should be strictly adhered to.

8. *Inadequate or over-reduction of occlusal surface:* Prior to the preparation appointments, the type of occlusal reduction (planar or rounded and smoother) should be first reviewed according to the requirements of the restoration being planned, e.g. Procera.

9. *Non-uniform reduction:* Lack of uniform/multiplane reduction, especially on facial surface may compromise with esthetics. The over-contoured palatal aspect of the restorations may result in loss of stable, holding contacts in occlusion and may lead to multiple deleterious effects on stomatognathic system.

10. *Inadequate lingual extension for laminate veneers in diastema closures:* In such cases, the lab technician may find it hard to make the contact between adjacent teeth in a natural, cleansable and esthetic location. For optimum results, the proximal reduction should be carried out in same way as for a complete crown.

11. *Undercuts in preparation:* These can be best analyzed on a cast than in an impression. A periodontal probe can be effectively used to see the severity of the undercut by placing its tip in the margin first and then pivoting the probe towards the preparation and stopping at the initial contact.

Bibliography

1. Anusavice KJ. Standardizing failure, success, and survival decision in clinical studies of ceramic and metal-ceramic fixed dental prostheses. Dent. Mater.: 2012;28:102–11.

2. Assif D, Pilo R and Marshak B. Restoring teeth following crown lengthening procedures. J. Prosthodont. Dent.: 1991;65:62–4.

3. Behr M, Rosentritt M and Handel G. Fiber reinforced composite crowns and FPDs: a clinical report. Int. J. Prosthodont.: 2003;16:239–43.

4. Blair FM, Wassell RW and Steele JG. Crowns and other extra coronal restorations: preparations for full veneer crowns. Br. Dent. J.: 2002;192:561–71.

5. Broseghini C, Broseghini M, Gracis S and Vigolo P. Aesthetic functional area protection concept for prevention of ceramic chipping with Zirconia frameworks. Int. J. Prosthodont.: 2014;27:174–6.

6. Chana H, Kelleher M, Briggs P and Hooper RJ. Clinical evaluation of resin-bonded gold alloy veneers. J. Prosthet. Dent.: 2000;83:294–300.

7. Cherukara GP, Davis GR, Seymour KG, Zou L and Samarawickrama DY. Dentin exposure in tooth preparations for porcelain veneers: a pilot study. J. Prosth. Dent.: 2005;94:414–20.

8. Denissen HW, ElZohairy AA, Van Waas MA and Feilzer AJ. Porcelain-veneered computer generated partial crowns. Quint. Int.: 2002;33:723–30.

9. DiTolla MC. A new metal free alternative for single and multi-unit restorations. Compend. Cont. Dental Educ.: 2002;23:25–33.

10. Dodge WW, Weed RM, Baez RJ and Buchanan RN. The effect of covergence angle on retention and retention form. Quint. Int. 1985;16:191–4.

11. Donovan TE and Chee WWL. Cervical margin design with contemporary esthetic restorations. Dent. Clin. N. Am.: 2004;48:417–31.

12. Donovan TE and Cho GC. The role of all-ceramic crowns in contemporary dentistry. J. Calif. Dent. Assoc.: 2003;31:565.

13. Esteves HJM, Costa N and Esteves ISB. Clinical determination of angle convergence in a tooth preparation for a complete crown. Int. J. Prosthodont.: 2014;27:472–4.

14. Galindo DF, Ercoli C, Funkenbusch PD, Greene TD, Moss ME, Lee HJ, Ben-Hanan U, Graser GN and Barzilay I. Tooth preparation: A study on the effect of different variables and a comparison between conventional and channeled diamond burs. J. Prosthodont.: 2004;13;1–14.

15. Gavilis JR, Morency JK, Riley ED and Sozio RB. The effect of various finish line preparations on the marginal seal and occlusal seat of full crown preparations. J. Prosthet. Dent.: 1981;45:138–45.

16. Gilboe DB and Thayer KE. Beveled shoulder concept: full good crown preparation. J. Can. Dent. Assoc.: 1980;46:519.

17. Gunay H. Tooth preparation using guide pin instruments and the biological width. Int. Dent.:9, 76–82.

18. Heintze SD and Rousson V. Survival of zirconia and metal-supported fixed dental prostheses: a systematic review. Int. J.Prosthodont.: 2010;23, 493–502.

19. Jacobsen PH, Wakefieldt AJ, O'Doherty DM and Rees JS. The effect of preparation height and taper on cement lute stress: a three dimensional finite element analysis. Eur. J. Prosthodont. Rest. Dent. 2006;14:151–7.

20. Jorgensen KD. The relationship between retention and convergence angle in cemented veneer crowns. Acta. Odontol. Scand.: 1955;13:35–40.

21. Kent WA, Shillingburg HT and Duncanson MG. Taper of clinical preparations for cast restorations. Quint. Int.: 1988;19:339–45.

22. Kimmich M and Stappert CFJ. Intraoral treatment of veneering porcelain chipping of fixed dental restorations. J.A.D.A.: 2013;144:31–44.

23. Kishimoto M, Shillingburg HT Jr, and Duncanson MG, Jr. Influence of preparation features on retention and resistance. Part II: three-quarter crowns. JPD: 1983;49:188–92.

24. Kois JC. Altering gingival levels: the restorative connection, part I: biologic variables. J. Esthet. Dent.: 1994;6:3–9.

25. Kois JC. New paradigms for anterior tooth preparation: rationale and technique. Contemp. Esthet. Dent.: 1996;2:1–8.

26. Kurtzman GM. Spinning down the tooth: Advances in crown preparation. Compend.: 2014;35:362–3.

27. Lakatos S, Rominu M, Negrutiu M and Florita Z. The microleakage between alloy and polymeric materials in veneer crowns. Quint. Int.: 2003;34: 295–300.

28. Lanning SK, Waldrop CT, Gunsolley JC and Maynard GJ. Surgical crown lengthening: evaluation of biologic width. J. Periodontol.: 2003; 74:468–74.

29. Leles CR and Compagnoni A. A simple method to detect undercuts during tooth preparations for fixed proshodontics. J. Prosth. Dent.: 2001;85: 521–2.

30. Liu Y, Liu G, Wang Y, Shen JZ and Feng H. Failure modes and fracture origins of porcelain veneers on bilayer dental crowns, 2014.

31. Maxwell AW, Blank LW and Pellen GB. Effect of crown preparation height on the resistance and retention of gold castings. Gen. Dent.: 1990;38: 200–2.

32. McLaren EA and Vigoren G. Crown considerations, preparations and material selection for esthetic metal-ceramic restorations. Esthet. Tech.: 2001;1:3–9.

33. Mizrahi B. The Dahl principle: Creating space and improving the biomechanical prognosis of anterior crowns. Quint. Int.: 2006;37:245–51.

34. Norlander J, Weir D, Stoffer W and Ochi S. The taper of clinical preparations for fixed prosthodontics. J. Prosth. Dent.: 1988;60:148–51.

35. Olivera AB and Saito T. The effect of die spacer on retention and fitting of complete cast crowns. J. Prosthodont.: 2006;15:243–9.

36. Parker MH, Ivanhoe JR, Blalock JS, Frazier KB and Plummer KD. A technique to determine a desired preparation axial inclination. J. Prosth. Dent.: 2003; 90:401–5.

37. Patel PB, Wildgoose DG and Winstanley RB. Comparison of convergence angles achieved in posterior teeth prepared for full veneer crowns. Eur. J. Prosthodont. Rest. Dent.: 2005;13:100–4.

38. Peumans M, Van Meerbeek B, Lambrechts P and Vanherle G. Porcelain veneers: a review of the literature. J.Dent.: 2000;28:163–77.

39. Pilathadka S and Vahalova D. Contemporary all-ceramic systems, part 2. Acta. Medica.: 2007;50: 105–7.

40. Poyser NJ, Porter PF, Chana HS and Kelleher GD. The Dahl concept: past, present and future. BDJ: 2005;198:669–76.

41. Sharma A, Rahul GR, Poduval ST and Shetty K. Short clinical crowns (SCC)—treatment considerations and techniques. J. Clin. Exp. Dent.: 2012; 4:e230–6.

42. Shenoy A, Shenoy N and Babannavar R. Periodontal considerations determining the design and location of margins in restorative dentistry. J. Interdisci. Dent.: 2012;2:3–10.

43. Siegel SC and von Fraunhofer JA. Dental cutting with diamond burs: Heavy-handed or light-touch. J. Prosthodont.: 1999;8:3–9.

44. Small BW. Optimizing clinical longevity in the anterior: direct composite veneer, porcelain veneer or full crown. Gen. Dent.: 2003;51:100–2.

45. Smith CT, Gary JJ, Conkin JE and Franks HL. Effective taper criterion for the full veneer crown preparation in preclinical prosthodontics. J. Prosthodont.: 1999;8:196–200.

46. Spitznagel FA, Horvath SD, Guess PC and Blatz MB. Resin bond to indirect composite and new ceramic/polymer materials: A review of the literature. J. Esthet. Rest. Dent.: 2014;26:382–93.

47. Syu JZ, Byrne G, Laub LW and Land MF. Influence of finish line geometry on the fit of crowns. Int. J. Prosthodont.: 1993;6:25.

48. Tjan AH, and Miller GD. Bio-geometric guide to groove placement on three-quarter crown preparations. JPD: 1979;42:405–10.

49. Walls AWG, Nohl FSA and Wassell RW. Crowns and other extracoronal restorations: Resin-bonded metal restorations. Br. Dent. J.: 2002;193: 135–42.

50. Yeh S and Andreana S. Crown lengthening: basic principles, indications, techniques and clinical case reports. NY State Dent. J.: 2004;70:30–6.

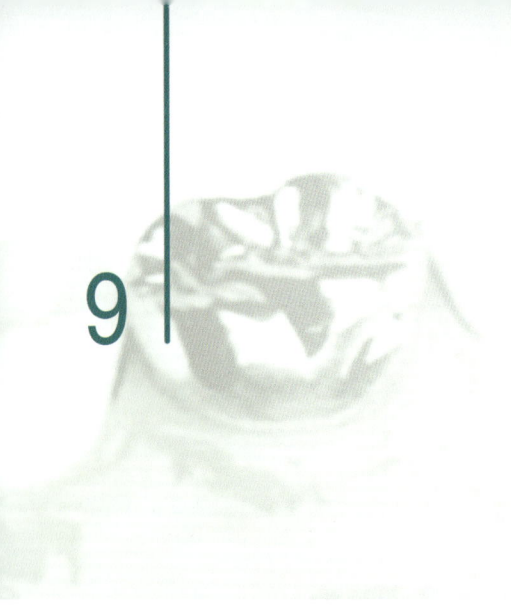

9

Laminates

The restoration of unaesthetic anterior teeth has always posed a challenge to the restorative dentist. The discoloration of enamel may be attributed to local factors, such as trauma and infection or to general factors, such as hereditary and congenital causes. The restoration of such teeth for achieving esthetics is widely accepted in dental practice. The discoloration is customarily treated with veneer crowns, which involves the loss of substantial tooth structure. Such a treatment modality becomes difficult in young patients, since crown cutting may lead to variable degree of pulpal damage. The placement of crown margins vis-à-vis the gingival margins also creates problems in young patients.

Mostly four types of treatment modalities are recognized to mask the discolored teeth, viz. (i) non-invasive (bleaching, microabrasion), (ii) minimal invasive (enamel recontouring, direct composites (iii) micro invasive (veneers) and macro invasive (crowns).

The other forms of treatment modalities to mask discolored teeth have also been tried, viz. bonding a denture tooth to the labial surface of the natural tooth, paint-on composites, vital bleaching, etc. These procedures were ineffective, mainly because of inherent limitations of the materials used. The advent of porcelain material overcomes the limitation of these modalities.

Full veneer porcelain crowns have been established as successful. Advances in porcelain material coupled with advances in bonding porcelain to enamel created the possibility of laminate veneers as an alternative to full crowns. Laminate is defined as a thin slice of acrylic/composite/porcelain fabricated in laboratory and cemented onto the teeth. A veneer is a layer of tooth colored material that is applied to a tooth to restore localized or generalized defects and intrinsic discolorations. The laminate veneer is a conservative esthetic restoration of anterior teeth to mask discoloration, restore malformed teeth, close diastemas and correct minor tooth alignment. Laminate is bonded directly to the prepared tooth.

Indications
- Discolored teeth
- Hypocalcification
- Diastemas
- Peg lateral incisors
- Chipped teeth
- Lingual-positioning (linguo-version)
- Malposed teeth

Contraindications
- Insufficient tooth structure (enamel) for bonding

- Labial version
- Excessive interdental spacing (broad diastemas)
- Parafunctional habits, viz. clenching, bruxism
- Crowding; moderate to severe
- Caries susceptibility
- Poor oral hygiene

Advantages

- Minimal tooth preparation required
- Reasonably stronger and durable
- Conservative treatment for incisal fractures
- Esthetically acceptable

Disadvantages

- Placement is technique sensitive
- Cannot be repaired easily
- Brittle margins
- Finishing is difficult, especially at margins
- Potential for overcontouring
- Not cost effective

The laminates/labial veneers are mainly fabricated in composite resin or porcelain.

COMPOSITE LAMINATES

Composite resin laminates can be fabricated directly or indirectly. Direct fabrication is also described for the convenience of reader.

A. Direct Composite Resin Veneers

Direct composite application on discolored teeth has been tried with success, though for short duration. It is a good treatment for fractured anterior teeth.

Direct veneers can be of the extra-enamel type (without preparation), intra-enamel (preparation limited to enamel) or the intra-enamel/dentin (preparation involving dentin). The treatment protocol is less invasive than full crowns. The longevity of direct application depends on factors related to patient, operator and the restorative material. The satisfactory longevity of success can be achieved by precision attention at each stage. The patient must be warned about the effect of smoking, drinking alcohol, consuming too much coffee and dye-containing foods. Maintaining proper hygiene also affects longevity. The patient must also be informed that these restorations can be repaired quickly and safely to extend the durability of these veneers.

A proper diagnosis and adequate planning is mandatory for placing direct veneer.

The teeth are usually classified according to the degree of discoloration:

- Teeth without color alteration, or presenting 'discrete' patches of discoloration
- Teeth exhibiting marked discoloration

The direct veneers will change the color and may also alter the size, shape and position of the tooth. Operator has to consider the expectations of the patient. Sometimes, the color created by composite is not satisfactory. This is because composite in lesser thickness permit light to pass through and may not mask the background color of the tooth. The deep preparation and increasing the composite thickness usually overcomes this problem. Use of opaquers can also be useful.

Restorative 'Try-in'

Veneers are usually restricted to labial surfaces of anterior teeth. On maxillary anterior teeth, they hardly interfere with function. However, on mandibular anterior teeth, especially when incisal angle is involved, veneers can affect the function. Alongwith achieving functions, the esthetic aspect (color, texture and shape) is also to be looked into. The 'Try-in' of the restoration is preferred to anticipate the final restoration, which can be conveyed to the patient. The restoration during 'Try-in' procedure should be finished and polished properly so as to simulate the final restoration in shape, size and color.

During diagnosis and planning, the clinician must be prepared to conduct surgical and restorative procedures. Properly articulated models, photographs and computer images of the case are a great aid in designing these restorations. These aids render visualization of the possible results much easier facilitating treatment decision.

The 'Try-in' restoration is preferably fabricated in laboratory over the cast. In case of partial veneering, composite can be cured near the defect to verify color. Since, the composite is cured over un-etched surface, it can be removed easily.

The patient's opinion of the restorative try-in is critical. Patient may consult his/her family members before finalizing the decision.

Operator should be careful as regard the proximal surface of teeth, which forms the embrasure. The proximal surfaces of teeth might not be perceived from the frontal view in certain cases. The visibility of gingival area is governed by the position of the lip, especially during smiling.

Principles of Preparation

The preparations of direct veneers on teeth, which exhibit discrete patches of color alteration should be shallow having well-defined chamfer finish lines. Occasionally, in the absence of color alteration and with a tooth in linguo-version, no preparation is necessary. In case of full veneer, covering total labial surface, the preparation is to be extended to proximal and gingival regions. Such a preparation is preferred to manage diastema and to improve the appearance of cone-shaped lateral incisors.

Preparation for direct veneers for severely discolored teeth follows the same principles. The depth of preparation depends upon the need of masking the background color. A restoration should have enough material thickness to prevent the background from negatively influencing the final appearance.

The important features to be considered during preparation are:
a. Depth of preparation
b. Extent of preparation

c. Gingival margin
d. Proximal margin
e. Incisal margin

a. Depth of Preparation

Enamel presents a mean thickness of approximately 1.0 mm on the labial surface of anterior teeth. Enamel offers variable thickness from the cervical to incisal regions, being thinner in the cervical and thicker in the incisal region. The preparation depth aims to offer enough space for a thickness of composite capable of masking a dark background color.

It is important to determine the cause of any discoloration before deciding the depth of preparation. A few teeth initially presenting lighter shade might darken after some time. To anticipate the depth of tooth reduction, it is also important to consider dynamics of color alteration.

The usual depth of preparation in teeth with slight discoloration should be approximately 0.4 mm in the cervical area and 0.5 mm at the middle third and incisal areas.

The labially positioned teeth are to be accordingly reduced even without the need for color change. In case of protrusion, the orthodontic realignment is mandatory before a veneer can be placed. The preparation, if required, should be carried out with care so as to achieve uniform reduction. Reduction of labial enamel on teeth with severe discoloration preferably be increased to 0.5 mm in the cervical region and 0.7 mm in the middle third and incisal areas. In cases of teeth with linguo-version, less reduction is needed. Preparations involving dentin should be avoided.

b. Extent of Preparation

The extent of preparation (boundaries of preparation) should not leave any dark area on the tooth structure.

The extent of preparation depends upon the following features:
• The height of smile line
• Degree of tooth discoloration

- Extent of lingual tilt
- Dimensions and location of proximal contacts
- Shape and size of embrasures
- Presence and extension of any fracture line
- Incisal function
- Need for crown lengthening
- Esthetic needs

c. Gingival Margin

The gingival margins are preferably placed supragingivally; however, in discolored teeth the margins are to be extended subgingivally.

The advantages of placing the margin supragingivally are:

- Isolation is easier; minimal chances of contamination during adhesive procedures.
- Easy access for the finishing and polishing.
- Injury to the gingival tissue is minimized.
- No impingement on biological width area.
- The marginal integrity can easily be evaluated.
- Minimizes the risk of undue exposure of dentin in the cervical region.

The gingival margin should be extended approximately 0.3 mm in the gingival sulcus in teeth exhibiting discoloration. The gingival finish line in all cases must be continuous and well defined.

d. Proximal Margin

The proximal surface is divided into two regions for extending the proximal finish lines.

  i. The surface that is in direct proximal contact (incisal-third area)
 ii. The surface that is extending gingivally from the contact area (gingival embrasure area)

The proximal finish lines are extended (labio-lingually short of contact area) on teeth free from discoloration or with discrete color patches only on labial surface. In teeth requiring color alteration, the margin is extended palatally to involve 0.2 mm of proximal contact area.

The proximal margin of the preparation in the sub-contact area is extended more towards palatal direction depending upon the size of the embrasures. This prevents direct visibility of tooth structure from an angle. The finish line must be a well-defined and continuous chamfer. On the teeth with severe color alteration, the proximal margin must be extended palatally halfway into the labio-lingual dimension of the contact area to prevent that margin from being visible.

The proximal margin in the sub-contact area must also be extended palatally until the unprepared tooth surface cannot be seen. To determine the margin finish line in the sub-contact area, the dynamic areas of visibility is to be kept in mind.

e. Incisal Margin

The incisal margin can be established on the labial surface (maintaining the incisal edge), at the incisal edge or extending on to the palatal lingual surface. Placement of incisal margin depends on tooth color, need to increase the tooth length, presence of sound tooth structure in the region and incisal function. In teeth free from color alteration, the incisal margin can be established on the facial surface as a knife-edge end. If the teeth need to be lengthened, finish line will be placed on the palatal surface as chamfered line. For teeth that exhibit discrete color alteration, the incisal finish line must be established at the incisal edge. The preparation finish lines must always be well-defined and continuous chamfers along their extension.

Clinical Technique

The veneer preparation involves the following steps:

a. Preparation of Matrix

The preparation is carried out using matrix or without matrix. The matrix is indicated in cases where the involved tooth presents color alteration with normal shape and position (no linguo-version, tipping or any other mal-positioning); however, if the tooth has altered shape and positioning, the matrix is not advised.

The matrix technique saves time and allows replication of form, contour and texture of the original tooth surface. The matrix technique can also be used for making provisional veneers. The matrix should preferably be prepared during the diagnostic/planning visit.

The preparation of matrix is carried out as follows:

i. The retraction cord with a diameter equal to the dimensions of the gingival sulcus is selected (No. 07 cord is considered ideal). The cord is carefully introduced into the gingival sulcus on the labial and proximal surface. A new smaller piece is then inserted on top of the first cord. Liquid vaseline is applied to the concerned tooth and the adjacent teeth. If any tooth involved in making the matrix has a composite restoration, it must be coated with vaseline.

ii. The powder and liquid of a colorless acrylic resin are placed in a separate dappen dishes. Using a No. 00 brush, the monomer is applied on the labial and proximal surfaces.

iii. A brush wetted in the monomer is dipped into the polymer and the mix is applied to the tooth surface. The application of acrylic resin should start from the gingival region to incisal area and then on to the proximal surfaces.

iv. The second cord is removed from the sulcus, leaving the first one positioned to keep the sulcus open. This procedure permits the acrylic resin to flow into the region. When placing resin on the proximal surface, it should cover the proximal surfaces and not extend palatally. (If acrylic resin is polymerized on the palatal surface, it will be difficult to remove the matrix.)

v. The matrix is removed gently with appropriate instruments.

vi. The internal surface of the matrix should be carefully inspected to detect air bubbles or other imperfections, which are rectified accordingly. Sharp edges in the incisal-palatal and proximal regions can be removed with a sand paper disc. The matrix is then tried in the mouth. If adequate, it is stored in water until the veneer is made.

vii. On the day scheduled to place the veneer, the matrix is taken out from the water, dried with air and lubricated with liquid vaseline on both its internal and external sides. Lubrication is necessary to prevent the restorative resin from uniting chemically with the matrix.

b. *Preparation of the Tooth*

Depth of preparation depends upon the degree of discoloration of tooth. For teeth free from discoloration or presenting only a discrete discoloration, the preparation depth is less; whereas in teeth with severe discoloration, the depth is accordingly increased depending upon the severity of discoloration. The tooth preparation is carried out as:

i. A central depth cut in a gingivo-incisal direction is made using the appropriate round bur. The 0.5 mm depth cut must be made at the center of the labial surface and 0.3 mm at the cervical area for non-discolored teeth. Depth cut is accordingly increased for discolored teeth and is slightly increased from middle-third to incisal area for both non-discolored and discolored teeth.

ii. Multiple depth cuts in a gingivo-incisal direction are made on the labial surface, maintaining the labial gingivo-incisal convexity by positioning the diamond point vertically at three or more different angles.

iii. After making depth cuts, the distal half of the labial surface is reduced following the gingivo-incisal convexity. Reduction should extend into the labial embrasure.

iv. For non-discolored teeth, preparation should extend short of proximal contact; whereas teeth with mild or severe discoloration require extension into the proximal contact by about 0.1–0.2 mm. It is advisable to check the embrasure areas from several angles to assure that the preparation includes all visible areas. After preparing the distal half on the labial surface and the proximal area, the prepared tooth should be evaluated for the preparation depth. If insufficient, depth should be increased.

v. After careful examination of the distal-proximal areas, the mesial half of the labial surface and the mesio-proximal surface is prepared. Particular attention should be given to the dynamic visibility area. The preparation should follow the labial surface convexity of the tooth to adequate depth.

vi. After the completion of labial and proximal reduction, the incisal finish line is defined. When lengthening the tooth is indicated, a chamfer will be prepared at the incisal edge. This chamfer must extend from mesial to distal including the proximal surfaces (Fig. 9.1).

vii. Finally, evaluate whether the margins are to be extended subgingivally or not. A round-ended diamond point is used to establish the subgingival extension, if required. A 0.1 mm extension is sufficient for non-discolored teeth; whereas, 0.3 mm is needed for severely discolored teeth.

viii. The finished preparation is examined to detect any darkened tooth surface, which might be visible when the tooth is restored. The finish line should be well-defined with continuous chamfer.

c. Isolation

The teeth to be prepared for veneer laminates should be isolated using rubber dam (absolute isolation). Alternatively, cotton rolls can also be used (relative isolation).

If the preparation has a subgingival extension, a retraction cord is placed in the gingival sulcus (Figs 9.2a–c) to prevent sulcus fluid from contaminating the conditioned tooth surface (Fig. 9.3). It also facilitates complete visualization of the cervical margin. A specially designed matrix can also be useful in achieving the isolation. This matrix offers a perfectly isolated field while permitting visual and mechanical access to cervical and proximal margins.

d. Matrix Try-in

After isolation of the field, the previously fabricated acrylic matrix is positioned onto the

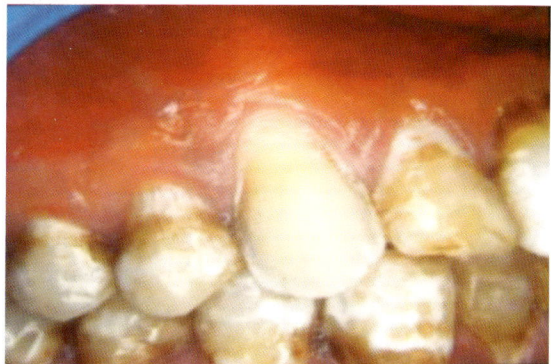

Fig. 9.1: Chamfer placement

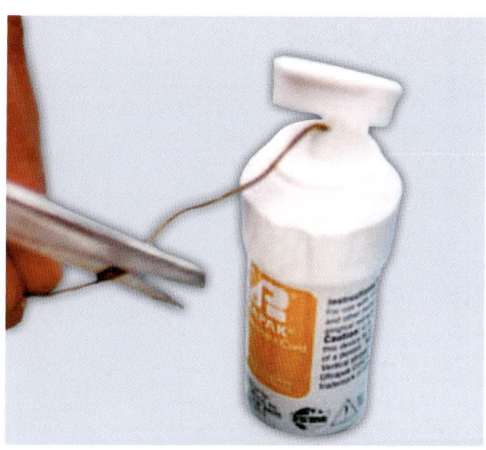

Fig. 9.2a: Gingival retraction cord

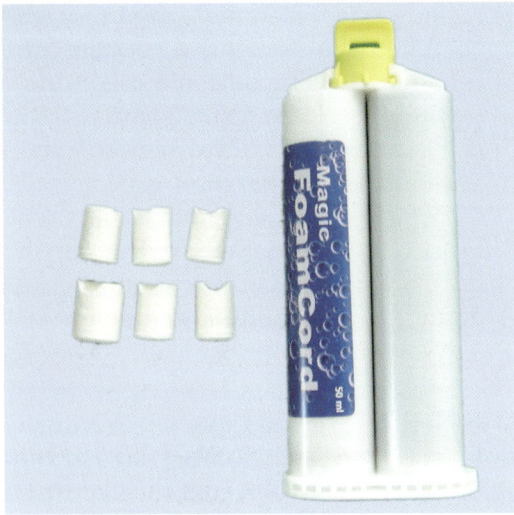

Fig. 9.2b: Foamcord retraction system

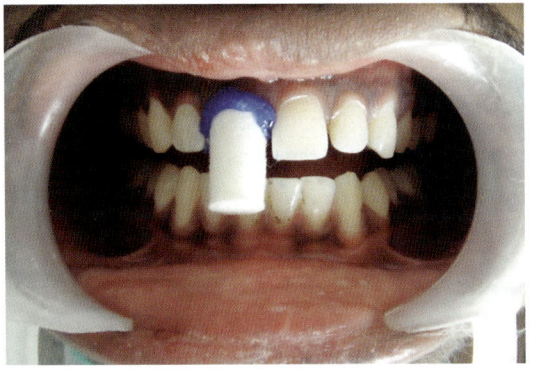

Fig. 9.2c: Clinical use of foamcord

prepared tooth and evaluated. The matrix must be positioned several times to facilitate its insertion and to check its extensions beyond the margins.

Since it is made before the preparation, it may extend beyond the finish lines causing difficulties with the restoration. To avoid such problems, the acrylic resin should be extended into the gingival sulcus when the matrix is made. A better idea of the final thickness of restoration is gained during the matrix try-in.

e. Acid Etching

After achieving the isolation, a Mylar strip is positioned in the inter-dental space of the concerned tooth and the adjacent tooth. To prevent the band from interfering with the procedural steps, its end should be passed to palatal surface through the inter-dental spaces of adjacent teeth.

The acid is applied to the prepared tooth extending about 0.1 mm beyond the margins onto the unprepared enamel. The acid should not flow too far beyond the prepared areas (Fig. 9.4).

Acid application must be performed with care to involve areas which need conditioning. After acid application for 15 seconds, the prepared surface is washed and air dried gently (Fig. 9.5). The acid etch is performed similarly over enamel and any exposed dentin. Drying is slightly different in enamel and

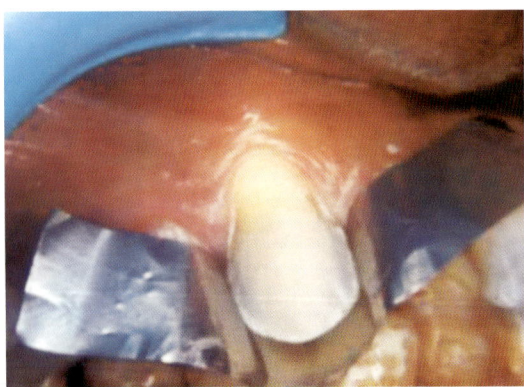

Fig. 9.3: Isolation of the tooth

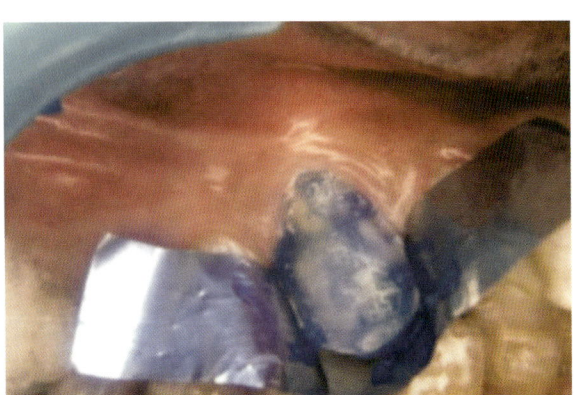

Fig. 9.4: Acid etching

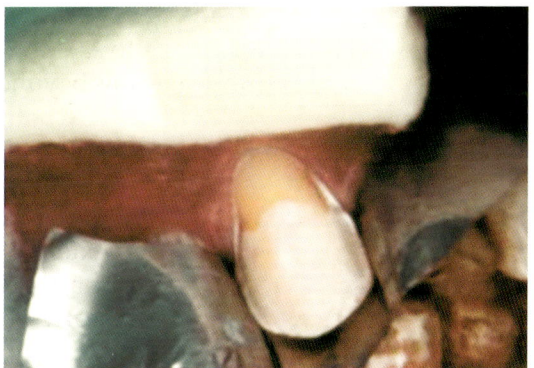
Fig. 9.5: Drying the preparation

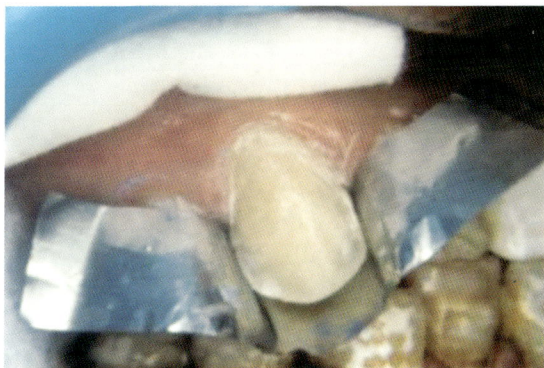
Fig. 9.6: Application of adhesive resin

dentin; an absorbent paper is used on dentin and air on the enamel.

f. Application of the Adhesive System

The manufacturer's recommendations should be followed properly. The sequence of use of adhesive components, if not followed, may lead to restoration failure. The adhesive application after acid etching is described here.

In case, where only enamel is involved, the primer is omitted; whereas primer is mandatory in case dentin is involved (dentin involvement may be limited to the discrete areas). Dentin may get involved in enamel free cervical areas. This usually happens where the tooth presents an associated erosion/abrasion lesion. The adhesive resin is applied with sponges or brushes. Resin is spread with a mild air jet and polymerized for 20 seconds (Fig. 9.6).

It is suggested that silane primers along with unfilled resins, enhance the bond between layers of the veneering material. Durability of the bond, however, depends on the composition of the bonding agent.

For veneering composite resin over metals, adhesives such as Metallite, Siloc etc. are used to improve the bond.

g. Insertion of Composite Resins

The choice of composite depends upon the preparation depth. Two types of composites are mainly used; hybrid is used for bulk internally and microfilled is used on the external surface. Two types of composites, facilitate teeth exhibiting different hues in the cervical, middle and incisal regions. Hybrid resin is responsible for producing these hues.

Different shades of resins are placed in layers so as to achieve uniform gradation of shacks in different regions of teeth. The cervical increment is extended over about 50% of the area targeted for the central increment. Next, the incisal increment is positioned over about 50% of the central increment also. The central increment is positioned last. These resin increments can be applied on the tooth surface with a syringe or a composite spatula. Each increment is 'spread' with a camel hairbrush or the spatula itself after application to the tooth surface (Fig. 9.7).

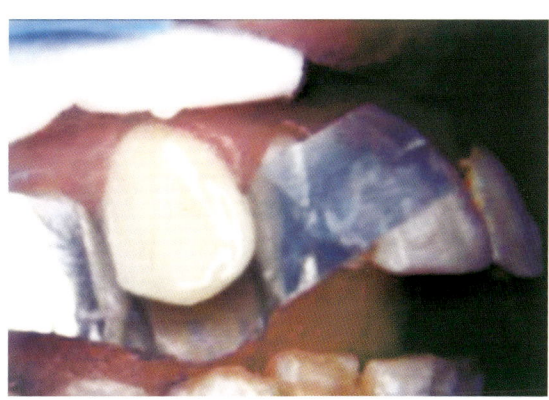
Fig. 9.7: Placement of composite resin

The hybrid region is spread evenly leaving uniform space for microfilled composite. Both are polymerized individually.

To polymerize hybrid resin increments, light is positioned from the palatal side of the tooth for 60 seconds for each increment. Since, resin shrinkage occurs in the direction of the light, it is intentionally directed towards tooth structure. Then the curing of each increment is carried out from labial side for 60 seconds.

After polymerization of the hybrid resin, only one increment of microfill resin is applied to cover the hybrid resin entirely and extending beyond the enamel margins.

The acrylic matrix is positioned to check the hybrid resin not impinging on the space to be filled with microfill resin. Liquid vaseline is used to lubricate the surfaces of the matrix after try-in process.

The excess vaseline is removed from the matrix by a mild air jet and the microfill resin is spread in the matrix. There should be thin increment of resin in the matrix according to the space available. Care is taken to avoid incorporation of air bubbles in resin. Matrix with microfill resin should be carefully positioned and properly seated. The excess resin must be removed with an explorer. The resin is light cured for 60 seconds from cervical to incisal region. Using a spoon excavator, matrix is removed carefully and resin is polymerized for an additional 60 seconds.

h. Finishing and Polishing

The finishing and polishing should ideally be carried out at a later appointment; allows hygroscopic expansion of the resin and result in better marginal adaptation. Primary finishing can be initiated with rubber dam still positioned or following its removal. The gingival margins are better finished if the rubber dam is removed. Protect the gingival tissues by retracting with a gingival retractor.

A No.12 scalpel blade is used to remove excess resin and adhesive from gingival areas and proximal embrasures. Fine diamond points can also be used. Do not 'clip' the resin at marginal area. The scalpel blade is used from resin towards the tooth. Functional contacts of restoration have to be adequately adjusted. Patient is instructed to avoid contact with the dyes particularly artificial ones.

The detection of white lines is indicative of deficient marginal adaptation. Deficient area is acid etched and sealed with the resin region. (The area of deficiency can be widened for better result.)

Final finishing and polishing can be carried out with or without water coolants. Water, though avoids overheating, may interfere with the visualization of tooth/resin interface.

It is established that dry polishing of composite resins elevate surface temperature to approximately 140–200°C, increasing surface hardness of resin and diminishing surface porosity by producing artificial 'resinous mud'.

Final polishing can be carried out with abrasive points/discs specially designed for composite resin. Decreasing order of abrasiveness is preferred. The finer grit disc should be used at a higher speed to give luster to the surface. After the discs have been used, minor intricacies of texture can be modified using a fine grit diamond point. Finishing and polishing on proximal regions is carried out with plastic backed discs. Inter-proximal finishing strips are effective for areas that cannot be reached by the discs (Fig. 9.8).

Use of Color Modifiers (Intrinsic characterization)

Various shades and degrees of translucency of composite resins are due to use of various color modifiers (dyes, pigments or tints). They are free flowing low viscosity composite resins (approximately 20% filled by weight). Titanium dioxide and ferrous oxides are added to achieve different shades.

The less viscous resins (color modifiers) can be used in two ways, viz.

i. Color modifiers incorporated in base paste or composite resin mix and

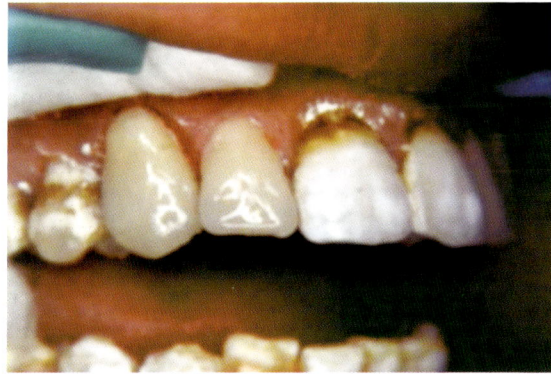

Fig. 9.8: Finishing the laminates

ii. As intrinsic characterizers applied and polymerized between layers of restorative resin. They should never be used on external surface of restoration. Mixing the color modifiers and restorative resin may incorporate air bubbles interfering with esthetic results. This creates a restorative resin with substantially lower filler particle content leading to lowered physical properties.

Limitations of Tints

- The depth and intensity of color of tooth
- The background thickness/depth of discoloration
- Depth of preparation
- Thickness of first layer of restorative composite resin applied
- Shading of restorative resin between the tooth and the tint

Advantages of Tints

- To mask a dark background (opaquers for darkened teeth)
- To mask white-opaque, yellow/brown tooth background (hypoplastic/fluorosed teeth)
- To mask a metallic post
- To replicate special features, viz. areas of hypoplasia, fracture lines and localized areas of color concentration

- To reproduce/create an incisal translucency
- To emphasize developmental sulci, inclines, and lobes on the tooth
- To characterize pit and fissure areas in posterior teeth

The tints are used with soft brushes in thin individually polymerized layers between increments of restorative resin; they should never be used on restoration surface.

The tints are mostly white, blue, red, yellow and brown. White is used to mask the dark background/hypoplastic areas. Blue is used to simulate the incisal translucency. Red is used to eliminate the bluish-gray color of teeth stained by tetracycline. Yellow and brown simulate gingival tones.

The composite resin shades like incisal (translucent), cervical (yellowish or brown), dentin (more opaque) and enamel (more translucent) satisfy majority of esthetic requirements of these restorations.

The incisal region presents voluminous enamel particularly in young teeth. This area warrants the need of translucency; however, incisal contour can be more or less uniform. The restoration of incisal contour varies from a uniform contour of whole incisal region to an irregular contour in-between the developmental lobes. Such details can appropriately be reproduced with tints.

Opaquers

The opaquers are the resinous materials applied as a thin film over the tooth surface facilitating blocking the passage of light onto the restoration. The opaquers can mask a dark background; achieving final shade as required for the final restoration.

There are two types of routinely used opaquers: (i) Opaque restorative resins (identified by the letter 'O') and (ii) Opaque tints (fluid resins similar to those used to provide characterization). Glass-ionomer cements, being opaque, can be used as direct opaquers. There is limited space available for the composite resin in a direct veneer;

therefore, an opaquer that can be easily applied as thin film is preferred.

The amount of opacification needed depends on background darkness to be masked and on the final veneer thickness. This is in turn related to the tooth position in the arch and color of the tooth. The darker the background, the more opaquer is required (tetracycline stains, very dark non-vital teeth).

Opaquer is applied preferably in one increment after the tooth preparation. It must be sufficient to mask the dark background of the tooth or metal post. Procedures to bond opaque to the tooth are same as adhesion. These materials must be fully cured when the restorative resin is inserted.

The opacification results can be evaluated by applying opaque in small areas and visualizing the masking effect. In case, the results are not satisfactory, the opaquer can be modified.

Liquid opaquers (tints) must be bonded between two cured adhesive resin layers and not applied on margins or on the incisal area. The opacification achieved by liquid opaquers and compatible resins generally give best esthetic results.

A material that is chemically compatible with resin composites should be used; the opaquer should be light curable and able to mask the dark tones with ease.

Two clinical cases depicting diastema and re-aligning anterior teeth are shown in Figs 9.9 a and b and 9.10 a, b and c.

B. Indirect Composite Resin Veneers

The indirect resin veneers have superior shade qualities and control of facial contours. As they are composed of microfill resins, they can be polished to a lustrous finish. The limited bond strength achieved with indirect veneers restricts their use to cases not involving heavy functional contacts (prone to chipping and fracture). These are beneficial in saving chairside time.

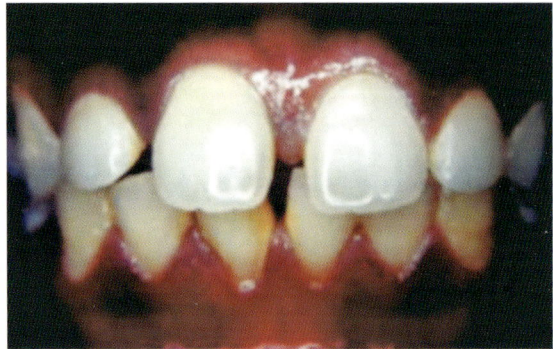

Fig. 9.9a: Diastema

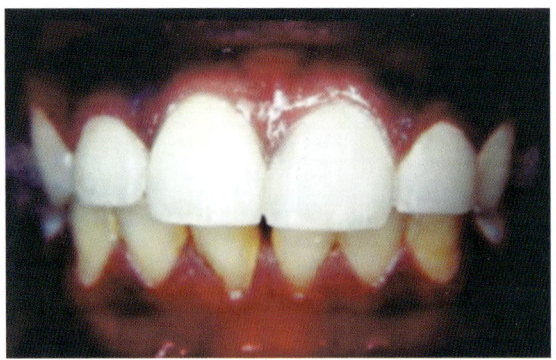

Fig. 9.9b: Postoperative

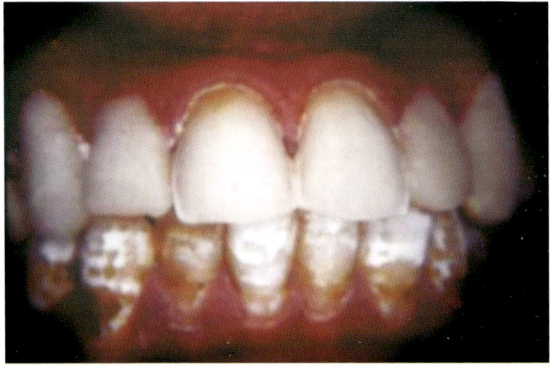

Fig. 9.10a: Preoperative

Clinical Technique

Indirect composite resin veneers are fabricated in a laboratory. Shade selection is carried out prior to isolation of the teeth in order to eliminate shade variations that can occur because of drying and dehydration of the teeth. Both body and incisal shades of

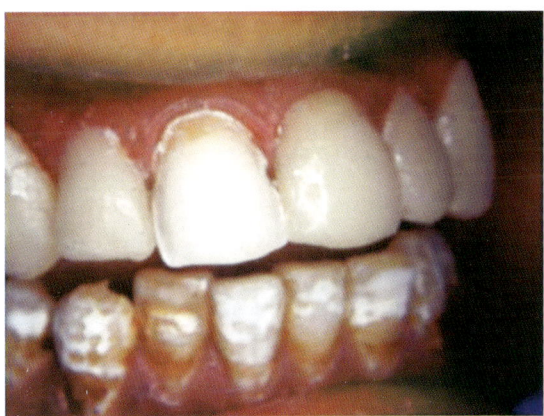

Fig. 9.10b: Prepared central incisor

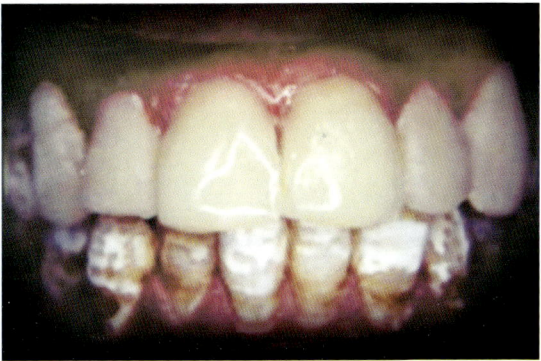

Fig. 9.10c: Postoperative

composite resin are available, which can be selected for final restorations.

Teeth are isolated with use of absorbent cotton rolls and gingival retraction cord. Carious lesions, if present, should be restored prior to initiating the veneer preparations. The defective restoration, if any, should also be replaced.

Teeth to be veneered are prepared with a bevel ended diamond point to a depth approximately equivalent to enamel thickness. The depth of reduction ranges from 0.5 to 0.6 mm midlabially to 0.2–0.3 mm along the gingival/cervical aspect of the preparation. Greater depth is required, in case, intrinsic stains are present. However, the entire preparation should preferably be restricted to enamel to facilitate better acid etching.

A no. ¼ round bur (0.4 mm in diameter), is suited for gauging the depth cuts. This allows inspection of remaining unprepared tooth structure in cross-section following preparation of only one-half of the labial surface. A moderate chamfer should be created along the margins of the preparation. The inter-proximal margins should be extended beyond the inter-proximal line angles of the tooth. Gingival margin is prepared at the level of free gingival crest or slightly subgingival. Subgingival extension should preferably be avoided. Incisally, preparation should be restricted to labial aspect of the incisal edge and should never be terminated in an area subjected to occlusal function.

An impression of the prepared teeth is made following removal of the gingival retraction cord. A working cast with individually removable dies of the prepared teeth is fabricated.

The prepared tooth/teeth are thoroughly cleaned with a flour of pumice or a fluoride-free cleansing agent. Teeth are once again isolated with cotton rolls. A try-in of veneer is a must to evaluate the fit. Minor adjustments can be carried out with suitable composite resin finishing instruments.

If the inner aspect of veneer is totally smooth, a coarse diamond point should be used to slightly roughen the underside of veneer, thus improving the potential for additional micro-mechanical bonding. Care must be taken not to contaminate the underside of veneer prior to bonding.

A thin film of bonding agent is placed on the etched enamel but not yet cured. The veneer is then loaded with a homogenous pre-selected resin, approximately 0.5 mm thick and is seated on the tooth. Veneer should be positioned first at gingival margin, allowing excess cement to extrude incisally as the veneer is fully seated. Care should be taken so as the air should not enter between tooth and veneer. The veneer should be held firmly in place till polymerization.

The underlying bonding medium is polymerized for 40 seconds from both labial and lingual directions. If a layer of opaque resin is added into the resin veneer, then curing time should be doubled. Excess material is removed using appropriate instruments. Gingival retraction cord should be removed to facilitate access and visibility. After polymerization, occlusion must be evaluated for any functional interferences. Protrusive and lateral functional contacts should preferably be restricted to enamel.

The surface glaze of unfilled resin on the labial surface of the veneer may wear away easily. A highly lustrous surface can be re-established through conventional chair side finishing and polishing techniques (Fig. 9.11a and b).

Conditioning Sequence for Tooth and The Veneer

i. For enamel surface pre-treatment
- Cleaning with pumice
- Rinsing with clean water
- Application of mylar strips around teeth to be conditioned
- Etching of enamel surface (37% phosphoric acid for 15 seconds)
- Rinsing with clean water
- Adhesive application

ii. For composite veneer pre-treatment
- Sandblasting with aluminium oxide particles
- Ultrasonic bath in ethanol to remove remnant particles
- Coupling agent application and evaporation
- Adhesive application
- Resin composite application on the inner surface of the veneer

COMPONEERS

Componeers are prefabricated composite veneers (Fig. 9.12), especially manufactured in thin shells that can be fixed onto the labial surfaces of teeth. The procedure is easy, immediate and economical. The indications are the same as for other veneers, such as correcting minor defects, gaps, tooth discoloration, broken edges, etc. The advantages are improved esthetics in one visit, customized

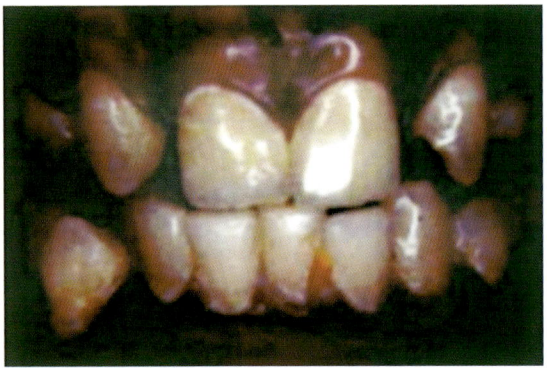
Fig. 9.11a: Preoperative

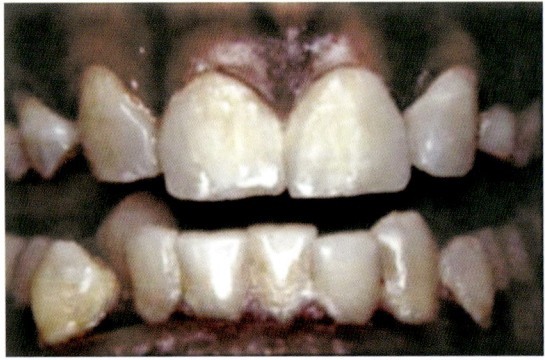
Fig. 9.11b: Postoperative

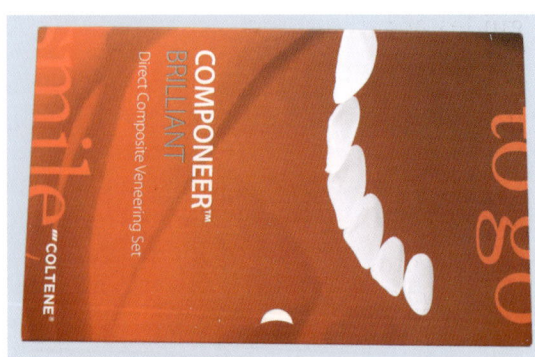
Fig. 9.12: Componeer kit

shaping of front teeth and economical. The shine of the veneer can be refreshed by polishing. The componeers are cemented using the same cementing agent, thereby improving bonding (Figs 9.13a-m).

Procedure

The procedure involves the following steps:

- The rubber dam sheet is cut from second premolar (15) to second premolar (25) and the clamps are fitted on the 1st molars (16 and 26) on both sides (use of split rubber dam). The rubber dam is fixed as shown in Figs 9.13a and b. The loose ends on the dam are attached to the mucous membrane area with the help of butyl cyanoacrylate.

- *Enamel preparation:* Minimal tooth preparation is required for componeers (thickness of componeer is 0.3 mm at the cervical margin, which increases to 0.5 mm at the middle and 0.7 mm at the incisal edge). Only roughening of the enamel is enough for patients who agree for a little protrusion, but if it is a single tooth component where arch form has to be maintained, the 0.3 to 0.5 mm of reduction is required (Fig. 9.13c). Inter-dental areas are also roughened to accommodate the thickness of composite. A diamond coated single sided re-contouring strip is required for inter-proximal preparation of enamel.

- *Size selection:* The size of the componeer is selected with the help of contour guides provided in the kit (Fig. 9.13d). The contour guides are transparent and light blue in color to complement the color of the tooth. The rule is that the componeer should cover the width of the tooth and if the componeer is longer cervico-incisally, it should be adequately trimmed (Fig. 9.13e).

- 37% phosphoric acid etching (Fig. 9.13f) is carried out for 15 seconds followed by rinsing for 10 seconds.

- After drying the tooth surface, appropriate gingival retraction cord is placed in the free gingival margin of prepared teeth.

- Two layers of 5th generation bond is applied to the prepared teeth (first one is rubbed for 15 seconds with nylon tufted brushes). After the application of 1st layer and air blowing it, mylar strips are placed between the teeth and then the second layer is applied (Fig. 9.13g). The bonding agent is light cured for 20 seconds lingually and then 20 seconds buccally. The same bonding agent is applied on the inner surface of the componeer, which is held with the help of componeer holder (provided in the kit) and air blown (this layer is not light cured).

- The chosen shade of composite is applied on the inner surface of componeer and the same composite is applied on the bonded tooth surface.

- The componeer is compressed on the tooth surface and pushed into its final position with the help of componeer placer (provided in the kit) which has a concave silicon tip (Fig. 9.13h). The extra composite (flash), which comes out, should be removed with MB-C Instrument (provided in the kit) (Fig. 9.13i). After the final placement of the componeer, it should be light cured for 30 seconds both lingually and buccally.

- The composite in the inter-dental areas should be removed with fine tapered instruments (Fig. 9.13j, k). The inter-dental polishing is carried out with composite polishing strips. The buccal surface of the

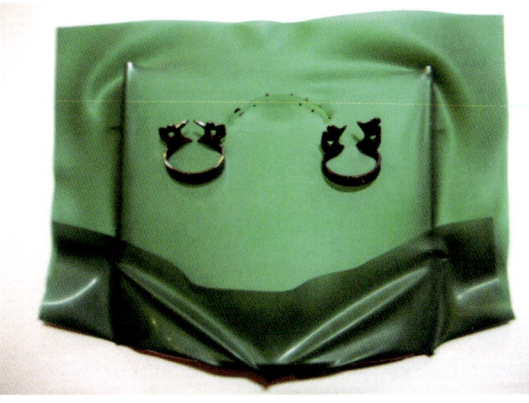

Fig. 9.13a: Rubber dam preparation

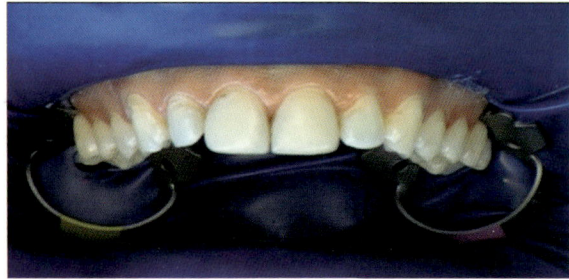

Fig. 9.13b: Rubber dam application

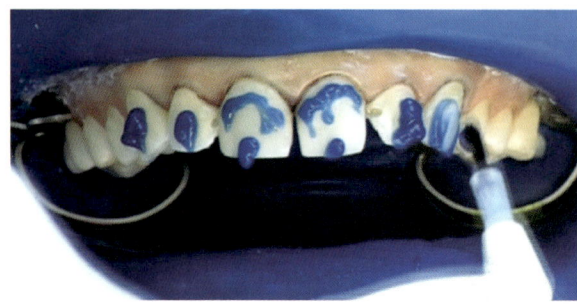

Fig. 9.13f: Etching

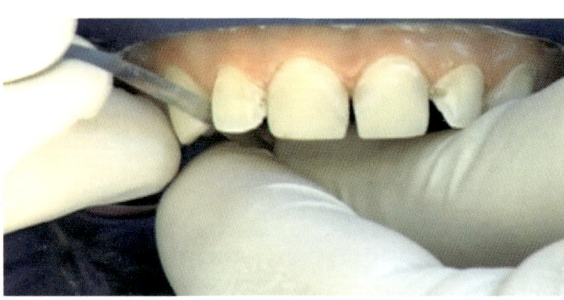

Fig. 9.13c: Enamel preparation

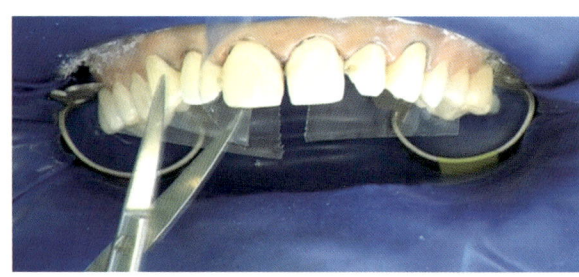

Fig. 9.13g: Mylar strip adjustment

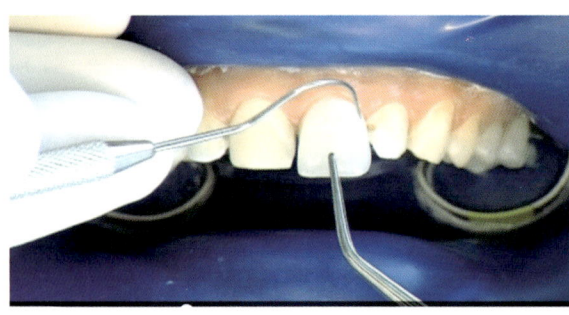

Fig. 9.13d: Selection of componeer

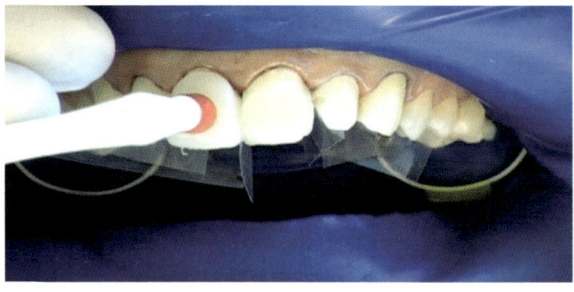

Fig. 9.13h: Compressing the componeer

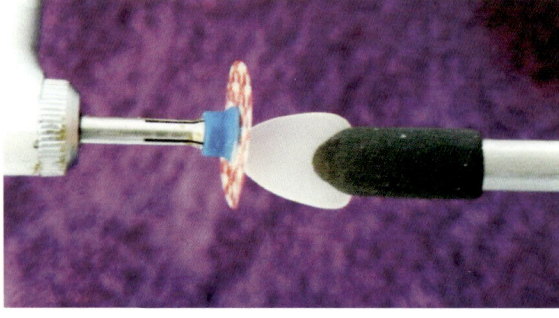

Fig. 9.13e: Minor adjustment (trimming componeer)

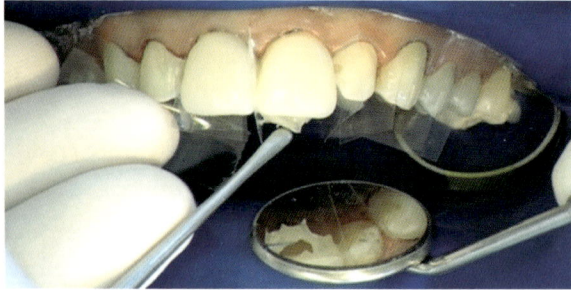

Fig. 9.13i: Removing flash

componeer is polished with pre-polisher
and high gloss silicon polishers provided
in the kit (Fig. 9.13l). The final occlusion is
checked (Fig. 9.13m).

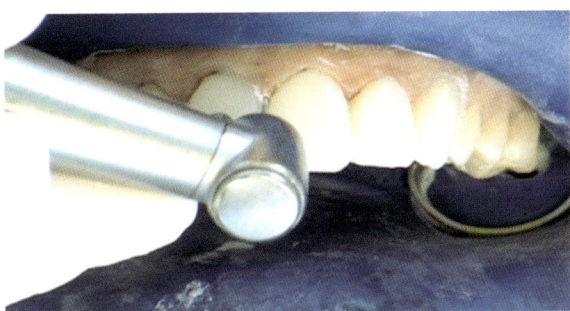

Fig. 9.13j: Finishing interdental areas

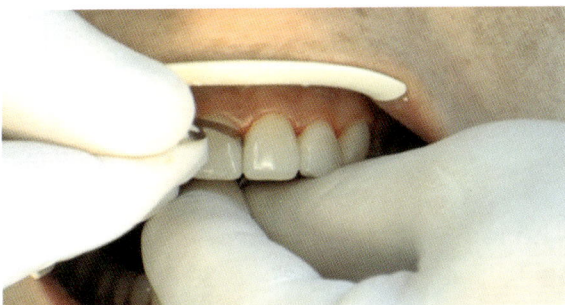

Fig. 9.13k: Finishing interdental areas

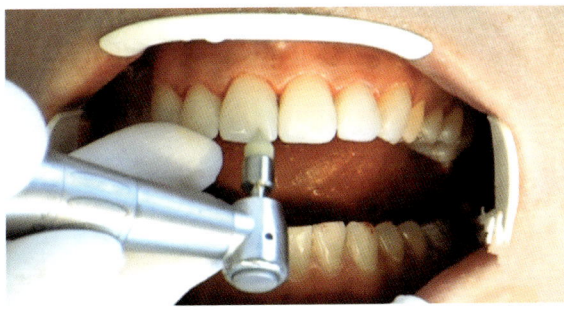

Fig. 9.13l: Polishing

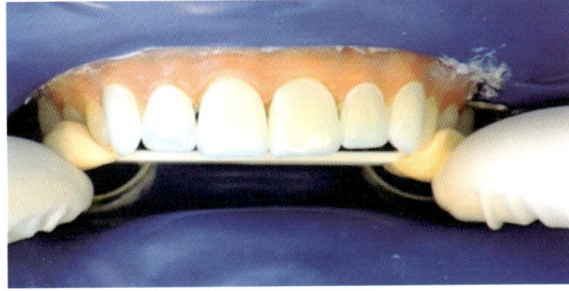

Fig. 9.13m: Final occlusion checking

Advantages

Componeers offer many advantages, such as:
- Minimal invasive, conservative tooth preparation
- No impression required
- Minimum application time required
- Cementation using the same material
- Highly polished surface, esthetically pleasing
- Cost effective

Limitations

The limitations of componeers are:

Two bonding interfaces are involved; first, the inner surface of the processed composite resin veneer and second, the acid-etched enamel. Tensile strength ranges from 2000 to 2750 psi.

The degree of polymerization is significantly greater with indirect resin veneers than that achieved by chair side conventional polymerization techniques; therefore, the potential for establishing strong chemical bonds between the processed veneer and resin-bonding medium is significantly diminished.

The preparations may involve considerable removal of sound tooth substance. The inherent nature of composite resins exhibiting polymerization shrinkage, dimensional changes, staining and poor wear resistance may also lead to poor prognosis.

The microfilled composite resins can achieve satisfactory appearance and shine. However, microfilled composites wear at twice the rate of conventional composites as a result of tooth brushing. To overcome this problem, it is suggested that conventional or hybrid composite should be used to form the bulk of the veneer and a thin layer of microfill composite be placed on the surface for appearance and surface shine. This superficial layer would have to be replaced at intervals.

The acrylic veneers could overcome some of these problems; however, the restored teeth being bulky, coupled with weak chemical bond between cement and veneer may lead to failure.

Both composite and acrylic veneers have a dull, monochromatic appearance. Low abrasion resistance leading to loss of contour and staining, and loss of surface luster, biological incompatibility with gingival tissue, limited bond between laminates and composite, were the major drawbacks of these resin veneers.

PORCELAIN LAMINATE

The development of porcelain veneers and the associated technique for their fabrication were developed in early 80s. Earlier, porcelain for veneering was built up in layers on a platinum foil matrix adapted to the cast. Etched silanated porcelain blocks have also been used to restore fractured incisors. At present, a number of systems have been employed including castable, pressable and glass infiltrated ceramics.

Components of Porcelain Laminate Veneer System

A cross section of the veneer system would reveal the following components:

a. Etched Porcelain

The etched unglazed porcelain has long been tried in class IV cavities. Etching the porcelain with 5 to 7% hydrofluoric acid, for varying length of time, increases the bond strength. The bond strength increases from 88 psi (6.0 Mpa) for no etch to 110 psi (7.5 Mpa) for a 20 second etch. In the unetched porcelain, bond failure occurs at the resin/porcelain junction; whereas in etched porcelain, fracture occurs in the body of porcelain.

b. Coupling Agent

Coupling agent is defined as 'an agent, which acts by adsorbing on to and altering the surface of a solid, to facilitate, either a chemical or physical process'. The usual mode of action of coupling agents is by chemically bonding to both the silica in the porcelain and the matrix of the composite resin (or acrylic).

The direct chemical bonding of porcelain teeth to acrylic denture bases by means of coupling agents has been tried. Since, the coefficient of thermal expansion varies, the bond gets deteriorated on bench cooling of heat-cured acrylic. The silane-coupling agents are being used as an integral part of the porcelain laminate veneer system. The bond formed between composite and porcelain is resistant to thermal cycling, owing to similar coefficients of thermal expansion of both porcelain and composite resins.

c. Luting Cements

The low viscosity luting agent with small particle size is required for good adaptation. The limited working time of the self-curing luting agents caused some seating problems with the earlier veneers. Light-cured cements provided longer working time with similar physical properties. Dual-cure cements (both chemical and light-cure systems), ensure maximum polymerization of the resin, while retaining the option of an extended working time. The details of luting cements are described in Chapter 12.

Advantages of Porcelain Laminates

Porcelain laminates offer the following advantages:

  i. *Color:* Since, the porcelains are available in different colors, they can be used in variable degrees of discoloration and offer better color control and stability.
 ii. *Bond strength:* The bond of etched porcelain veneer enamel is considerably stronger than any other veneering system.
iii. *Periodontal health:* The highly glazed porcelain surface resists deposition of plaque, thus maintaining periodontal health.

iv. *Resistance to abrasion:* The wear and abrasion resistance is exceptionally good.

v. *Inherent porcelain strength:* Porcelain has good compressive strength but poor flexural strength. The strength, however, increases considerably after the restoration is bonded to the tooth.

vi. *Resistance to fluid absorption:* Porcelain absorbs less fluid than any other veneering material.

vii. *Esthetics:* The esthetics is significantly better than any other veneering material because ceramic has the ability to control color and the surface texture.

Disadvantages of Porcelain Laminates

The disadvantages of porcelain laminates are:

i. *Technique sensitive:* The placement of veneers is technique sensitive.

ii. *Repair:* The veneers cannot be easily repaired once they are luted to the enamel.

iii. *Time:* The process of placing veneers require two visits; preparation/ impression making and luting.

iv. *Color:* It is difficult to modify the color once the veneers are luted in position on the enamel surface.

v. *Tooth preparation:* Precisional preparation is required to avoid overcontouring.

vi. *Fragility:* The veneers are fragile, especially, when pre-bond adjustment is required.

Indications

The indications for ceramic laminate veneers are:

i. Tooth discoloration (fluorosis, endodontically treated teeth and tetracycline staining) resistant to bleaching procedures. The color changes due to irreversible process of aging can also be masked by porcelain laminates.

ii. The teeth requiring morphologic modifications.

- Conical teeth (peg laterals)
- Closure of diastemas
- Elongation of incisal edges
- Various types of enamel hypoplasias

iii. Rehabilitation of compromised anterior dentition.

- Extended coronal fractures
- Congenital and acquired malformations
- *Malpositioned teeth:* Developing the esthetic illusion of straight teeth where orthodontists have limitations due to prolonged treatment time.
- *Malocclusion:* The configuration of anterior teeth can be changed to develop incisal guidance or centric holding contacts in malocclusion, especially, in periodontally compromised teeth.
- *Poor restorations:* Teeth with unesthetic restorations on labial surfaces can be restored with laminates.
- *Wear patterns:* Porcelain laminates are useful in those cases that exhibit slow progressive wear patterns.

Contraindications

The contraindications are:

i. Teeth with poor quality enamel or insufficient sound enamel. There should be enamel around the whole periphery of the laminates for good bonding.
The sufficient enamel should be available for bonding, because bonding to dentin provides much less retention than to enamel. If the tooth lacks enamel and is composed predominantly of dentin, then ceramic crowns will be the treatment of choice.

ii. Rotated or overlapped teeth present problems in the placement of the veneers. Broken down teeth also offer limited support for veneers.

iii. Patients with oral habits, such as bruxism or habit of rubbing foreign objects to teeth are not suited for veneers. The porcelain veneer may not bear the shearing stress created by such habits.

Types of Ceramic Veneers

The types of ceramic veneer include:

i. *Conventional powder-slurry ceramic (feldspathic porcelain):* This type of porcelain is layered on the refracting dies in the laboratory.

ii. *Heat-pressed ceramic:* The products are melted at high temperature and pressed into a metal using the lost-wax technique (IPS Impress).

iii. CAD/CAM, machineable ceramic (CEREC)

Pre-restorative Evaluation

The color transparencies provide a useful reference for characterization in the laboratory and for future reference. The shade of the existing teeth and the proposed shade of the restored teeth should be decided upon and recorded. The shade should be thoroughly discussed with the patient before finalizing.

The patient's static and dynamic occlusal relationships should also be assessed. Contact relationships between the incisors and canines in centric occlusion and during excursive movements will be a major determining factor for deciding the positions of porcelain finish line at the incisal level.

Presence of incisal facets may lead to unsupported porcelain on incisal edges, especially on canines. Loss of posterior support with anterior posture of the mandible; edge to edge or class III incisor relation, will influence the choice of treatment modality.

Fundamental Principles

A number of clinical studies involving ceramic veneers observed satisfactory success rates. In order to achieve better results with ceramic veneers, the following fundamental principles must be considered:

i. Bonding to Enamel Substrate

In spite of considerable improvement in the field of dentin bonding, the longevity of ceramic veneer is accepted to be dependent upon the amount of enamel substrate supporting it. The difficulty of dentin bonding vis-à-vis ceramic veneer is the disparity in flexibility between a rigid veneer and elastic dentin. The selection of teeth without labial enamel or removal of enamel for veneers is an attempt to match the high elastic modulus porcelain with lower elastic modulus dentin. The functional loading of the veneered tooth will transfer this energy to the porcelain-tooth interface resulting in debonding or cracking of the porcelain. It is established that greater the amount of dentin involved during laminate preparation, the greater will be chances of opting full veneer crowns.

ii. Replaced Old Restorations/ Restore Minor Teeth

The old restorations should be removed prior to bonding in order to ensure better bonding to the luting agent. The removal can be carried out at the time of cementation of the veneer. The fresh substrate without any contamination is preferred for better bonding. Minor defects are also prepared in similar way; deeper defects, however, can be filled with composites.

iii. Avoid Heavy Occlusal Loads

It is accepted that the veneers gain considerable strength after bonding; however, its brittle nature cannot be overlooked. A relative brittle veneer is vulnerable to heavy occlusal loading. In case of heavy occlusal loading and/or parafunctional habits leading to tooth wear, full veneer crown is recommended. Alternatively, high strength porcelains, such as Procera, can be used, compromising esthetics to some extent (thickness may display opaque look).

iv. *Inability to Mask Deep and Intense Discoloration*

Veneers become less useful, in case, the discoloration is deep and intense. The veneer needs to be of sufficient thickness in order to mask the color effectively, which means cutting a deeper preparation than usually recommended for ceramic veneers. This results in preparation in dentin, which is not conducive for laminate success. In addition, as preparation reaches deeper and deeper, its shade becomes increasingly dark, making it difficult to mask. High opaque porcelain (Procera) is selected in such cases, compromising with esthetics.

v. *Avoid Veneer in Crowding*

Veneers are successfully used to treat spacing; however, in case of crowding, the selection of veneer should be judicious. In case of crowding, it is likely that the tooth preparation may involve dentin, which should be avoided by all means. The crowding should be treated orthodontically and the minor correction, if need be, can be carried out by veneers.

Similarly, restoring mandibular anterior teeth with veneers is technically difficult due to their small size and thin enamel available, coupled with inadequate access. Full crowns are better choice in such cases.

Tooth Preparation

There is no single and ideal way to prepare teeth for porcelain laminates. The choice of tooth preparation depends upon multiple factors. The decision whether to reduce the enamel or not; if to reduce, then to what extent, should depend on the following features:

- Esthetics
- Relative position of the tooth in the arch
- Depth/extent of discoloration
- Placement of margins
- Age of the patient
- The potential for periodontal problems
- Maintaining oral hygiene

The enamel is prepared or reduced achieving the features such as:
- To provide an adequate space for the porcelain material.
- To provide a path of insertion; the incisal or the inter-proximal extensions are to be included in the veneer. The best path of insertion would require the least amount of enamel reduction.
- To provide space for the opaquer.
- To prepare a receptive enamel surface for etching and bonding the laminate.
- To facilitate sulcular margin placement in severely discolored teeth.

The tooth may and may not require enamel reduction. In the young patient or where teeth are in linguo-version or retro-inclined or of abnormal shape like peg-shaped laterals, reduction of enamel can usually be avoided. However, where there is a need to mask out discoloration or modify the contours, a reduction of the enamel surface is mandatory.

Armamentarium

The armamentarium required for preparation:
- Basic instruments, like handpiece, lip retractor, mirror, etc.
- High speed diamond points
- Three-tier depth cutting burs (LVS-I: 0.3 mm depth and LVS-2: 0.5 mm depth)
- High speed two-grit burs (LVS-3 and LVS-4)
- Dental floss
- Sharp, dark pencil
- Retraction cord and associated instruments
- Abrasive finishing and polishing discs

Procedure

The preparation is carried out following the sequence as:
1. Labial reduction
2. Inter-proximal reduction/extension
3. Gingival/sulcular extension
4. Establishment of finish line/margin
5. Incisal reduction
6. Lingual reduction

1. Labial Reduction

Labial preparation and the amount of reduction should facilitate the placement of the restoration. Preparation should remain within the enamel and should include all the peripheral margins to ensure an adequate seal to enamel. The minimum reduction of enamel virtually eliminates the need of temporary cover. In certain cases, to facilitate cosmetic alignment, some amount of dentin is to be exposed by the preparation of tooth. This may not be critical if it is limited to only small areas and the peripheral margins remain on enamel. Reduction is usually carried out without local anaesthesia.

The operator decides the depth of enamel reduction and selects the appropriate diamonds burs. Usually, LVS No. 1 (0.3 mm diameter) is used cervically and LVS No. 2 (diameter of 0.5 mm) incisally (Fig. 9.14). Depth cuts should be 0.5–0.7 mm for maxillary teeth. Cervical to incisal reduction is increased accordingly. Lingually positioned teeth also require less reduction. This type of preparation provides enough surface for the dentin, enamel and translucency layer of porcelain at the cervical end. LVS is drawn gently across the labial surface of the tooth in a mesial to distal direction. This will develop the depth cuts as horizontal grooves, leaving a raised chip of enamel in between (Fig. 9.15). Then, this remaining enamel is removed by using round-ended taper fissure diamonds to

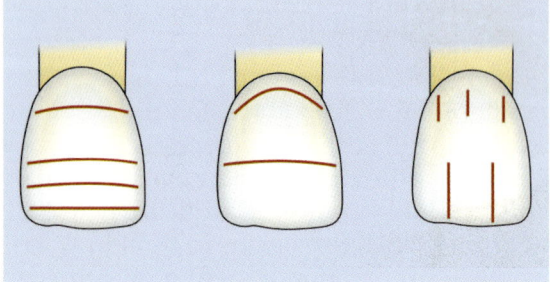

Fig. 9.15: Horizontal and vertical grooves placement

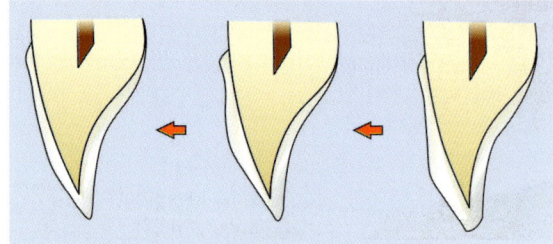

Fig. 9.16: Three plane reduction

the depth of the original grooves. This would reduce the tooth to the desired depth (Fig. 9.16). (To prevent over-reduction, pencil lines are drawn into the prepared depth guide. The labial reduction is completed when the pencil marks are removed by the action of the reduction bur.)

The remaining enamel must be removed up to the depth of the initial cuts.

At the marginal area, it is desirable to use a fine grit diamond that will create a definite smooth finish line to enhance the seal at the periphery.

Move the diamond across the labial surface from a mesial direction, following the contour of the gingiva from top of the mesial inter-proximal aspect to distal inter-proximal aspect. Finish line should preferably be at the gingival margin (Figs 9.17a–c).

2. Inter-proximal Reduction/Extension

The margin of the porcelain laminates should generally be hidden within the embrasure area. Depending on the individual form of the tooth, it is usually desirable to extend this

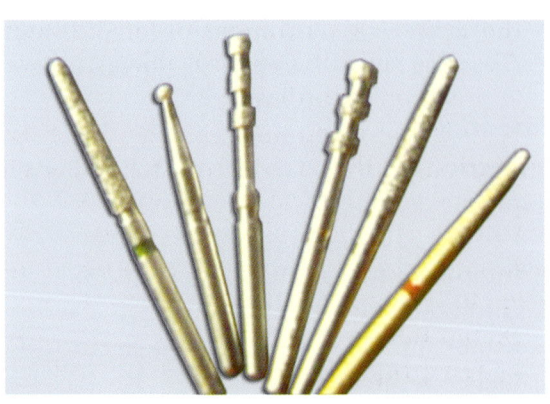

Fig. 9.14: Diamond points

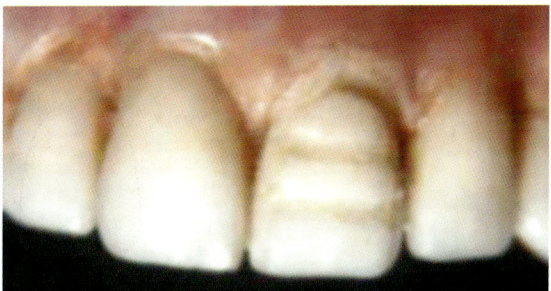

Fig. 9.17a: Horizontal grooves

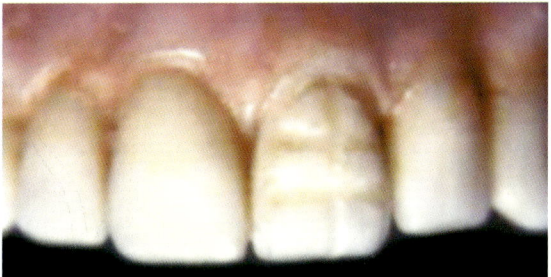

Fig. 9.17b: Vertical grooves

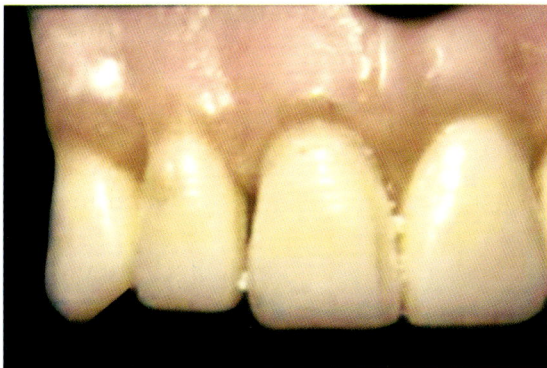

Fig. 9.17c: Prepared tooth

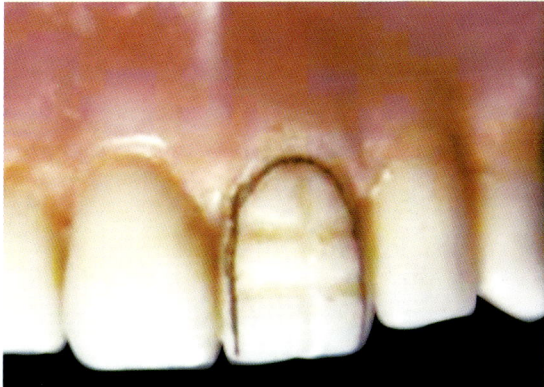

Fig. 9.18: Inter-proximal extension

given to mask the underlying color; unprepared area will display the unesthetic margins.

The proximal reduction depends upon the morphology of contact area and also the need of making the underlying color of the tooth.

- In case of diastema, the finish line should terminate as far as the lingual aspect as possible without creating an undercut area. It should extend from the incisal edge to the point adjacent to the height of the gingival papilla.
- For no diastema and no color change, prepare the proximal chamfer line with LVS-3 and LVS-4 diamond bur, extending 0.2 mm facial to the contact area (the subcontact area is prepared accordingly).
- For teeth exhibiting color changes, prepare proximal chamfer line with LVS-3 and LVS-4 diamond burs, extending one half to the labio-lingual dimension of the inter-proximal contact area (the subcontact area is prepared accordingly).

It is considered useful to have extra reduction in the embrasure area so as to facilitate the addition of porcelain bulk in this region as it improves the strength of the laminate around the whole periphery and also, to achieve a good color control for proximal translucencies.

When preparing a tooth for proximal reduction, operator has three options to

margin about half way into the inter-proximal contact area. Extension of the laminate beyond the proximal contact to the proximo-lingual line angle ensures the wrap-around effect (Fig. 9.18).

The proximal subcontact area (inter-proximal tooth structure immediately gingival to the contact area with the adjacent tooth) should be taken care of. Since, this area is not visible by direct viewing, it is usually left under-prepared or un-prepared. It is essentially important when laminates are

position the proximal margins; (i) labial to the proximal contact, (ii) halfway through the contact, and (iii) lingual to the contact.

i. When the proximal margin of the ceramic veneer is placed labial to the proximal contact of the adjacent tooth, access for finishing is restricted. There is probability of visible stain forming along this margin in future. Such stains, being difficult to remove, make the veneers unesthetic.

ii. Placing the proximal margins halfway through the contact area makes it difficult to section the model to make dies, leading to inaccurate reproduction of the margins.

iii. Placing the proximal margins on lingual surface after breaking the contact, provides benefits as:
- Margins are more accessible for finishing
- Margin stains, if any, in future, will not be visible
- Greater resistance to labio-lingual flexion because of curvature
- Dies can easily be separated without damaging the margins
- Impression making is easier
- Facilitate positioning and seating during cementation
- Veneer display improves proximal contours and esthetics

In case, it is difficult to break both the proximal contacts, it is advisable to involve one contact (placing the margins lingual to that contact) to allow seating of the veneer from the labial side.

3. Gingival/Sulcular Extension

The preparation is usually extended up to the gingival margin; however, in some cases it is extended just within the sulcus. In routine, there is no need to hide the margin subgingivally as in cases of crown bridge procedures. The porcelain with the underlying composite resin will blend harmoniously with the rest of the tooth without showing a cement line. In case, extension is required, there is no need to extend more than 0.05 to 0.1 mm into the sulcus; otherwise, supragingival laminates are preferred if a dramatic color change is not a priority.

The supragingival finish lines are considered advantageous because that increases the likelihood of the margin to end in enamel only; however, the major disadvantage is the subsequent staining or color change at the margins. The supragingival margins are preferred where the area is concealed by lip during smiling; whereas when the entire clinical crown is included in the facial display, the gingival margin is extended 0.1–0.2 mm into the free gingival margin.

Place a gingival displacement cord in the sulcus for about two to three minutes.

Margins first prepared at the gingival margins are visible now, which can be extended into the gingival sulcular area without disturbing the gingival tissues.

This sulcular preparation does not disturb the biologic width area, so there is a little potential of subsequent gingival inflammation. The margin must remain at a point where it will be visible for finishing of the porcelain laminate and will not lead to tissue displacement. The fine grit diamond points cut very slowly, thus reducing the risk of over preparation, especially during extension into the sulcular area.

4. Establishment of Finish Line/Margin

A confluent finish line is established during labial and proximal reduction. The ideal choice of finish line is chamfer or radial shoulder. Customarily, shoulder finish line is preferred for all-ceramic restorations. However, in porcelain laminates, chamfer is preferred. A feather or knife-edge finish line, though conservative, but not advised because it is difficult to accurately fabricate porcelain to the required degree of thinness. The thin margin invariably produces poor marginal fit and potential laboratory problems in delineating the exact end of preparation finish line. Therefore, chamfer is the most acceptable finish line. Finish lines are extended proximally and gingivally by means of a round-ended tapered diamond point. Alternatively, a round bur of 1.2 mm diameter can also be used. When the round bur is held at 45 degree to the surface of the tooth, it creates such a finish line.

Proximal finish line is extended into the embrasures, but kept short of the contact point. The contact is never broken in case finish line extends half way up to the contact area. Rarely, the contact is broken to establish esthetic proximal translucency and is extended to the proximo-lingual line angle. Cervically, the finish line is in level with the contour of the free gingival margin. In absence of any discoloration, the finish line may even be left in a supragingival position; but when the tooth is discolored, it is necessary to extend the finish line subgingivally by 0.5–1.0 mm. The increase in depth of subgingival preparations may result in gingival inflammation and subsequent periodontal tissue loss.

5. Incisal Reduction

The incisal reduction should be at least 1.0 mm, if it is desired to restore the original length. If teeth are to be lengthened, rounding the incisal edge without vertical reduction is sufficient. If incisal edge is to be included, it is useful to increase the horizontal tooth reduction at the periphery of the preparation (inter-proximal areas). The fabrication of a porcelain veneer overlapping the incisal edge makes placement of the restoration much easier. This incisal overlap can be fabricated purely as a positioning device and later can be removed once the veneer is bonded in place. This latter type of incisal extension does not require crown type preparation (Figs 9.19a and b). A butt joint finishing line provides for the proper porcelain thickness at the margin to prevent fracture. The finishing line should slope

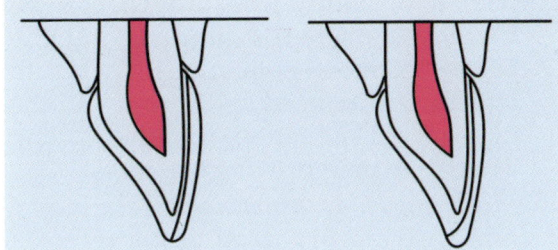

Fig. 9.19a: Incisal reduction

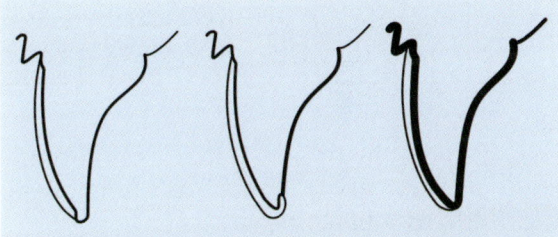

Fig. 9.19b: Incisal reduction with and without overlap

gingivally (75° from the facial). This provides resistance to facial displacement of the restoration.

The preparation may vary at the incisal end. Usually, three types are recognized:

 i. *Incisal chamfer (interlock) preparation:* The incisal edge is not reduced in length. The natural guiding palatal surface is preserved, which is important functionally. A chamfer (0.5 mm) is created along the facial incisal margin using the tip of tapered diamond point. This provides additional space for porcelain at the incisal area (Fig. 9.20).

 ii. *Incisal Butt-joint preparation:* This type of preparation is carried out to increase the

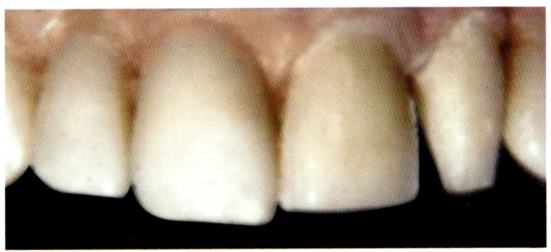

Fig. 9.20: Beveling the incisal edge

length of tooth (the length can be increased up to 2.0 mm). Using the tapered diamond points, the incisal tooth structure is reduced by 0.5 mm and the facial incisal line angle is rounded leaving a butt-joint margin along the incisal edge.

iii. *Incisal lingual-wrap preparation:* The incisal lingual-wrap preparation is preferred because of its ease of handling by the operator (positive seating during placement). The incisal surface is prepared as in butt-joint preparation. The mesio-incisal and the disto-incisal corners are additionally reduced by 0.5 mm. Then, the incisal chamfer so prepared is extended to the palatal surface. The lingual chamfer line should be above or under the centric occlusal contact to avoid occlusal contact on the porcelain-tooth interface. The contact should be on porcelain or on the tooth structure.

In general, never end the incisal edge where excursive movements of the mandible will cause shearing stress across the junction of porcelain laminate and tooth. The incisal line angles must be rounded to reduce internal restorative stresses.

6. Lingual Reduction

Any reduction of the incisal edge necessitates lingual enamel modification so as to create chamfer and not the butt joint at the incisal-lingual junction (Fig. 9.21). This modification will help to prevent the porcelain from shearing away from the incisal edge during occlusal function. It also ensures increased thickness of porcelain in this area that is being used for incising and guidance. The bonding

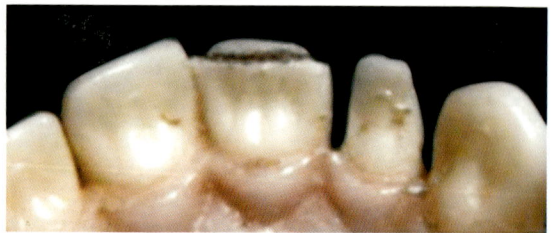

Fig. 9.21: Lingual view

of enamel is at right angles to the porcelain on the incisal edges, thus increasing the strength of the restoration. Excessive buccal convexity of a tooth may make it difficult to overlap the incisal edge and maintaining the incisal path of insertion. An excessive amount of labial tooth structure may have to be removed to facilitate the path of insertion, resulting in exposure of dentin.

The smooth enamel surface is prepared with fine diamond points with a light sweeping motion, followed by polishing with small diameter flexible discs. The discs are also used to round off sharp angles left in the preparation; for example, the preparation of the incisal bevel. Any defects in the surface of preparation may be filled with composite, or if dentin is exposed, glass-ionomer cement can be preferred.

Tooth preparation is evaluated thoroughly keeping in mind achieving the following features:

- Even and adequate reduction, as per need
- Definite and smooth finish lines
- Gingival extension as per need
- A single path of insertion
- Rounded line angles
- Modification of the contact and subcontact areas

Temporization

Temporization is not necessary; the preparation is usually maintained intra-enamel. Minor irregularities, if any, are filled with composite resin. Patients seldom experience sensitivity as a result of the preparation, which do not necessitate the need of temporary cover. The temporary cover, if placed, may lead to chronic inflammation and migration of the gingival tissues; subsequently, the esthetics of the final restoration is compromised. With no temporary cover, patients usually do not feel difficulty in maintaining good oral hygiene. The impression making and cementation can be carried out conveniently. The temporization is preferably avoided.

Impression Techniques

A special impression tray is optional; however, stock tray modifying the labial flange can produce good impression. The addition of acrylic stops in the tray helps to prevent penetration of the prepared incisal edges through the impression material.

Retraction cord is used only when the finish line has been carried subgingivally. If simple blowing with an air syringe reveals the finish line, then low viscosity impression material can be carried into the sulcus without any retraction.

The details of impression materials and impression making is described in Chapter 10.

Laboratory Techniques

Impression is poured in type IV dental stone and accurate die(s) is prepared. Duplicate dies, if required, can be prepared with duplicating materials. The veneer can be fabricated by two techniques in the laboratory.
a. Incremental technique with platinum foil matrix
b. Direct build-up on refractory dies

a. Incremental Technique with Platinum Foil Matrix

Individual dies are made from the stone cast onto which the platinum foil is adapted. Porcelain is built up incrementally on closely adapted platinum matrices. The margins are trimmed to achieve a flush relationship with finish lines. The thickness of porcelain veneer varies from 0.5 to 1.0 mm. It is vital that the chroma, hue and intensity of the porcelain should be closely matched. Blank pieces of porcelain of similar thickness may be constructed for shade matching and along with different resin shades and can be tried before final glazing. The veneers are finished and glazed, and the platinum matrices are removed. The labial surfaces of the veneers are then coated with clear varnish and sticky wax.

The veneers are placed in a 10% solution of hydrofluoric acid for 15 minutes with ultrasonic agitation (follow manufacturer's recommendations). On removal from the acid, the veneers are thoroughly washed in water and soaked in a dilute bicarbonate solution to neutralize any residual acid. They are then transferred to an acetone bath, kept there for several hours to remove the varnish and wax. The internal surface appears frosted at this stage.

b. Direct Build-up on Refractory Dies

Porcelain veneers made directly on refractory dies are less likely to distort during the firing process, thus, providing much better adaptation. The veneers can be fabricated with feldspathic, pressable and castable ceramics. Presently, pressable ceramic is a preferred choice for veneers.

The cast is modified to exaggerate the finish line and also to block out the undesirable undercuts. A duplicate cast can be made after the modifications (Fig. 9.22). Following the manufacturer's directions, a slightly gray shade cast is preferred; however, white refractory cast also serves the purpose. Margins are marked on the refractory cast with a marking pencil. The margins must be protected during the burn-out procedure. The thin marking line can only be seen with magnification, especially after the porcelain is fired.

The most important requirement is that the coefficient of thermal expansion of the refractory and the porcelain should match (manufacturer's provide the refractory and

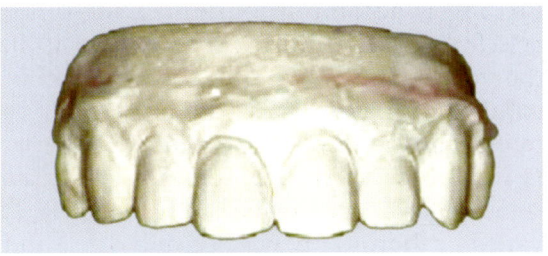

Fig. 9.22: Refractory cast

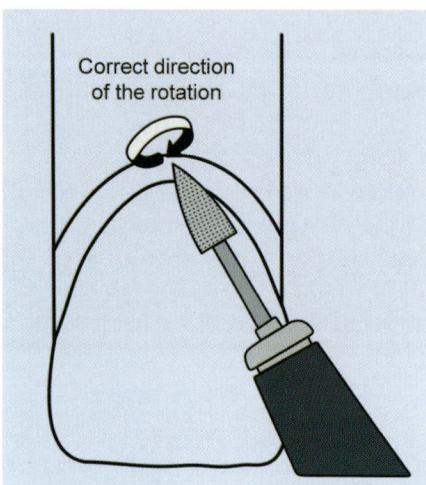

Fig. 9.23: Polishing (diagrammatic)

porcelain of the same nature). Porcelain is built up in layers on the individual refractory die and baked according to the precise firing program. A second layer of porcelain compensates for the shrinkage of the first firing and restores the veneers to full contour. The contour and surface texture is created before the final glaze, and the contacts are evaluated for insufficiencies. The veneers are made as smooth as possible with sandpaper disks and porcelain polishing wheels (Fig. 9.23). Insufficient contacts are corrected and the veneers are glazed. Shaping, staining, trimming and glazing are completed on the refractory die and the refractory is removed by air-abrasion. The dies are divested using carborundum points. Air abrasive can also be used at lower pressure, which avoids damaging the margins.

Veneers are prepared for etching by covering the labial surface with sticky wax. Etching is accomplished with hydrofluoric acid for 30 seconds in an ultrasonic unit. Then the veneers are washed and neutralized in a solution of baking soda and water for one minute in the ultrasonic cleaner. Sticky wax is chilled with fluoromethane spray and removed from the veneer. After etching, the veneer is thoroughly washed and dried and a silane coupling solution is applied.

Veneer Try-in Procedure

The veneers are fragile and should be handled carefully with fingers. A color contrasting surface such as a dark paper napkin should always be used. Fit and contour is checked on the model. Where several veneers are being fitted, all must be tried on the model together to ensure that there is no binding at the contact; in case of any overlaps, or insufficiency, the same should be corrected. Adjustments are made with fine diamond points, always holding the veneer in the fingers. The teeth for veneer placement are cleaned with pumice/water slurry and are isolated with cotton rolls. The veneers are tried wet, first individually to check the fit, then together to confirm that there is no proximal binding. The general shape and contour are assessed. Minor alterations of shape/length can be adjusted after cementation, when the veneers are supported and less prone to accidental fracture. Veneers are removed, cleaned with isopropyl alcohol, dried and kept aside.

Appropriately, luting agent is also selected at the time of try-in process. Different shades may be tried until the desired effect is achieved. The trial paste is removed by peeling it out with a nylon/plastic instrument, soaking the veneer for a few seconds in acetone or ethyl acetate and washing with clean water. Special effects such as crack lines, white hypoplastic patches and translucent incisal edges are normally incorporated into the porcelain during build up in the laboratory, but slight staining modifications may be made at the chairside with colored composites. The color match of both porcelain and composite resin should be checked; if not satisfied, the same can be modified (Fig. 9.24).

Veneer Placement

The placement of veneer involves the following steps:

a. Preparation of Veneer

The fitting surface of the veneer is coated with silane coupling agent and is allowed to dry

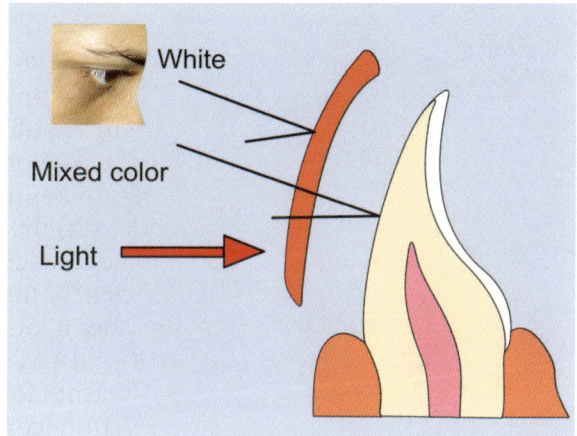

Fig. 9.24: Selecting color

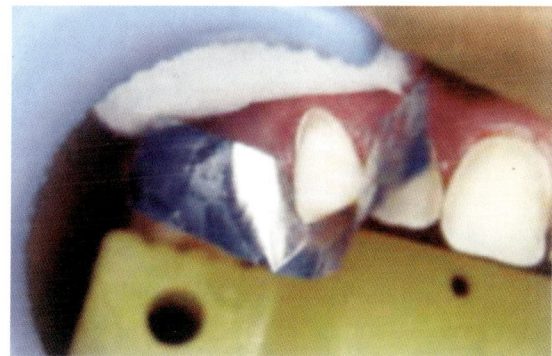

Fig. 9.25: Etching and drying of prepared tooth

for one to two minutes. Excess is blown off and clear bonding agent is applied on the silane-treated surfaces. A few authors do not prefer application of bonding agent to etched porcelain surface. Excess bonding agent is also blown off. The silane coupling agent facilitates chemical attachment to the etched porcelain and the resin matrix of the composite cement and bonding agent.

If the etched surface is contaminated, it should be soaked in acetone and cleaned. Cotton wool should not be used to wipe the surfaces dry, because it leaves tags. The procedure of silane and bonding agent application is repeated.

b. Preparation of the Tooth

The tooth is isolated preferably using rubber dam. This is essential for moisture control and manipulation of veneers. The prepared tooth is washed thoroughly. The selected tooth is separated from the adjoining teeth with mylar strips. The tooth is etched with ortho-phosphoric acid for 60 seconds, washed for 30 seconds and dried with an oil and water-free air supply.

A thin film of light-cure bonding agent is applied to the etched enamel and the excess blown off. The bonding agent is cured accordingly. Thick films of cured bonding agent may prevent proper seating of veneer.

It can also cause fracture arising from loss of congruity of the fitting surfaces. If any dentin is exposed, a dentin adhesive may be used (Fig. 9.25).

c. Cementation

The selected shade of cement is placed evenly on the porcelain to cover the whole fitting surface without trapping air. The veneer is seated gently, starting with the cervical end to incisally using even pressure. Fresh matrix strips may prevent excess cement blocking the contact area and also allow shaping of the proximal surfaces. The excess cement is removed using appropriate instruments. After the veneer has been properly positioned, a 10-second spot cure of the cement is carried out before final polishing.

A clinical case showing step-wise preparation of laminates on maxillary canine is depicted in Figs 9.26a–l. The treatment of fluorosis with laminates is shown in Figs 9.27a–e.

LUMINEERS

Lumineers are ultrathin porcelain veneers that can be bonded directly over the tooth structure to enhance esthetics. Conventional veneers are also considered 'conservative', though, many a times, substantial tooth tissue needs to be compromised. A true conservative approach, Lumineers, were developed with significant advantages. The approach referred to as 'no

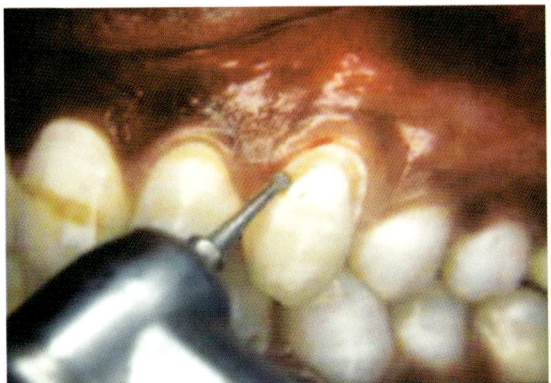

Fig. 9.26a: Repairing cervical margin

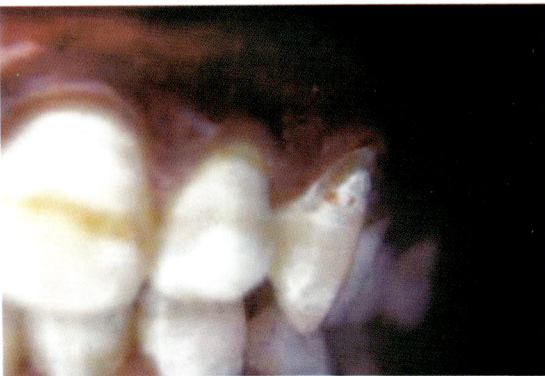

Fig. 9.26d: Proximal view

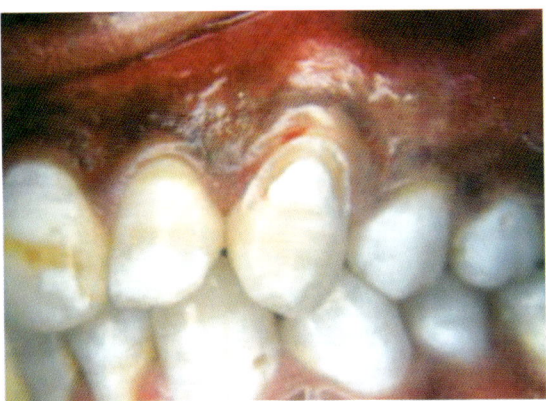

Fig. 9.26b: Prepared cervical margin

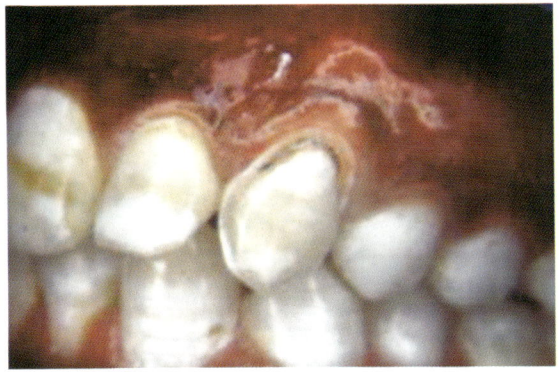

Fig. 9.26e: Prepared tooth margins

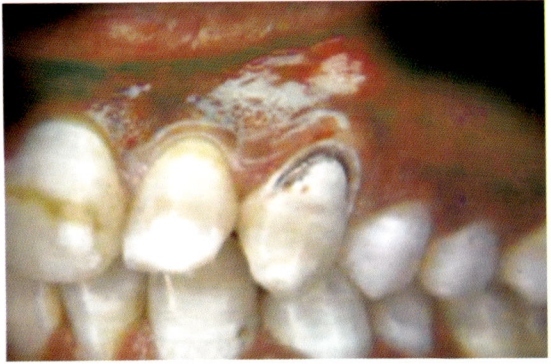

Fig. 9.26c: Highlighting cervical margin

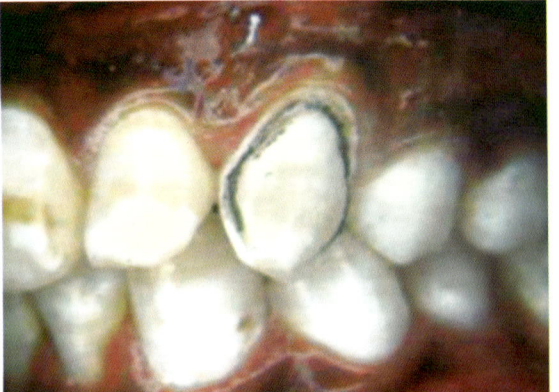

Fig. 9.26f: Highlighting tooth margins

prep technique' is characterized by no preparation or very minimal preparation of the teeth.

The no preparation technique was possible only because of advances in bonding system and also in porcelain technology allowing ultrathin veneers with sufficient strength. Approximately, 0.3 mm thick veneers are created, which can be bonded to the labial enamel without any preparation. Such a thin

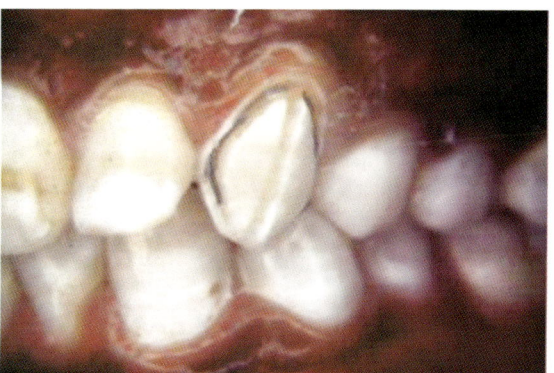

Fig. 9.26g: Vertical groove

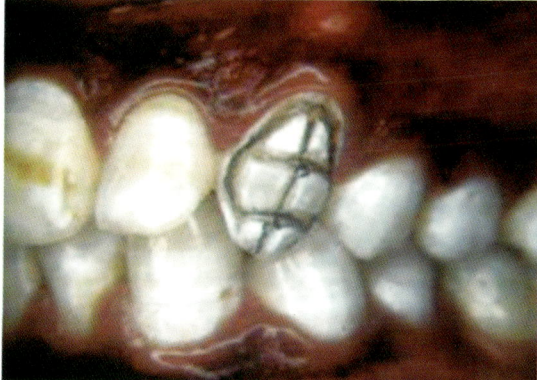

Fig. 9.26j: Highlighting horizontal groove

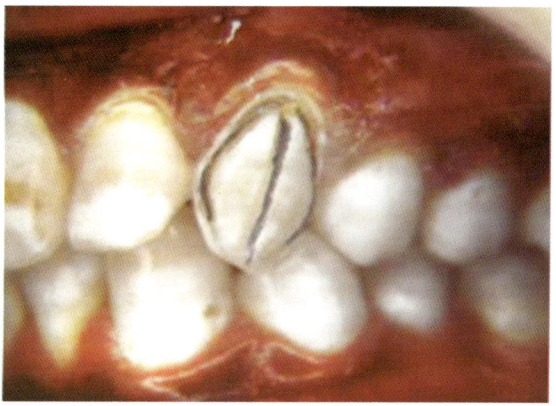

Fig. 9.26h: Highlighting vertical groove

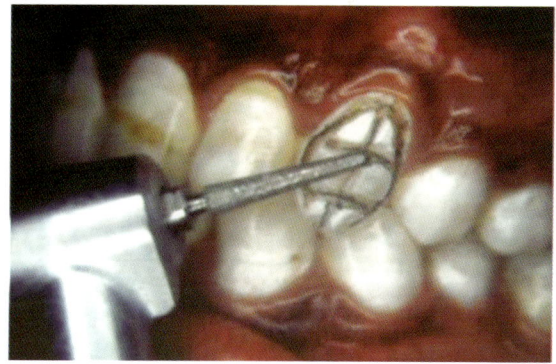

Fig. 9.26k: Preparing tooth

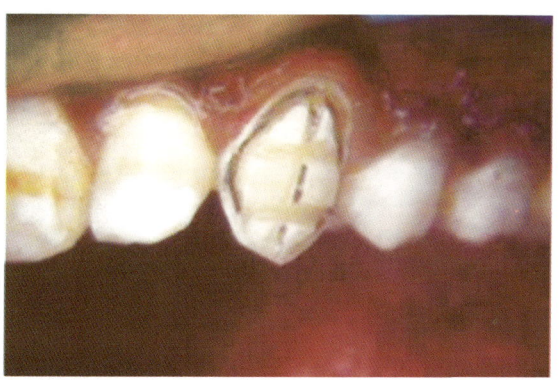

Fig. 9.26i: Horizontal groove

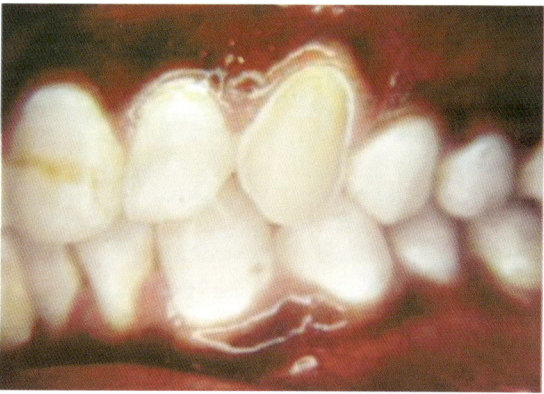

Fig. 9.26l: Prepared tooth

veneer does not lead to overcontouring. Lumineers, also available as Vivaneers, Durathin, etc. are recommended for eliminating gaps, correction of color and restoring minor fractured teeth. Lumineers offer advantages such as no need to prepare the teeth (no local anaesthesia) and no temporary cover. These can be placed over the existing restorations, improving the overall esthetics.

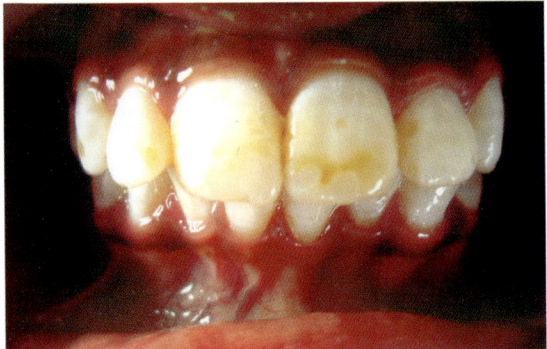

Fig. 9.27a: Preoperative

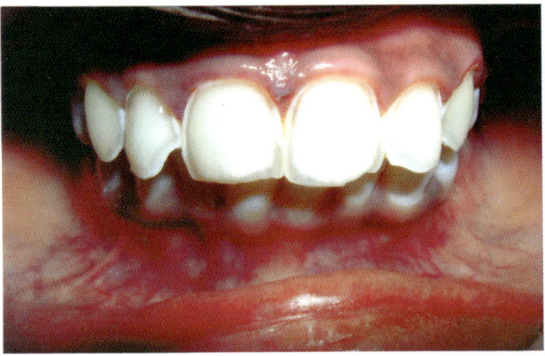

Fig. 9.27b: Tooth preparation

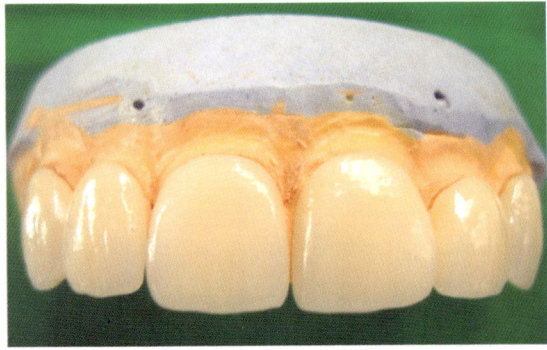

Fig. 9.27c: Laminate on cast

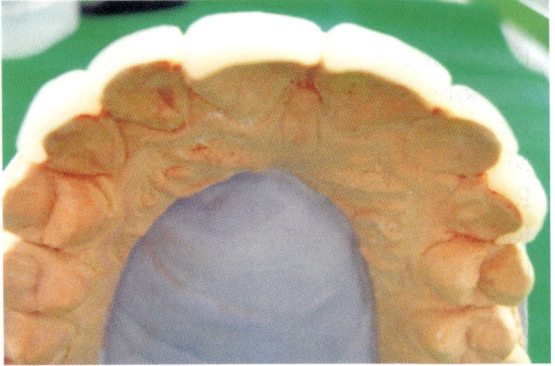

Fig. 9.27d: Lingual view

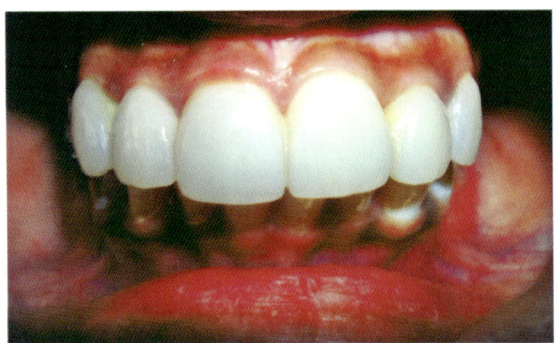

Fig. 9.27e: Laminates (postoperative)

- No postoperative sensitivity and pulpal involvement
- Long-lasting bonding (bonding to enamel only)
- Esthetically pleasing (patient acceptability)
- No need for provisional restorations
- Can be placed over unesthetic crown without replacing the same
- In case patient dislikes, it can be removed and the surface is polished to achieve the same tooth.

The lumineer technique provides excellent results, with many benefits for the patient and the operator. Highly favourable results have been substantiated by many clinical studies.

Advantages
- Fast and painless technique
- Conservative (preserve tooth structure)
- Tissue management not required

Disadvantages
- May appear bulky and overcontoured (a few authors prefer preparing tooth surface, especially the convexities)
- Overcontouring may harm periodontal tissues
- The width and length may not be altered significantly
- Color masking is not proper

Indications

- Enhancing esthetics/appearance of patients
- Masking milk color changes (small discrete wear of color change)
- Masking existing restorations
- Restoring small chipped teeth
- Refreshing existing ceramic restorations
- Reshaping small diastemas

Contraindications

- Severe/moderate discoloration
- Insufficient enamel substrate
- Large defects, especially at the incisal edges
- Rotated/malposed teeth

Examples

- Cerinate porcelain lumineers (by Den-Met)
- Vivaneers (by Glidewell lab)
- MAC Veneers (advanced cosmetics)
- Lithium disilicate veneers
- Durathin veneers

Porcelain versus Resin Veneers

- Superior strength and retention is possible with porcelain veneers. Due to this advantage, they are preferred in cases requiring lengthening of teeth or modifying functional contacts.
- Surface texture of glazed porcelain is superior to that of polished resin because of its durability and high luster. (However, polishing is difficult in local-isolated areas after veneer placement.)
- Porcelain veneers are more durable than resin veneers.
- Resin veneers are easily repaired and replaced; whereas it is difficult with porcelain veneers (need for repair/ replacement is less with porcelain veneers due to their superior bond strength and retention to etched enamel).

Bibliography

1. Alhekeir DF, Al-Sarhan RA and Al Mashhan AF. Porcelain laminate veneers: clinical survey for evaluation of failure. The Saudi Dent. J.: 2014;26:63–7.
2. Barghi N and Overton JD. Preserving principles of successful porcelain veneers. Contemp. Esthet.: 2007;11:48–51.
3. Barreto MT and Bottaro BF. A practical approach to porcelain repair. J.Prosth.Dent.: 1982;48:349–51.
4. Beier US, Kapferer I, Burtscher D and Dumfahrt H. Clinical performance of porcelain laminate veneers for up to 20 years. Int. J Prosthodont: 2012;25:79–85.
5. Belsser UC, Magne P and Magne M. Ceramic laminate veneers: continuous evolution of indications. J. Esthet. Dent.: 1997;9:197–207.
6. Brunton PA and Wilson NHF. Preparation for porcelain laminates veneers in general dental practice. BDJ: 1998;184:553–6.
7. Cagidiaco MC, Ferrari M, Garbroglio R and Davidson CL. Dentin contamination protection after mechanical properties for veneering. Am. J. Dent.: 1996;9:57–60.
8. Calamia JR and Calamia CS. Porcelain laminate veneers: reasons for 25 years of success. Dent. Clin. N. Am.: 2007;51:399–417.
9. Christensen GJ. What is a veneer? Resolving the confusion. J. Indiana Dent. Assoc.: 2005;846:9–12.
10. Clyde JS and Gilmour A. Porcelain veneers: A preliminary review. BDJ: 1988;164:9–14.
11. Coyne BM and Wilson NH. Indirect laminate veneers: a review. Evidence Based Dent. 2004;5:43.
12. Culp L and McLaren EA. Lithium disilicate: the restorative material of multiple options. Compend. Contin. Educ. Dent.: 2010;31:716–20.
13. Denry I and Holloway JA. Ceramics for dental applications: a review. Materials: 2010;3:351–68.
14. Dietschi D and Devigus A. Prefabricated composite veneers: Historical perspectives, indications and clinical application. Eur. J. Esthet. Dent.: 2011;6:178–87.
15. Dumfahat H. Porcelain laminate veneers. A retrospective evaluation after 1–10 years of service. Part I, Clinical procedures. Int. J. Prosthodont.: 1999;12:505–13.
16. Dumfahat H and Schaffer H. Porcelain laminate veneers. A retrospective evaluation after 1–10 years of service. Path II Clinical results. Int. J. Prosthodont.: 2000;13:9–18.
17. Duune SM. A longitudinal study of the clinical performance of porcelain veneers. BDJ: 1993;175:317–21.

18. Fahl Junior N. The direct/indirect composite resin veneers: a case report. Pract Periodontics Aesthetic Dent.: 1996;8:627–38.

19. Fradeani M, Redemagni M and Corrado M. Porcelain laminate veneers: 6–12 years clinical evaluation: A retrospective study. Int. J. Periodontics and Restorative Dent.: 2005;25:9–17.

20. Friedman MJ. A 15-year review of porcelain veneer failure. A clinician's observation. Comp. Contin. Educ. Dent.: 1998;19:625–8, 30, 32.

21. Friedman MJ. Porcelain veneer restoration. A clinician's opinion about a disturbing trend. J. Esthet. Restorative Dent.: 2001;13:318–27.

22. Garber DA. Porcelain laminate veneers: to prepare or not to prepare? Compend. Contin. Educ. Dent.: 1991;XII:178–82.

23. Garber DA. Direct composite veneers versus etched porcelain laminate veneers. Dent. Clin. North Am.: 1989;33:301–4.

24. Goldstein MB. No-prep/minimal-prep: the perils of oversimplification. Dent. Today 2007;26:10.

25. Gomes G and Perdiago J. Prefabricated composite resin veneers-a clinical review. J. Esthet. Resto. Dent.: 2014;26:302–13.

26. Gresnigt MM, Ozcan M, Muis M and Kalk W. Bonding of glass ceramic and indirect composite to non-aged and aged resin composite. J. Adhes. Dent.: 2012;14:59–68.

27. Guess PC, Schultheis S, Bonfante EA, Coelho PG, Ferencz J and Silva NRFA. All-ceramic systems: laboratory and clinical performances. Dent. Clinic North Am.: 2011;55:333–52.

28. Gurel G. Porcelain laminate veneers: minimal tooth preparation by design. Dent. Clin. North Am.: 2007;51:419–31.

29. Gurel G. Influence of enamel preservation on failure rates of porcelain laminate veneers. Int. J. Prosthodont.: 2013;33:31–9.

30. Harasani MH, Isidor F and Kaaber S. Marginal fit of porcelain and indirect composite laminate veneers under in-vitro conditions. Scand. J Dent. Res.: 1991;99:262–8.

31. Hedge TK. Minimal prep veneers: a conservative alternative. Pract. Proced. Aesthet. Dent.: 2008;20: 475–7.

32. Heymann HO. Indirect composite resin veneers: Clinical techniques and two-year observations. Quint. Int.: 1987;17:111–8.

33. Horn RH. Porcelain laminate veneers bonded to etched enamel. Dent. Clinic North Am.: 1983;27: 671–84.

34. Ikeda M, Nikaido T, Foxton M and Tagami J. Shear bond strengths of indirect resin composites to hybrid ceramic. Dent. Mater. J.: 2006;24:238–43.

35. Javaheri D. Considerations for planning esthetic treatment with veneers involving no or minimal preparation. J. Am. Dent. Assoc.: 2007;138:331–7.

36. Lang SA and Clifford BS. Castable glass ceramic for veneer restoration. J.Prosth.Dent.: 1992;67: 590–4.

37. LeSage B. Establishing a classification system and criteria for veneer preparation. Compend. Contin. Educ. Dent.: 2013;34:104–17.

38. Mague P and Belser UC. Novel porcelain laminate preparation approach driven by a diagnostic mode-up. J. Esthet. Restorative Dent.: 2004;16: 7–16.

39. Magne P and Douglas WH. Porcelain veneers—dentin bonding optimization and biomimetic recovery of the crown. The Int. J Prosthodont.: 1999;12:111–21.

40. Mangani F, Cerutti A and Putignano A. Clinical approach to anterior adhesive restorations using resin composite veneers. Eur. J. Esthet. Dent.: 2007;2:188–209.

41. Malcmacher L. No-preparation porcelain veneers—back to the future! Dent. Today: 2005;24:865, 88, 90–1.

42. Maneenut C, Sakoolnamarka R and Tyas MJ. The repair potential of resin composite materials. Dent. Mater.: 2011;27:e20–7.

43. Marshall SJ, Bayne SC, Baier R, Tomsia AP and Marshall GW. A review of adhesion science. Dent. Mater.: 2010;26:e11–6.

44. McLaren EA. Porcelain veneer preparations: to prep or not to prep. Inside Dentistry: 2006;76–9.

45. McLaren EA and LeSage B. Feldspathic veneers: what are their indications? Compend. Contin. Educ. Dent.: 2011;32:44–9.

46. Migliau G, Besharat LK, Sofan AA, Sofan EA and Romeo U. Endo-restorative treatment of a severely discolored upper incisor: resolution of the "aesthetic" problem through Componeer veneering System. Ann Stomatol.: 2015;6:113–8.

47. Mizrahi B. Visualization before finalization: a predictable procedure for porcelain laminate veneers. Pract. Proced. Aesthet. Dent.: 2005;17: 513–8.

48. Newsome P and Greenwall L. Management of tetracycline discolored teeth. Aesthetic Dent. Today: 2008;2:15–20.

49. Newsome P and Owen S. Ceramic veneers in general dental practice. Part five: Aftercare and dealing with failure. Aesthet. Dent.: 2008a;2:9–12.

50. Newsome P and Owen S. Longevity of ceramic veneers in general dental practice. Aesthetics: 2009;3:6–10.

51. Peumans M, Van Meerbeek B, Yoshida Y, Lanbrechts P and Vanherle G. Five-year clinical performance of porcelain veneers. Quint. Int.: 1998;29:211–21.

52. Pini NP, Aguiar FHB, Lima DAN, Lovadino JS, Terada RSS and Pascotto RC. Advances in dental veneers: materials, applications and techniques. Clin. Cosmet. Invest. Dent.: 2012;4:9–16.

53. Pneumans M, Van Meerbeek B, Lambrechts P and Vanherle G. Porcelain veneers: A review of literature. J. Dent.: 2000;28:163–77.

54. Pneumans M, De Munch J, Fieuws S, Lambrechts P, Vanhule G and Van Meerbeek B. A prospective ten year clinical trial of porcelain veneers. J. Adhes. Dent.: 2004;6:65–76.

55. Priest G. Proximal margin modifications for all-ceramic veneers. Pract. Proed. Aesthet. Dent.: 2004;16:256–72.

56. Radz GM. Minimum thickness anterior porcelain restorations. Dent. Clin. North Am.: 2011;55:353–70.

57. Rickman LJ, Padipatvuthikul P and Chee B. Clinical applications of preheated hybrid resin composite. Br. Dent. J: 2011;211:63–7.

58. Schwartz JC. Vertical shoulder preparation design for porcelain laminate veneers. Compendium: 2000; 12, 316, 18, 20 passim.

59. SRe D, Augusti G, Amato M, Riva G and Augusti D. Esthetic rehabilitation of anterior teeth with laminates composite veneers. Case Reports in Dentistry: Article ID849273, 2014;1–9.

60. Shaini FJ, Shortall AC and Marquis PM. Clinical performance of porcelain laminate veneers: A retrospective evaluation over a period of 6.5 years. J. Oral Rehab.: 1997;24:553–9.

61. Strassler HE. Minimally invasive porcelain veneers: indications for conservative esthetic dentistry treatment modality. Gen. Dent.: 2007;55:686–94.

62. Swift EJ and Friedman MJ. Critical appraisal: porcelain veneer outcomes. Part II. J. Esthet. Restor. Dent.: 2006;18:110–3.

63. Turgut S, Bagis B. Effect of resin cement and ceramic thickness on final color of laminate veneers: an in vitro study. J. Prosth. Dent. 2013; 109:179–86.

64. Wakiaga J, Brunton P, Silikas N and Glenny AM. Direct versus indirect veneer restorations for intrinsic dental stains. Cochrene Database Syst. Rev.:1, CD004347; 2004.

65. Wittenben JG, Wright RF, Weber HP and Gallucci GO. A systematic review of the clinical performance of CAD/CAN single-tooth restorations. Int. J. Prosthodont.: 2009;22:446–71.

10 Impression Making

The main requisite in successful fabrication of indirect restorations is to transfer an accurate replication of the patient's hard and soft tissues to the dental laboratory. Impression making is a blend of art and science. The ability to analyze dental impressions and to understand how to avoid inaccuracies is the key to successful restorations. Impression making would be easy if impressions of non-vital objects are to be made. The problem arises in the oral cavity since the soft tissues, which vary in thickness and rigidity are displaceable under pressure. The operator is to 'make' the impression and not to 'take' since manipulation of vital tissues, an important aspect, is to be carried out by the operator. The choice of the impression material also depends upon the variability of the tissues to be included in the impression.

An impression can be defined as 'the negative replica/imprint of any object'; whereas dental impression is defined as 'the negative replica or imprint of teeth, the alveolar ridge and the adjoining tissues'. Negative replica of nose, tongue and cheeks are also made in various fields of dentistry and plastic surgery. The negative replica so obtained is converted into positive replica using various materials. The positive replica of single tooth is known as 'Die' and the positive replica of whole arch or the part of it is known as 'cast' or 'model'.

The impression material should possess certain qualities so as to produce an accurate replica of the concerned objects and tissues. The material should have sufficient flow so as to reach every corner of the tooth or tissues to be recorded in impression and at the same time it should be viscous enough to remain adapted to the tray. The impression material should have sufficient working time for mixing, loading and placing the tray in the oral cavity. In oral cavity, it should set early, since movement of tray during setting will lead to distortion. The impression should also be dimensionally stable for sufficient time after its removal.

Impression materials, methods and techniques are constantly changing. There are reports of impression making as early as in seventeenth century. Impression trays were reportedly used in early eighteenth century. Earlier, plaster of Paris, waxes and gutta-percha were widely used as impression materials. Not going in detail regarding the history of the impression materials, the main concern will be the clinical aspects of the routinely used materials coupled with techniques used to make impressions.

Requisites of Impression Material

The clinical requirements of an impression material are:

- A pleasant odour, taste and acceptable color
- Adequate shelf life for storage and distribution
- Easy manipulation
- Sufficient consistency and texture
- Sufficient elasticity (free from permanent deformation under strain)
- Adequate strength (should not break or tear during removal from oral cavity)
- Dimensionally stable, consistent with temperature and humidity
- Compatible with die material; the contact angle of the impression material with the die material is important (lower the contact angle, fewer the voids).
- Non-toxic and non-irritant
- Cost effective

Properties of Clinical Significance

The properties of clinical significance are:

i. *Yield strength/elastic recovery:* Yield strength determines the ability of the impression material to withstand stress without permanent deformation; elastic recovery implies that the impression should be sufficiently elastic so that it will return to its original dimensions without distortion. Polyvinyl siloxane has the best elastic recovery, followed by polyether and polysulfide. The strain at yield point indicates the amount of undercut that the impression material can overcome without permanent elastic deformation.

ii. *Tear strength:* The tear strength indicates the resistance of the impression material to tear after setting. The values of tear strength should not be superior to the yield strength. In such cases, the impression might be resistant to tear but may easily be distorted. The ideal impression material should absorb most of the energy, prior to critical point of permanent deformation (0.04%). The material, which tears before this critical point, is more suitable for dental impressions. Polyethers are considered best having highest tear strength; whereas hydrocolloids are having least tear strength.

iii. *Wettability:* Wettability implies the ability of impression material to flow into small areas. The wettability in an impression material results in fewer voids and less entrapment of oral fluids providing better impressions. Minute details are required in fixed prosthodontics.

iv. *Contact angle; ability to reproduce details:* Impression material with low contact angle facilitates flow producing bubble-free casts. A few impression materials, such as polyvinyl siloxane, require surfactants to lower the contact angle before pouring casts. Polyethers and polysulfides have relatively low contact angles.

v. *Dimensional stability and accuracy:* The dimensional stability of an impression material is the ability to maintain the accuracy over a period of time. The polymerization/setting shrinkage should be less, which allows the impression to be poured days after making the impression. Polyethers and polyvinyl siloxanes have better dimensional stability as compared to alginate, which has low dimensional stability. Polysulfides also distort over time (important, if impression is sent to laboratory for pouring).

Polyether and polyvinyl siloxane impression materials remain dimensionally accurate for one to two weeks. Polysulfide impression material is dimensionally accurate if poured within one to two hours (important for clinicians to pour the impression within time frame).

vi. *Hydrophilic/hydrophobic nature:* Impression materials, which can tolerate moisture, are hydrophilic. Hydrophilic or hydrophobic nature of an impression material has an effect on the surface quality of the polymerized impression material. Presence of moisture results in impression with voids/pitted surfaces and the detail reproduced is inferior. Polyethers and polysulfides are hydrophilic; whereas polysiloxanes are hydrophobic. New hydrophilic siloxanes are also introduced. The hydrophilization is increased with the incorporation of non-ionic surfactants. Moisture control is critical in predictable clinical results (polyether and polysulfide are compatible with inherent moisture present in mucosal tissues). Hydrocolloids are the most hydrophilic material.

vii. *Flexibility:* Flexible impressions are easier to remove from the oral cavity after impression making. It is established that viscosity of the impression material is the most important factor in producing impressions and dies with minimal bubbles and maximum details. Alginates are considered as the most flexible impression materials; whereas polyethers are the least flexible.

viii. *Ease of handling:* The manufacturers supply the impression material with respect to setting criteria as fast-set or standard-set. The handling of the impression material is to be taken care of by the operator following manufacturer's instructions. Apart from the handling characteristics, the impression material should be well tolerated by the patients.

IMPRESSION MATERIALS

The types and characteristics of commonly used impression materials are:

1. Hydrocolloids

The impression material should be elastic, i.e. the material should transform from a semisolid state to solid state under the conditions of oral environment. Two systems are utilized; one involves flexible gels having characteristics of colloids, where bonds are established between the individual components of the dispersed phase and the second involves elastomeric polymers, where the setting reaction produces an optimal amount of cross-linking between the molecules.

The colloidal state is in between the state of suspension and solution (e.g. sugar completely dissolved in water is 'solution'; whereas sand particles suspended in water is 'suspension'). In the colloids, molecules or combination of molecules (dispersed phase) are present in the dispersion medium. In case, the dispersion is water, the material is known as hydrocolloid. These exist in two different forms known as 'Sol' and 'Gel'. 'Sol' is practically the liquid state and 'Gel' is the semisolid state. Gel is produced by a reaction, known as 'Gelation'. The temperature at which the sol is converted into gel is the 'gelation temperature'.

Depending upon gelation, the hydrocolloids are divided into two:

a. *Reversible hydrocolloids:* Where the gel once formed can be converted back to sol by heating at specific temperature (for example, agar-agar).

b. *Irreversible hydrocolloids:* When the gel once formed cannot be converted back to sol (for example, alginate).

a. Reversible Hydrocolloids (Agar-Agar)

Agar-agar impression material is composed of agar, borates, potassium sulphate and certain waxes and is supplied in collapsible tubes. The fluid impression material is supplied in jars, which can be used with syringes.

Manipulation: The agar material is heated in a specially designed equipment between 75 and 100°C. Then, it is cooled down to 45–55°C in a similar tempering bath. The special rim lock trays with water circulating devices are used. After the tray is loaded and inserted, water is circulated at 15–20°C through the tray until the gelation occurs. The time for gelation is usually three and half minutes. After the gelation process is over, the impression is removed with a single stroke. The impression is to be poured immediately since dimensional changes occur very soon. In case, storage is unavoidable, it can be stored up to one hour in hundred percent humidity. The stone/plaster cast must be removed promptly, since the impression will dehydrate and also the prolonged contact of plaster/stone with the impression material will result in rough surface on the cast.

In a modified technique known as 'wet field technique', the area to be recorded is flooded with warm water. The syringe material (fluid agar) is applied over the teeth in sufficient bulk. The tray material (algniate) is then inserted onto the liquid material. The hydraulic pressure allows the material to move into every corner of the segment.

Advantages
- Good elasticity.
- Well tolerated
- Do not distort easily.
- Relatively cheap.

Disadvantages
- Flow is not appropriate.
- Tears easily, requires more bulk especially at edges.
- Electroplating is not feasible.
- Although the impression materials can be reused but the reused material does not exhibit the same properties.

The reversible hydrocolloid, though an excellent impression material, has been replaced by irreversible hydrocolloids mainly because of their manipulation difficulties.

b. Irreversible Hydrocolloids

The irreversible hydrocolloids (alginate) were developed to overcome the disadvantages of the agar material. Alginates are composed of diatomaceous earth, potassium alginate, calcium sulfate, zinc oxide and potassium titanium fluoride. Sodium phosphate acts as retarder, whereas potassium titanium fluoride acts as accelerator. The concentrations of sodium phosphate and potassium titanium fluoride are adjusted so as to produce regular and fast setting alginates. Alginates are simple to manipulate, comfortable for the patient and do not require any special equipment. The newer alginates contain 1–3% sodium silicofluoride (Na_2SiF_6), which improves surface quality of dental stone poured into set alginate (Fig. 10.1).

Alginate impression materials are supplied in powder form, which is mixed with water. A plastic scoop is supplied with powder pack and another scoop is provided for measuring accurate amount of water.

Certain modified alginates are also available in the form of sol, which contains water but no calcium ions. The calcium ions in the form of plaster of Paris are added as reactor. These components can be available in two parts: one containing alginate sol and other, the reactor.

Quaternary ammonium salts have also been added to the alginate powder to make it bactericidal; however, it was not very effective against viruses and tubercle bacilli.

The gelation time is three to four minutes under optimal environmental conditions. In

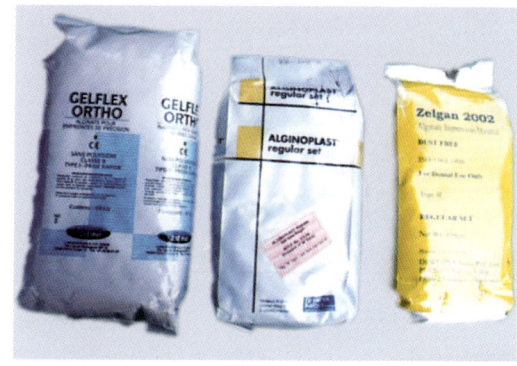

Fig. 10.1: Alginate (conventional and improved)

case of changed environment condition, i.e. too hot and too cold weather, the gelation time can be altered by using cold water in hot summer days (prolong the gelation time) and warm water in cold winter days (reduce the gelation time). The mixing spatula and the bowl can also be accordingly cool or warm to adjust the gelation time. The water/powder ratio in no circumstances should be changed to adjust the gelation time; since by doing so the properties of set alginate are invariably changed.

Manipulation

The correct amount of powder and water, as instructed by the manufacturers, is taken. The powder is stirred well (fluffing the powder by rotating the can) before use so as to uniformly distribute the filler contents, otherwise filler contents may settle down. The scoop is dipped in the powder, taken out and tapped gently with spatula to level the powder. A scoop of water, as instructed by the manufacturer, is also taken. The powder is poured first in the bowl and then the water is added slowly. The mixing is carried out in the plastic/rubber bowl using stainless steel spatula. The rubber bowl is preferred so as to completely plasticize the material (Fig. 10.2). As the water is added into the powder, start spatulating against the walls of bowl. The spatulation is carried out in the figure of eight manner, facilitating wiping out of air bubbles from the mix and making it smooth and even. A mixing time of 45 seconds to one minute is generally sufficient. The mix should be smooth and creamy that does not drip off the spatula when it is raised from the bowl. Certain mechanical devices (auto mixing) are also utilized for this purpose. Auto mixing decreases the contamination and eliminates the void formation; however, other physical properties remain the same.

The manipulation is described in the following subheads:

i. *Selection of Tray*

The routine stock trays are used for making alginate impressions. The stock trays are usually made of stainless steel or plastic and are available in different sizes. The tray should cover all the teeth leaving 3.0–4.0 mm space free buccally/labially and lingually. The peripheral part should not impinge upon the tissues (Fig. 10.3). The posterior part of the tray should just cover the posterior palatal seal (Fig. 10.4). The wider tray should be avoided mainly because of two reasons; first, the chances of distortion are more and second, the impression material near pharyngeal area may cause nausea to the patient. Too narrow trays should also be avoided as the teeth/tissues may touch the sides of the tray giving faulty impression (Fig. 10.5).

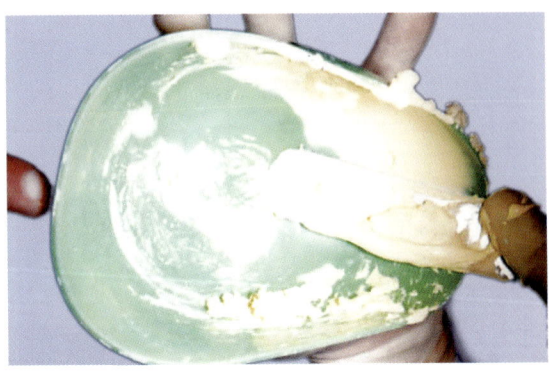

Fig. 10.2: Mixing alginate in rubber bowl

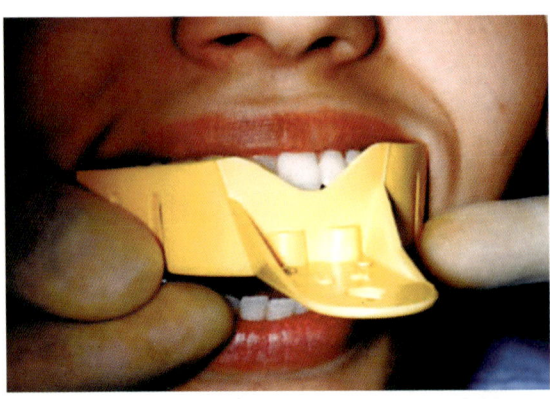

Fig. 10.3: Selection of tray (tray should not impinge the vestibule)

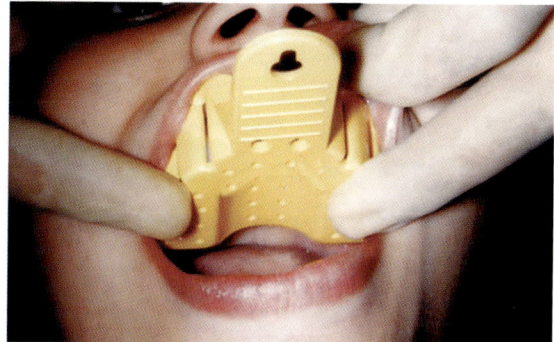

Fig. 10.4: Selection of tray (tray should cover the posterior palatal seal)

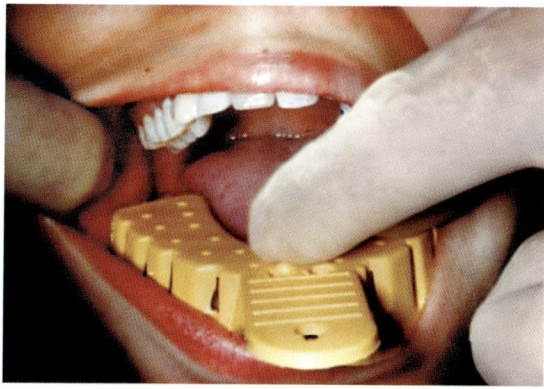

Fig. 10.6a: Correct positioning of tray (one side)

In lower arch, the tray should cover the last tooth along with the retromolar area, without impinging the lingual and labial/buccal folds (Figs 10.6a and b).

Occasionally, it is necessary to change the shape of the tray. The metal trays can be bent and the plastic trays can be modified by gently heating the edges. The height of the flanges and the length can be modified using tracing wax. Similarly, for high arched palate, tracing wax can be added in the center of the tray. Tracing wax is preferably used for modifying the tray.

The stock trays are usually perforated to allow flow of excess alginate and also to provide retention to the tray. Many a times, the perforations are insufficient to overcome displacing forces during withdrawal. It is essential to apply adhesive to retain the set

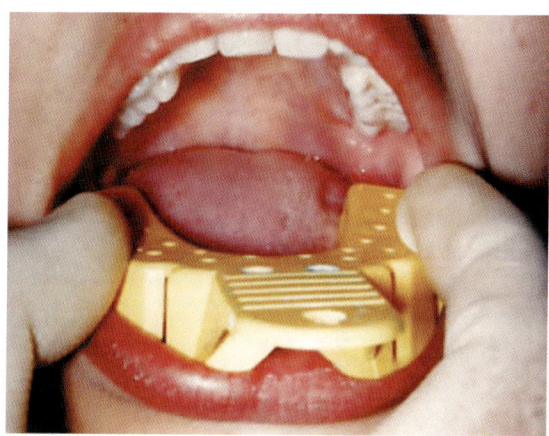

Fig. 10.6b: Correct positioning of tray (both side)

impression material. The adhesive is applied in thin layers on all internal surfaces of the tray. In addition, the adhesive should cover 2.0–3.0 mm beyond the peripheries of the tray.

ii. *Loading of Tray*

The material is then loaded in the tray and evenly distributed (Figs 10.7a and b). The excess material at the posterior palatal seal area is to be avoided since alginate if pushed towards pharynx causes nausea and discomfort to the patient. The outer surface of the mix may be smoothened by applying wet finger over it. The thickness of the alginate should be 3.0–4.0 mm all around the teeth so as to avoid rupture or tear of the material.

Before making the impression, instruct the patient to rinse the oral cavity thoroughly.

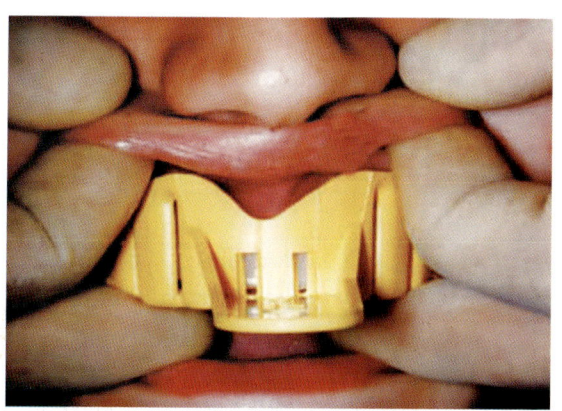

Fig. 10.5: Narrow tray

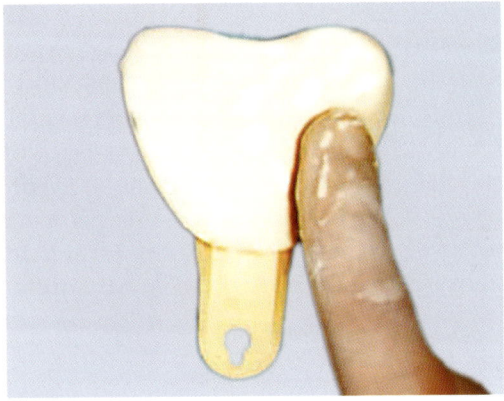

Fig. 10.7a: Loading of upper impression tray

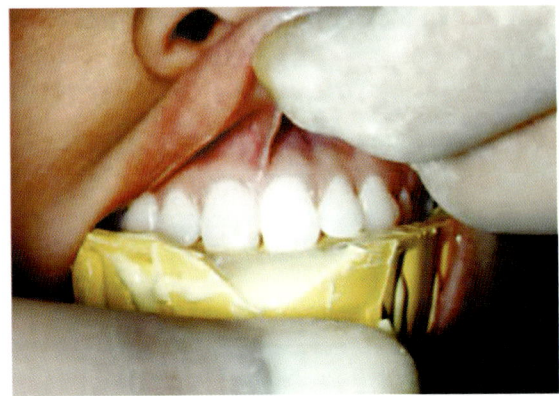

Fig. 10.8: Placement of upper impression tray

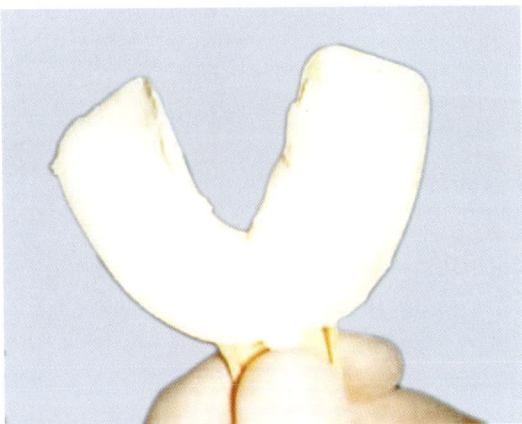

Fig. 10.7b: Loading of lower impression tray

This will aid in removing debris and other foreign particles, which can hinder the impression making. The occlusal surface is dried with three-in-one syringe in order to minimize the attached debris. The details of occlusal surfaces can be improved by 'buttering' the teeth with alginate prior to tray insertion. Similarly, the prepared tooth (inlay, onlay or crowns), lower lingual and labial hamular notch and the palatal vault should be filled with alginate to ensure that the adequate quantity of material is present, to accurately record the relevant anatomy of these areas. While making upper impression, retract the lips thoroughly with the operator's left hand and push the tray slowly (Fig. 10.8). Make the patient sit in upright position,

slightly moving the head down towards the chair side. The patient is requested to breathe deeply from nose. All these features avoid nausea and discomfort to the patient, since the setting/gelation might take approximately five minutes. Sufficient setting can be estimated by placing a blunt instrument on the surface and exerting light pressure. If the depression made by the instrument instantly disappears, it shows sufficient setting of the material. The alginate material should be kept in place even after setting for at least two to three minutes (Fig. 10.9). By doing so, the material gains strength and elasticity. The tray, all along the procedure, should be kept at one place putting equal pressure (Fig. 10.10). Distortion occurs if the tray is moved or unequal pressure is exerted during setting of the impression material.

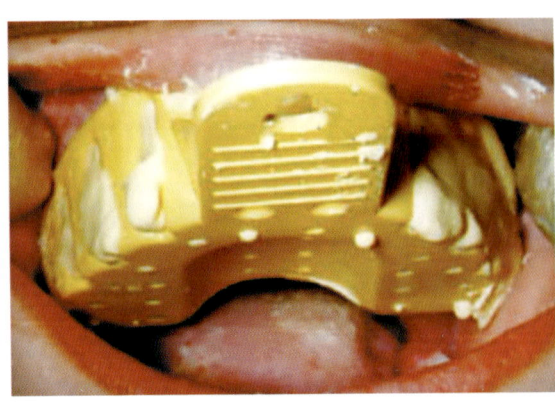

Fig. 10.9: Final set impression

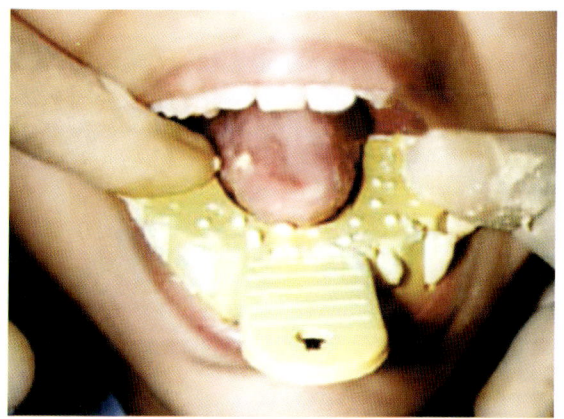

Fig. 10.10: Putting equal pressure on tray

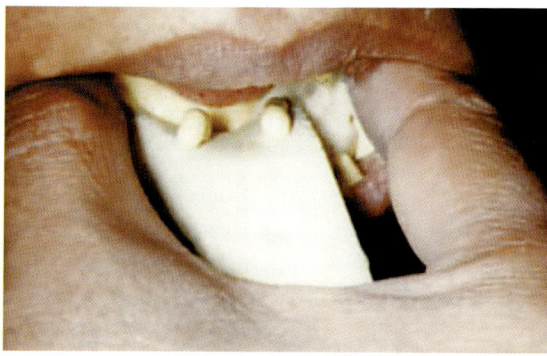

Fig. 10.12a: Breaking the peripheral seal (upper)

iii. Removing the Tray

The set impression is to be removed with a jerk or snap (Fig. 10.11). To and fro movement of tray is to be avoided. Usually, the alginate develops very effective peripheral seal. This seal is to be freed by running the fingers all along the periphery and pulling the tray off the periphery (Figs 10.12a and b). To break the seal, air can be blown from three-in-one syringe into the posterior buccal sulcus adjacent to the tray. Then, the tray can be removed accurately and quickly.

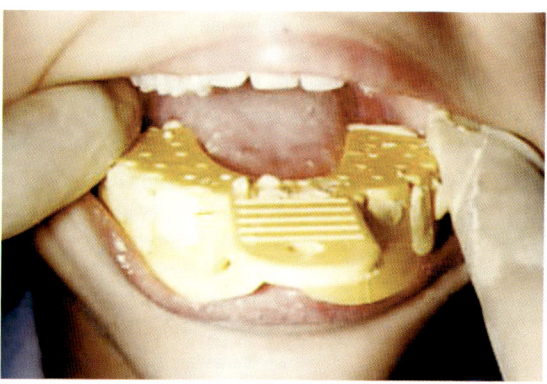

Fig. 10.12b: Breaking the peripheral seal (lower)

iv. Examination of the Impression

The impression is examined under good visibility as regard any rupture, voids etc. In case, the faults are affecting the quality of cast, the impression is rejected and the process of impression making is repeated.

The set material is washed thoroughly to remove oral fluids from the impression surface. The excess water is wiped off; however, the impression should not be unduly dry. The dry surface may lead to syneresis and distortion and also the gel may adhere to the surface of the cast. A cast with rough surface will result if water droplets are left. The fluid exudate appears on the surface of the impression as the polysaccharide chains are drawn further together. This results in shrinkage of the impression. In contrast, if the impression is left immersed in water for too long, it will absorb water by a process known as imbibition. Imbibed water pushes the polysaccharide chains apart and causes the impression to swell. The cast should be formed immediately. In case, storage is necessary, the impression is to be covered with wet napkin

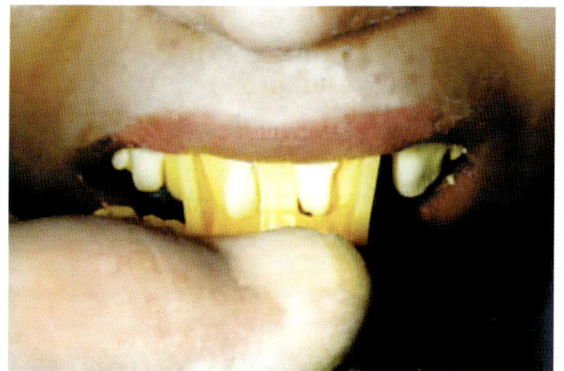

Fig. 10.11: Removal of tray with jerk

and covered with a bowl. The storage in no case should be more than one hour. The impression is disinfected by 2.0% glutaraldehyde spray or dipping in 5.0% sodium hypochlorite solution.

The stone plaster or plaster of Paris cast should be removed from the impression after setting (usually 30–60 minutes depending upon the environmental conditions). In case, the cast is allowed to remain in contact with impression material, a chalky surface may be produced. With prolonged contact, the set stone start absorbing water from the impression, resulting in poor surface details of the cast.

Advantages
- Manipulation is easy.
- Setting reaction not affected by latex gloves.
- Comfortable to patient.
- Fairly accurate.
- Produces good surface details.
- Good elasticity and flexibility.
- Two paste system alginates may provide better dimensional stability.

Disadvantages
- Poor dimensional stability (imbibition and dessication problem)
- Metal dies cannot be prepared.
- Not accurate for fixed prosthesis, especially long span bridges.
- Distortion; must be poured within 5–10 minutes (mishandling also leads to distortion).
- Multiple casts cannot be prepared.
- Lead salts present (0.0007–0.095%) are toxic when inhaled (acceptable limit of lead is 0.45 mg/m³).
- May tear at subgingival areas.
- May stick to dry teeth (moist teeth preferred for impression). The teeth are hydrated, especially when multiple impressions are required.

Newer Alginates
a. *Dustless alginates (Two paste form):* The powder of dustless alginates is coated with glycol. This is available in two paste system: Base with usual ingredients (silicone oil and water) and the catalyst (water and calcium salts). It overcomes disadvantages associated with powder–water system, such as evolution of dust during manipulation and the inconsistency in dispersing accurate amount of water and powder. They exhibit better tear resistance and good dimensional stability.
b. *Extended pour alginates:* Extended pour alginate also called '100-hour alginate' is designed as alginate material, which enables delayed pouring under storage of up to 100 hours. Manufacturers claim better dimensional stability, which is however not proved.
c. *High viscosity alginates:* Incorporation of hydrophobic agents and surfactant to the material enabling increase permeation speed of water. It also solves problem of gagging.
d. *Chromatic alginates:* Conventional alginates were modified by adding pH indicators to show a color change. Most pH indicators show color change above pH 8 which is immediately after mixing but the pH decreases below 8 during gelation. To overcome this problem, a combination of inorganic and/or organic pigment along with pH indicator has been incorporated. In this case, the color of alginate after setting is the color created due to pigments.

Common Errors

The various types of errors in the alginate impression material and the causes related to each error are tabulated in Table 10.1.

2. Rubber Base Impression Materials (Elastomers)

The irreversible hydrocolloids (alginate), though widely used, are not considered

Table 10.1: Types of errors and their causes (alginates)

Type of error	Causes
1. Distortion	• Movement of tray during gelation • Unequal pressure during gelation • Premature removal from oral cavity • Improper removal from oral cavity • Impression not poured in time
2. Bubbles	• Air incorporated during mixing • Rough outer surface during insertion
3. Grainy surface	• Improper mixing/prolonged mixing • Water–powder ratio too low
4. Tearing	• Inadequate bulk • Premature removal from oral cavity • Excessive moisture
5. Rough stone casts	• Excess water left in impression • Premature removal • Leaving model in impression for longer period • Inadequate cleaning of impression

adequate mainly because of their poor dimensional stability. Another group of impression material, known as rubber base impression materials or elastomers were developed and are still being modified to overcome the weak links of alginates. The elastomers are basically polymers, which when mixed with catalyst become rubber like materials. The basic chemical reaction is the polymerization/vulcanization of the polymer and the catalyst.

Four types of elastomers are commonly available:

a. Polysulfides
b. Condensation silicones
c. Addition silicones (polyvinyl siloxane)
d. Polyether

All these types of elastomers are further classified into four categories, viz. light body, medium body, heavy body and putty, depending upon the viscosity and the flow characteristics (the relative amount of material, which flows under a given weight).

a. Polysulfides

The polysulfide impression materials are supplied as two paste system. The base consists of polysulfide polymer, titanium dioxide, zinc sulfate, silica, etc. The catalyst (accelerator) consists of lead dioxide with other substances, such as dibutyl phthalate, sulfur, magnesium stearate, etc. The basic reaction is the cross-linking of the ingredients used (oxidation of -SH group results in chain lengthening giving it elastomeric properties). It is not a rigid material and the impression is easier to remove than with polyether and polyvinyl siloxanes.

Properties

• Unpleasant odour and color; stains the linen.
• Bitter taste.
• Long setting time (8–12 minutes), causes discomfort to the patient.
• Hydrophobic; less hydrophilic.
• Produces excellent surface detail.
• 3–5% deformation, which improves with time (impression should be poured after 30 minutes).

- Good flexibility and tear resistance.
- Not affected by latex gloves.
- Exhibit some degree of cellular toxicity.
- Does not adhere to itself, which makes it unavailable for border moulding.

b. Condensation Silicones

The condensation silicones were developed to improve upon the qualities of polysulfides and to overcome the drawbacks of odour, taste, etc. The dimensional stability and the setting time have also been improved.

The condensation silicone contains base and accelerator; the setting is by polymerization as a result of cross-linkage between the two components (Fig. 10.13).

Properties

- Pleasant taste, odour and color; no staining.
- Setting time is 6–8 minutes.
- Hydrophobic, the field should be completely dry.
- Surface details are excellent.
- Stiffer than polysulfides and good tear resistance.
- Low dimensional stability (impression to be poured immediately). The permanent deformation is up to 3.0%.
- Exhibit some degree of cellular toxicity.

c. Addition Silicones

The addition silicones or polyvinyl siloxanes are improved variety of condensation silicones. Both the base and the catalyst are supplied in different tubes and jars. Since, viscosity of both base and the catalyst is same, the mixing is much easier than the condensation silicone (Figs 10.14a and b). Once mixed (1:1 ratio of base and catalyst), the addition silicones rapidly develop elasticity and should be used as soon as possible. The usual addition reaction takes place after mixing. Normally, the two agents remain in balance except the release of hydrogen as a by-product. Palladium black and polymer fibers are used as hydrogen absorbers.

They are inert after setting and can be poured in any die material; however, before setting they are susceptible to contamination. The contamination is usually of sulfur or sulfur compounds, especially from latex gloves. The polyethylene gloves are preferred over latex gloves.

Properties

- Pleasant odor, taste and color (available in different flavors).
- Better dimensional stability (permanent deformation is between 0.05 and 0.1%): Allows multiple pours.

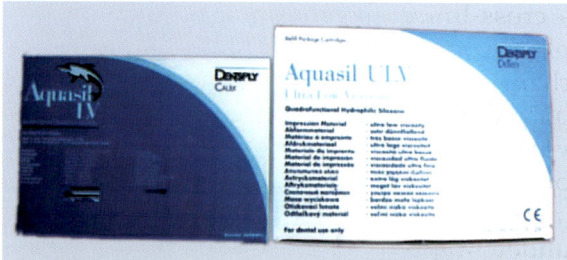

Fig. 10.14a: Addition silicone (Aquasil ULV)

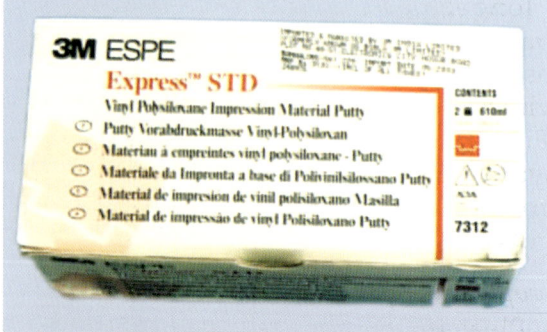

Fig. 10.14b: Addition silicone (Express STD)

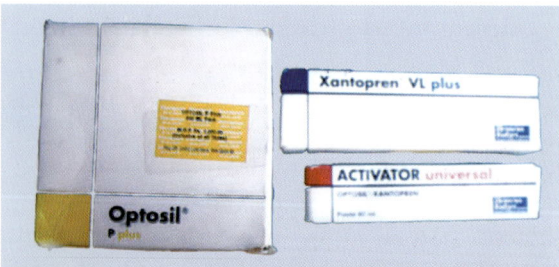

Fig. 10.13: Condensation silicon impression material

- Storage temperature does not influence the dimensional stability up to temperature 40°C. Beyond this temperature, distortion may occur.
- Better surface details.
- Good tear strength (tear strength better than hydrocolloid, but less than polyether.
- Low flexibility.
- Setting time is 4–5 minutes.
- Hydrophobic, the field should be dry before impression.
- Can be electroplated.
- Fairly inert after pouring with any die material.
- Foreign body reactions have been reported.
- Do not adhere to themselves after setting and cannot be used in border moulding.

d. Polyether

The polyether impression materials are usually available in two tubes; the base and the catalyst (accelerator). The base paste consists of polyether copolymer along with fillers and plasticizers. The catalyst paste has a cross-linking agent along with filler and plasticizers. The reaction after mixing causes chain lengthening and cross-linking to form a polyether rubber. The polyethers available are very stiff; however, proper viscosity polyethers are also marketed. Proper impression material should be applied in the undercut areas. The stiffness affects the ease of removal from the mouth.

Polyethers, after mixing, remain plastic for a longer period. This is desirable since impression can be distorted if the material is inserted into patient's oral cavity at a stage when it has already developed elasticity (Fig. 10.15). Because of being moderately hydrophilic, disinfection guidelines should be strictly followed. The material adheres to itself and can be used in border molding.

Properties

- Pleasant odour and taste (flavoured materials available).

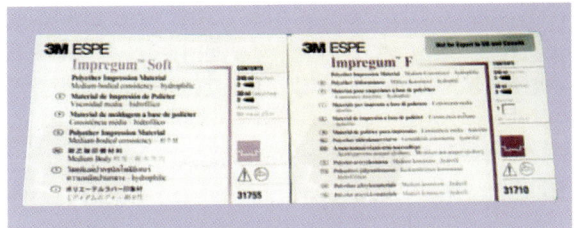

Fig. 10.15: Polyether impression material

- Dimensional stability is good (permanent deformation is around 0.1–0.2%). Allow multiple pours, at least in two weeks. Polyethers may absorb water, compromising die accuracy upon storage at high humidity.
- Storage temperature does not influence the dimensional stability. However, beyond 40°C, distortion may occur.
- Very stiff. (Final stiffness is twice that of addition silicones.)
- Setting time relatively short (3–5 minutes).
- Moderately hydrophilic (moisture in the impression field may not affect).
- Can be electroplated.
- Do not tear easily; allows the operator to get good subgingival details without tearing.
- The material is not affected by latex gloves.

Manipulation of Elastomers

The manipulation of Elastomers depend upon the type of material being used vis-à-vis its viscosity. The surface area (tissues) to be incorporated in the impression is also important. The manipulation is described under the following subheads.

i. Selection of Tray

In case, the impression is to be made in putty and the light body, the routine stock trays can be utilized. The stock trays are usually made of stainless steel or plastics and are available in different sizes. The selection and placement of tray in the oral cavity is similar to what is followed in making impression with alginate. The chances of material flowing into the pharyngeal area are less with rubber base putties; the posterior palatal seal area is properly covered in the impression.

ii. *Preparation of Special Tray*

In case the impression is to be made with medium body (putty and the light body are not used), a special tray is to be fabricated for impression making. The tray is usually fabricated in self-cure acrylics, though thermoplasticized trays are also used.

Requirement of custom tray
- The tray should be stable in form when exposed to oral environment
- It should be resistant to moisture
- High modulus of elasticity (rigid)
- The chemical/mechanical adhesion to the tray should be long lasting.

Advantages of custom trays
- Less impression material is required.
- Usually the tray is used once, sterilization is not a problem.
- Pre-selection of tray is not required.
- A uniform thickness of impression materials minimizes distortion resulting from curing shrinkage.

Disadvantages of custom trays
- Construction is time consuming.
- The residual monomer may irritate some patients.
- The tray should 'age' at least 24 hours before use.

Procedure
The impression of the teeth and surrounding tissues is taken with alginate or even impression compound and cast is prepared (Fig. 10.16). The prepared cast is coated with plaster of Paris filling all the undercuts (Figs 10.17a and b). The coating should be approximately 2.0–3.0 mm thick. Alternatively, pink wax (double fold) is adapted over the cast (Fig. 10.18).

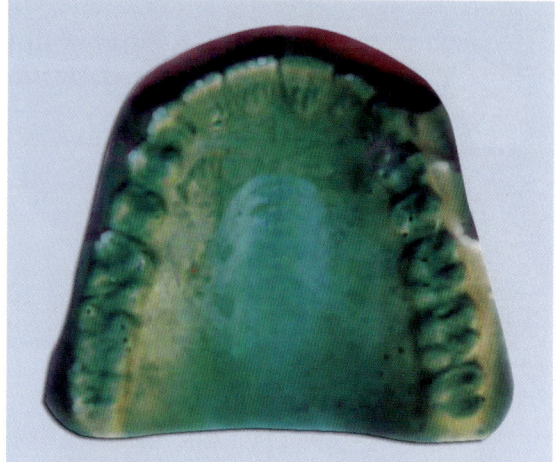

Fig. 10.16: Cast for making custom tray

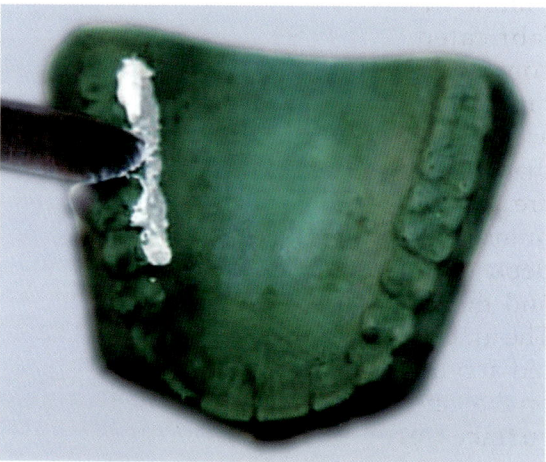

Fig. 10.17a: Filling undercuts for plaster

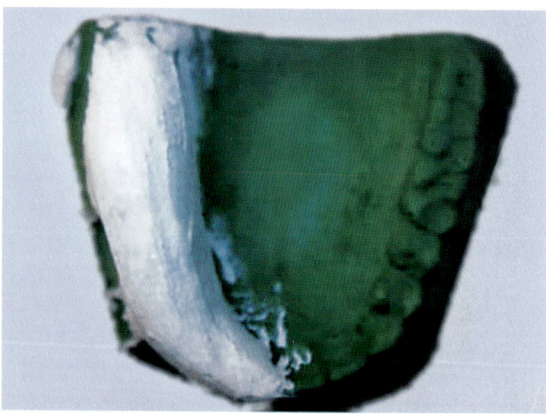

Fig. 10.17b: Filled undercuts

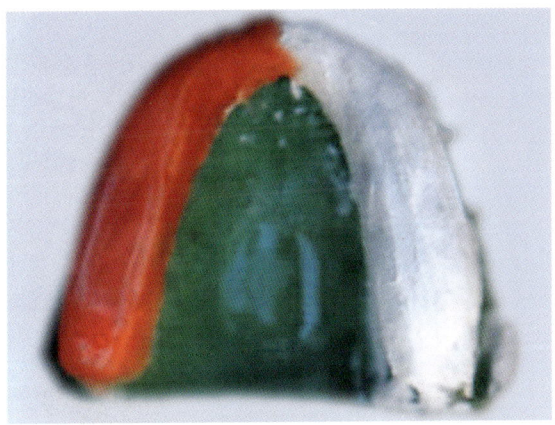

Fig. 10.18: Pink wax adapted

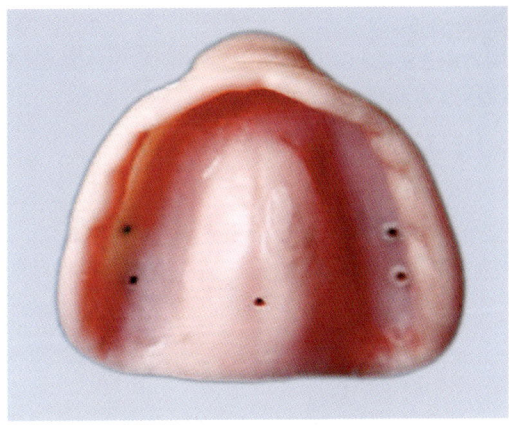

Fig. 10.19b: Holes drilled in custom tray

The tray is made in self-cure acrylics in routine though thermoplastic trays are also fabricated. A handle is also fixed. After complete polymerization and aging, the margins of the tray are finished. Small holes are prepared with acrylic burs. The usual diameter of the hole is 2.0 mm and the holes are 4.0–5.0 mm apart (Figs 10.19a and b). The number of holes and the diameter can vary depending upon the viscosity of the material and the need for pressure during insertion. The inner surface is roughened with large and old acrylic burs. Though adhesive is applied on the inner surface of the tray, yet the rough surfaces provide better retention of the material. Such techniques do not allow the impression to move freely, subsequently leading to distortion. The acrylic trays shrink 0.06% every 24 hours. The impression should be poured immediately.

iii. Gingival Retraction

The gingival tissues need to be retracted during impression making. The retraction process becomes more important if the finish lines of the preparation is subgingival. Various techniques and materials are being used to retract gingiva during impression making (mechanical, chemical and surgical means) (Fig. 10.20). Table 10.2 summarizes the techniques/materials used to visualize the gingival finish lines in impression making.

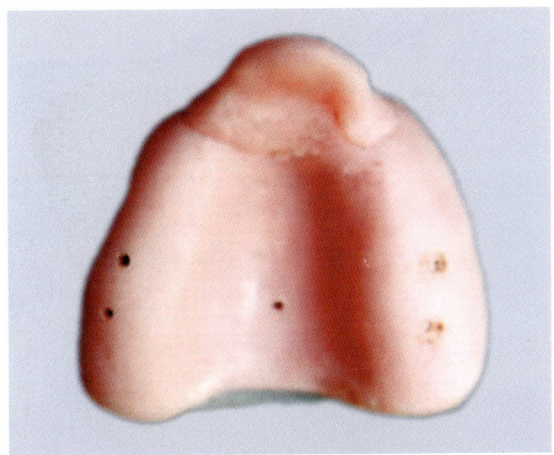

Fig. 10.19a: Prepared custom tray

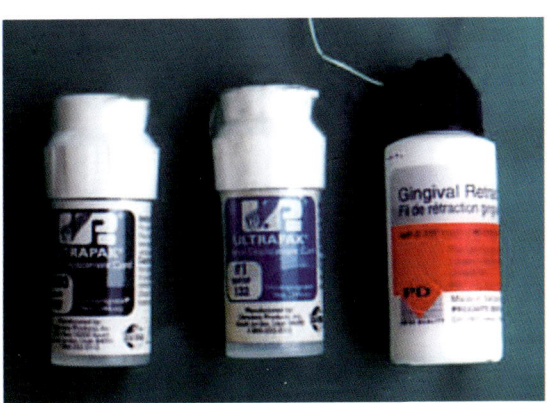

Fig. 10.20: Retraction cord

Table 10.2: Techniques/materials used to visualize subgingival finish lines in impression making

Material used	Uses	Hazards
Retraction cord (Normal, twisted or knitted)	Single cord or double cord can be used depending upon the need. In case, two cord technique is preferred, the first small diameter cord is left in place during impression recording (the cord tags should not protrude from the sulcus). Wetting the cord just before removal helps control haemorrhage. Usually, the first cord provides sufficient retraction and the second cord is not needed.	Excessive packing pressure may lead to recession or trauma to gums. Cord contaminated by gloves may prevent impression from setting, especially at gingival sulcus.
Chemical soaked cords (Solutions include: Epinephrine (1:1000 conc.), Alum (e.g. Aluminium potassium sulphate), Ferric sulphate (15.5%)	Ferric sulphate is considered better haemostatic agent than epinephrine but needs to be rubbed onto bleeding gingival sulcus. The solutions used should be washed off before impression making.	Concentrated solutions of Alum can cause severe inflammation and tissue necrosis. Ferric sulphate may stain the gums. Epinephrine may raise blood pressure and heart rate.
Electrosurgery	• Controlled tissue destruction by heating from electric current passing through the tissues • Widen gingival sulcus (troughing) before cord placed. • Gingivectomy for overgrown tissue or to crown lengthening • Coagulation (ball electrode) but produces most tissue destruction and slow healing.	Contraindicated in patients with cardiac pacemakers. Use in thin gingiva may result in recession.
Local curettage	• Palatal tissue respond better than thinner buccal tissues. • For subgingival preparation in healthy gingivae. Gingival sulcus depth must not exceed 3 mm and there should be adequate keratinized gingivae.	• A slightly deepening of the sulcus may result. • May damage attached gingiva • Not suitable in thin gingiva

Gingival Tissue Management

The management of gingival tissues, their retraction and deflection is mandatory for recording margin details of the preparation in impression making. The selection of method and materials for gingival retraction mainly depend upon the clinical situations, viz. inflammation/fibrosis gingiva, hemorrhage at the site, etc. The operator should carefully select the retracting material considering potential benefits and disadvantages.

Gingival retraction is defined as a process of exposing margins when making impressions of the prepared teeth. It is the deflection of the marginal gingiva away from a tooth. The gingival sulcus is deepened to expose the cervical portion of the tooth in order to have proper marginal finish to the restoration. The main goal of gingival retraction is to reversibly displace the gingival tissues, so that low viscosity impression material can be introduced into the sulcus, capturing the margin details without tearing the impression.

Need for Gingival Retraction

1. To provide access for impression material into the subgingival margins, recording the finish line properly.
2. Undermine caries can be treated easily.
3. The margins on the prepared tooth can be evaluated and modified, if need be.
4. Helps in easy removal of cement without damaging the gingiva.
5. The marginal fit of the restoration can be assessed.
6. To gain surface area, it may be necessary to extend the restoration below the gingival margin.
7. Facilitates finishing and polishing of the restoration, especially at margins.

Indications
- Presence of subgingival caries.
- Cervical abrasion and erosion.
- Gingival polyp at the margins.
- Subgingival finish line.
- Decreased crown:root ratio.

Contraindications
- Poor oral hygiene.
- Gingival recession.
- Bone Loss.
- Systemic diseases affecting gingiva.

The following features should be considered prior to gingival retraction:

a. The periodontium should be sound, especially around the prepared tooth and the adjoining teeth.
b. The crest of free gingiva should be at its normal position relative to the tooth surface with no recession.
c. Any hyperplastic/fibrosed tissue, if present, should be treated prior to restoration.
d. Crevicular fluid and bleeding should be arrested to achieve accessibility and effective manipulation.
e. The retraction at the gingival crevice area should be accomplished without detaching the apically located epithelial attachment and periodontal ligament.
f. Gingival retraction should not cause any irreversible damage to the gingiva/ periodontium.

Methods

The principal methods available for gingival retraction are:

a. Mechanical
b. Chemo-mechanical
c. Surgical/electrosurgical
d. Miscellaneous

a. Mechanical methods: The gingiva is displaced mechanically both laterally and apically away from tooth surface. The mechanical methods are generally employed where the gingiva is healthy with good vascular supply and adequate bone support.

The various materials used for mechanical retraction are:

i. Wooden wedges (used for depressing the inter-proximal gingiva)

ii. Cotton twills (forcibly introduced into the gingival sulcus; mechanical retraction achieved in 20–30 minutes)

iii. Cotton twills with fast setting zinc oxide eugenol (Thin mix of zinc oxide eugenol wrapped in cotton rolls is inserted into the gingival sulcus; provides better retraction and effective tissue tolerance, however, if kept for longer time, leads to loss of periodontal attachment)

iv. Rubber dam material (Heavy -0.010 inch or 0.25 mm, Extra heavy-0.012 inch or 0.30 mm and Special heavy-0.014 inch or 0.35 mm) is usually employed: effective in limited number of teeth; however, cannot be used with elastomeric impression materials.

v. Copper band (slight oversized band filled with modeling wax is effective in pushing the gingival sulcus; excess pressure should be avoided).

b. Chemomechanical methods: Certain chemical agents soaked in cotton or cords are utilized to achieve effective gingival retraction. The commonly used chemical agents are:

i. Epinephrine/nor-epinephrine (vaso-constrictors)

ii. Alum/aluminium chloride/tannic acid (biological fluid coagulants)

iii. Zinc chloride/silver nitrate potassium hydroxide (surface tissue coagulants)

iv. Concentrated zinc chloride/concentrated potassium hydroxide (chemical cantery)

i. *Epinephrine/nor-epinephrine (vasoconstrictors):* The chemical agents physiologically restrict the blood supply by decreasing the size of the blood capillaries (vasoconstriction), producing hemostasis. The retraction is achieved in 10 minutes; however, their use should be limited because of their systemic effects.

It is established that the amount of epinephrine absorbed from 2.5 cm of retraction cord during 5–15 minutes in gingival sulcus is 71 µg.

Contraindications
- Hypersensitive to epinephrine.
- Cardiovascular disorders.
- Hypertension
- Hyperthyroidism
- Diabetes
- Patients on β-blockers and anti-depressants

ii. *Alum/aluminium chloride/tannic acid (biological fluid coagulants)*
Biologic fluid coagulants locally coagulate blood and tissue fluids, effectively retracting the surface layer. 10% Alum solution is considered superior to epinephrine. 20–40% tannic acid is best effective than epinephrine, but shows good tissue recovery.

iii. *Zinc chloride/silver nitrate/potassium hydroxide (surface tissue coagulants):* Usually, 6–8% zinc chloride is used to coagulate the surface layer of sulcular and free gingival epithelium along with any fluids present in sulcus; however, these agents may cause ulceration and necrosis, when applied for prolonged time.

iv. *Concentrated zinc chloride/concentrated potassium hydroxide (chemical cautery):* 40% zinc chloride is used to chemically cauterize the local gingival tissues.

Retraction cords: *Retraction* is the downward and outward movement of the free gingival margin, achieved by different retraction materials and the techniques.

Relapse is the tendency of the gingival cuff to revert to its original position; influenced by the elasticity of the gingival cuff and the rebound forces of adjacent attached gingiva.

Displacement is a downward movement of the gingival cuff, usually caused by heavy consistency impression materials.

Collapse is the tendency of the gingival cuff to flatten under forces associated with the use of closely adapted customized impression trays. Retraction can also be classified as:

1. Cotton/synthetic
2. Braided/twisted/knitted
3. Coarse/fine
4. Impregnated/non-impregnated

The color coding indicates relative thickness of cords.

- Black – 000 (extra small)
- Yellow – 00 (small)
- Purple – 0
- Blue – 1
- Green – 2
- Red – 3 (extra large)

Ideal requirements of cord
- Should be dark in color
- Should effectively retract the gingival tissues
- Should not have any systemic effect
- Effects should be reversible
- Should not stick to the soft tissues
- Should provide effective hemostasis

Retraction cord insertion—guidelines
- Exact length to be incorporated into sulcus
- If using several inserts, start with small diameter followed by the larger one
- Start packing from one end to other
- The ends of cords should fall at axial angles of the tooth, rather than facial and lingual
- Packing instrument should be blunt preferably with serrations
- Load cords directed apically at an angle
- The packed material should be removed in hydrous field
- In double cord technique; larger diameter cord is removed, keeping the small diameter cord in the sulcus, and the impression is made.

Technique
In case of single cord, the cord is cut according to the need, moistened in the selected chemical agent (pre-soaked cords are also available) and inserted into the gingival sulcus area applying slight pressure at the apical direction.

The instrument should be inclined towards the area already tucked by the cord. Occasionally, it is necessary to hold the cord with one instrument while packing with the second. The instrument must be angled slightly towards the root to facilitate the subgingival placement. Excess cord is cut off in the mesial inter-proximal area.

In case of double cord technique, a small-diameter cord is placed in the sulcus followed by a second cord soaked in the hemostatic agent above the small diameter cord.

Diameter of the second cord should be the largest diameter that can be placed into the sulcus. After 8–10 minutes, the second cord is soaked in water and removed. The preparation is dried and impression is made with primary cord in place. After impression making, the small diameter cord is soaked in water and removed from the sulcus.

Advantage of placing double cord is that the first cord remains in place, thus reducing the tendency of gingival cuff to recoil and displace partially set impression material.

2.0% ferric sulphate has been used to control bleeding, when directly placed at the gingival sulcus. When hemostasis is required, retraction cord soaked in the ferric sulfate solution is packed into the sulcus following conventional guidelines.

It is advised to make multiple impressions in case more teeth are to be involved, especially, the anteriors. Gingival retraction of alternate teeth should be carried out and impression is made; followed by retracting the gingiva of remaining teeth and impression making.

c. *Surgical/electrosurgical*
i. *Surgical curettage:* A surgical curettage using rotary instruments is carried out to remove epithelial tissue in the sulcus along with creating a chamfer finish line in the

preparation. The technique is also known as 'gingitage' and is used where adequate gingiva is present and the sulcular depth is less than 3.0 mm.

Disadvantages
- There is poor tactile sensation when using diamonds points on gingival sulcular walls.
- May lead to destruction of periodontium.

ii. *Gingivectomy:* Gingivectomy, the excision of the gingiva, has also been preferred to remove hypertrophic gingiva.

Indications
- Interfering gingival tissue during any impression/restorative procedures.
- Gingival polyps seen in proximal caries.
- For crown lengthening procedures.
- For apical repositioning of whole periodontal attaching apparatus to create a healthy, safely manipulated, easily retractable free gingiva.

iii. *Electrosurgical:* Electrosurgical method is defined as the surgical reduction of sulcular epithelium by using electrode of high frequency. Electrosurgery produces a controlled tissue destruction to achieve the desired results.

Various types of electrosurgical electrodes are used in routine; such as, coagulating, diamond loop, round loop, straight loop, small loop, etc. The electrosurgical actions can be:
a. Electrosectioning/cutting (precise cutting with minimum tissue involvement)
b. Electrocoagulation (create coagulation of tissues, their fluids and oozed blood)
c. Fulgeration (involves deeper tissues, accompanied by carbonization)
d. Dessication (massive tissue involvement; uncontrolled action)

Guidelines to be followed during Electrosurgery
  i. The operational area should be moist.
  ii. Use fully rectified, undamped current with minimum energy output.

iii. Use light pressure touch and rapid strokes with a five seconds lapse between two strokes. (Always keep cutting electrode in the internal wall of sulcus, maintaining biologic width area.)
iv. Metallic restorations should not be touched (can create short circuit and damage surrounding structures).
  v. Always clean debris on the electrode tip with alcohol soaked gauge.
vi. After the impression, a blood clot is created with curetting the area for better healing.
vii. Avoid electrosurgery in patients with pacemaker.

Advantages
- Immediate hemostasis
- Better healing of the tissues
- Improved accuracy of the impression (margins visible)
- Decreased chair time and stress
- Minimal postoperative discomfort

Disadvantages
- Technique sensitive
- May lead to apical migration of marginal gingiva.
- Inaccurate current setting may cause tissue damage.
- Difficult to control lateral dissipation of heat

d. *Miscellaneous:* The newer agents used to achieve effective gingival retraction are:
  1. Magic foam
  2. Merocel strips
  3. Expasyl
  4. Gingitrac (Centrix)
  5. Lasers
  6. Stay-put retraction cord
  7. Comprecap
  8. Racegel
  9. Matrix impression system
  10. Cryosurgery
  11. Newer agents

1. *Magic foam:* Magic foam is the expanding vinyl polysiloxane material, designed for easy and fast retraction of the gingival sulcus without the potentially traumatic and time consuming packing of retraction cord. It is a non-hemostatic cordless retraction system consisting of foam and cartridges. The material in a syringe is delivered around the crown margins and a cap is placed to maintain pressure. After five minutes, the cap and the foam are removed and the preparation is ready for final impression.

Advantages
- Non-traumatic, application with minimum pressure
- Easy and fast application
- Comfortable to the patient
- Efficient, especially in multiple preparations

Disadvantages
- No hemostatic action
- Expensive

2. *Merocel strip:* Merocel strip (hydroxylate polyvinyl acetate) is a synthetic material that expands by absorption of oral fluids and exerts pressure on surrounding tissue. Placement of strips do not require local anaesthesia; ensures effective gingival retraction. The absence of fibers in the strips decreases the risk of post-operative complications. Merocel is soft and adaptable to surrounding tissues, not abrasive and can easily be shaped according to need.

Advantages
- Can be easily shaped and adapted around tooth.
- Effective in absorption of oral fluids.
- Significantly superior to retraction cords
- Strips are free of any fiber or debris (not damaging to tissues)

3. *Expasyl:* Expasyl is a chemo-mechanical technique for gingival retraction. The Expasyl material is Kaoline incorporated into an organic binder with aluminium chloride as hemostatic agent. It is supplied in syringe as viscous paste, which is injected into gingival sulcus, exerting a stable and non-damaging pressure. When left in place for one minute, this pressure is sufficient to achieve 0.5 mm of gingival retraction.

Advantages
- Effectively achieve hemostasis
- Minimum pressure required (atraumatic)
- Minimal tissue damage
- Helps in controlling bleeding
- Sufficient retraction in two minutes
- Less time consuming

Disadvantages
- Thickness of paste pose problems in pushing into sulcus
- Not cost effective
- Metal tips may not be suitable for interproximal areas

4. *Gingitrac (centrix):* Gingitrac is available as paste system; applying the paste around the margins using preloaded syringe. The paste contains aluminium sulfate, a mild natural astringent. It utilizes patients bite pressure to push material into gingival sulcus and achieve retraction. A cap can be used in single tooth preparation. The paste is removed prior to impression making.

Advantages
- Works in less than five minutes
- Gently retracts the gingiva with no tissue trauma
- Natural astringent controls bleeding
- Works on single or multiple crown preparations

5. *Lasers:* Soft tissue lasers have been tried for gingival retraction using flexible optical fibers.

Lasers work through photo-ablation and produce blood-free incisions followed by rapid healing without any inflammation. The laser technique is a little slower; however, produces controlled tissue retraction, free of hemorrhage and pain.

The common lasers employed are:
- *CO₂ (carbon dioxide):* Absorbs less energy near the tissues, with minimal increase of temperature.
- *Nd:YAG (Neodymium:yttrium-aluminium-garnet):* Preferred for retraction of hyper-trophied tissues; produces heat
- *Er:YAG (Erbium:yttrium-aluminium-garnet):* Fairly safe; not good in hemostasis
- *Argon:* Safe to use.

Advantages
- Their use requires minimal or no anaes-thesia; relatively painless.
- They do not harm dental tissues, including pulp
- Can be used around dental implants
- CO₂ laser provides better hemostasis
- Healing is rapid

Disadvantages
- Er:YAG is not good for hemostasis
- May not provide tactile feedback (CO₂ laser), leading to damage to attached gingiva.

6. *Stay–put retraction cord:* Stay–put is a unique combination of softly braided retraction cord and ultra fine copper filaments. When the stay–put cord is shaped, it remains in shape and does not deform. It is usually available as non-impregnated; however, aluminium chloride can be used for impre-gnation.

Advantages
- Can be easily adapted
- Can be shaped
- Does not deform in the sulcus
- Non-impregnated; can be impregnated with an astringent or hemostatic solution, if need be.

7. *Comprecap:* The use of aluminium chloride in conjunction with comprecap compression caps, is effective in controlling bleeding and providing tissue retraction. It holds the retraction cord deep in the sulcus, opening it even wider. After placing the retraction cord, the cap is placed over the prepared tooth and pushed into the sulcus. Patient is asked to bite on the cap for sometime; after that it is removed along the retraction cord.

Advantages
- It ensures a dry and clean area.
- Less technical skill required.
- Stops bleeding naturally by compression.

Disadvantages
Aluminium chloride used in conjunction with comprecap may interfere with setting of polyether/polyvinyl siloxane impression material.

8. *Racegel:* Racegel, a new hemostatic agent, available in gel form, controls bleeding and absorbs crevicular fluid prior to impression making. The gel contains 25% aluminium chloride, oxyquinol and excipients. Racegel can be used with or without gingival retraction cords.

The material's viscosity increases when in contact with the gingival tissue providing access to the gingival margin (thermodynamic property).

It facilitates access of the gingival crevice, reduces bleeding and oozing. Due to its consistency, it can be rinsed quickly, leaving no residual material.

Advantages
- Effective hemostatic agent
- Can easily be removed
- Can be used with or without retraction cord

Disadvantages
- May irritate eyes and skin
- Allergic reaction reported because of oxyquinol

9. *Matrix impression system:* The matrix impression system requires series of three impressions using three viscosities.

A matrix of occlusal registration rubber base material (semi-rigid) is made over the tooth preparation prior to gingival retraction.

The matrix is trimmed as per need and the retraction cord is removed. An impression is made with high viscosity rubber base impression material. After seating of the matrix impression, a stock tray filled with medium viscosity impression, material is seated over the matrix and the remaining teeth to make impression of the entire arch. Matrix impression system maintains retraction by trapping a highly viscous material in the sulcus when the matrix is seated.

Advantages
- Eliminates chances of tearing of sulcular flange
- Cleans blood and debris from sulcus area
- Delivers impression material in sulcus with accuracy
- Open sulcus for longer period of time.

Disadvantage
- Increased chairside time.

10. *Cryosurgery:* Cyrosurgery is preferred in cases of interfering and fibrosed gingival tissues. It is also indicated for apical repositioning of whole periodontal apparatus to create a healthy, retracted free gingiva. A sharp, cold knife is used to remove the tissues at 320–340°F using liquid nitrogen. The tissues freeze and shrink when in contact with nitrogen.

Advantage
Effective in fibrosed gingival tissues.

11. *Newer agents:* Nasal and ophthalmic decongestants show favorable results in gingival retraction. The commonly used agents are:
- 0.25% Phenylephrine hydrochloride (Neo-synephrine)
- 0.05% Oxymetazoline hydrochloride (Afrin)
- 0.05% Tetrahydrozoline hydrochloride (Visine)

Their use is limited because other techniques are more effective in achieving gingival retraction.

iv. *Mixing and Loading*

The tray is coated with the adhesive, which is supplied by the manufacturer (Figs 10.21a and b). Allow the adhesive to set, which takes usually 3–5 minutes. In case, the adhesive is not applied, it leads to concentric shrinkage, i.e. away from the tray and if adhesive is applied, the shrinkage is eccentric, i.e. towards the tray.

The adhesive is not interchangeable with different companies manufacturing their own adhesive compatible with the impression material. The adhesive with polysulfides contain butyl rubber, styrene acrylonitrile and volatile solvents. The adhesive supplied with addition silicone contains polydimethyl siloxane and ethyl silicate.

Impression Techniques

Various impression techniques for indirect restorations are:

1. *Single impression technique:* The impression tray is inserted into the patient's mouth only

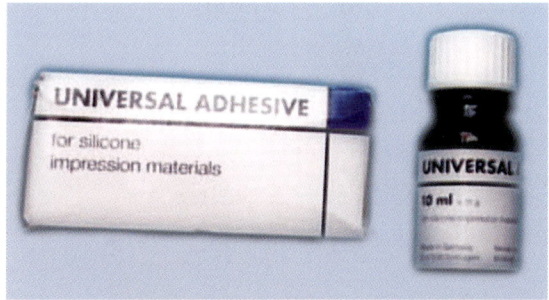

Fig. 10.21a: Adhesive for coating the tray

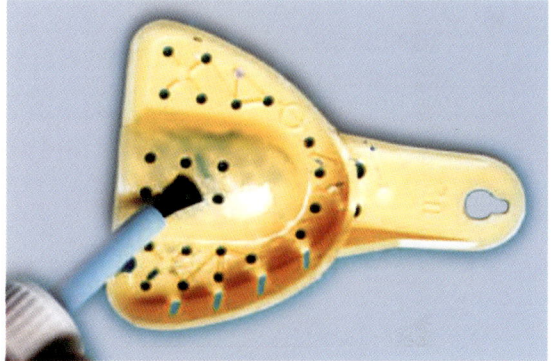

Fig. 10.21b: Coating uniform layer of adhesive

once using this technique. The technique may be further subdivided into two types, i.e. single mix or double mix depending on whether one or two viscosities of impression material are used.

a. *Double mix technique:* The process begins with fabrication of a custom tray in autopolymerizing acrylic resin using a 3.0 mm base plaster wax spacer and four tissue stops in non-functional areas of teeth. After the final setting of the resin, the wax spacer is removed and the intraoral correction of custom tray extensions is made.

   Tray adhesive is painted on the tissue surface and border of tray and the light body material is injected onto the prepared teeth; simultaneously, the custom tray is loaded with the putty material.

   The tray is seated in the mouth and held immobile until it polymerizes. The tray is removed with a snap after the final set of the material.

b. *Single mix technique:* The procedure is similar to the above method except that the same regular body or monophase material is used both as a tray and as a syringe material.

2. Double impression technique

a. *Using putty and light body in stock trays with polyethylene spacer:* Equal amount of base and the catalyst is taken from the jars

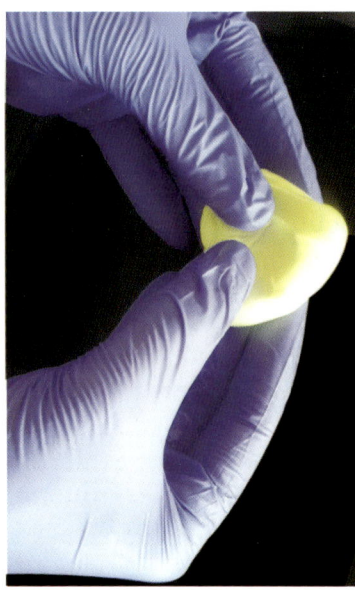

Fig. 10.23: Kneading of putty

(Fig. 10.22). Use the scoop given by the manufacturer for this purpose. For convenience, different color of scoops and jars are provided to easily identify base and the catalyst. The two are then mixed by doughing and rolling between the fingers (Fig. 10.23). The mixed putty is rolled into the impression tray (Fig. 10.24). The latex gloves should not be worn while the two putties are being mixed. The latex gloves prolong the setting time or the material may not set at all. The compounds used in vulcanization of latex gloves (sulfur

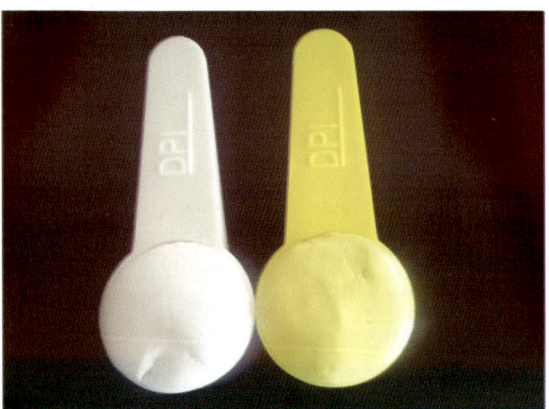

Fig. 10.22: Equal scoops of base and catalyst putty

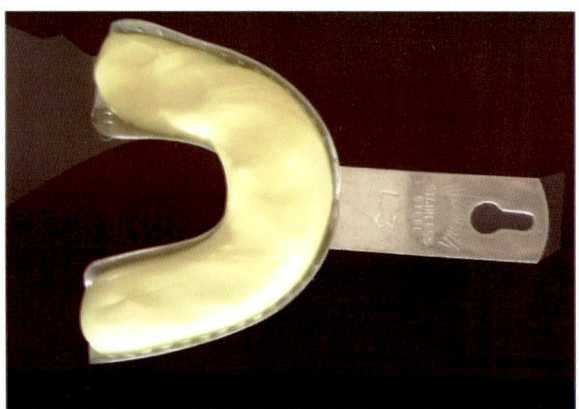

Fig. 10.24: Loading of putty in tray

compounds), migrate to the mix and contaminate the chloro-platinic acid catalyst, resulting in retarded or no polymerization. Thorough washing of gloves with detergent and water just before mixing decreases this effect. Alternatively, vinyl gloves can be used which do not have such effect. The latex gloves affect only addition silicones; the latex gloves, however, do not affect the other impression materials.

A spacer, usually a polyethylene sheet, covers the putty (Fig. 10.25). The single or double sheet is covered all along the arch if full complement of teeth is required in final impression and a part of the arch if that particular area is required. In case, the sheet is not available or operator does not prefer, the impression can be taken as it is and the surface of putty is scrapped from the area which is required for final impression. Special types of knives are available for the purpose; alternatively, sharp carvers, blades can also be used (Fig. 10.26).

The tray once inserted is kept at the same position keeping uniform pressure on all the sides (Fig. 10.27). Excessive pressure is avoided, which may tear the putty and

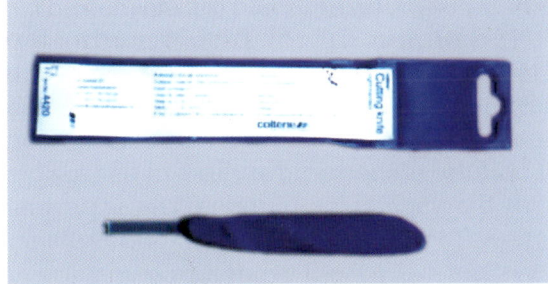

Fig. 10.26: Knife for scraping

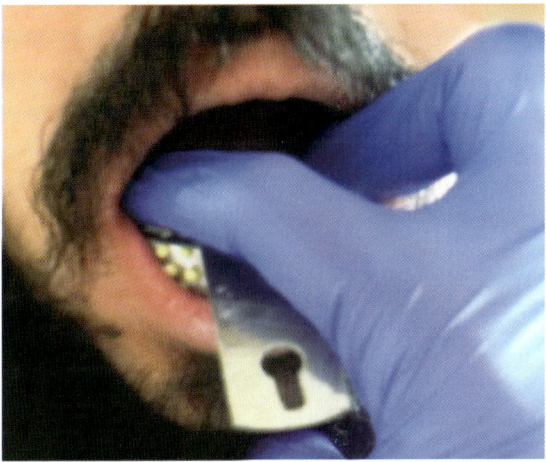

Fig. 10.27: Tray insertion in patient's oral cavity

hinder with the elastic nature of the material. When the fingernail impression rebounds completely, the putty is all set and the tray is to be removed with minimum sideward movements (Fig. 10.28).

The spacer is peeled off. The impression is checked for any gross abnormality. If so, the putty impression is repeated, otherwise the tray and the impression is covered with napkin and kept aside for final impression. For final impression, either equal amount of two parts of light body is mixed on a clean slab or a gun provided by the manufacturer does the mixing (Fig. 10.29a and b). Usually, the gun is utilized which mixes both the tubes in exact amounts and the narrow needle on top help in pushing the material into the inaccessible areas. Care should be taken to completely dry the area

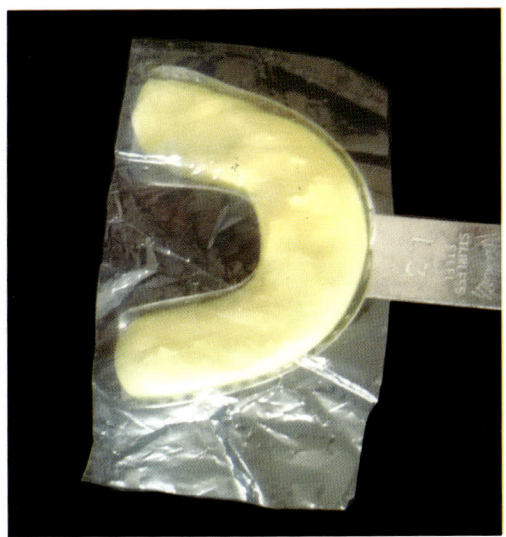

Fig. 10.25: Polyethylene spacer

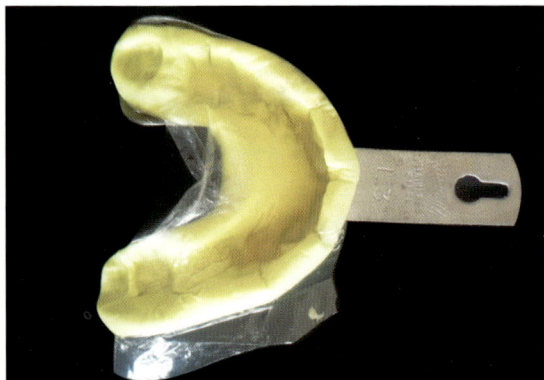

Fig. 10.28: Impression with spacer after removal from mouth

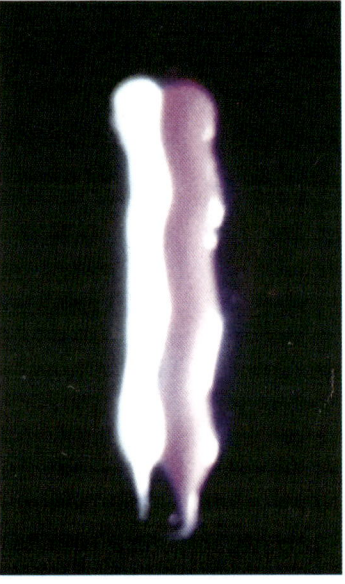

Fig. 10.29a: Light body: Base and catalyst

before making impression. Light body should be loaded on the tray (Fig. 10.30).

Stabilize the tray in position and keep it there with minimum pressure. The manufacturers usually instruct regarding the setting time of the material. The environmental factors should be taken care of. The tray removal should be parallel to the preparation path of withdrawal. The viscoelastic nature of the impression material warrants the material to be removed rapidly from the oral cavity. Unnecessary movement should be avoided. The peripheral seal on the buccal folds should be broken with the help of fingers; removing the tray with minimum movements. Rinse the impression with water and dry with air. The oral cavity should be checked for any remnant of the material, and cleaned. The thin chips should be thoroughly removed from interdental and other areas since the material has the potential of damaging tissues (Fig. 10.31).

b. *Using putty and light body is stock trays by scraping:* In this technique, the putty material around the prepared tooth in the interdental spaces is scraped out using a "putty cutter" or a surgical blade to provide space for the light body material.

3. ***Triple tray technique/dual-arch impression/ closed mouth technique:*** These techniques are indicated for single-unit, less extensive

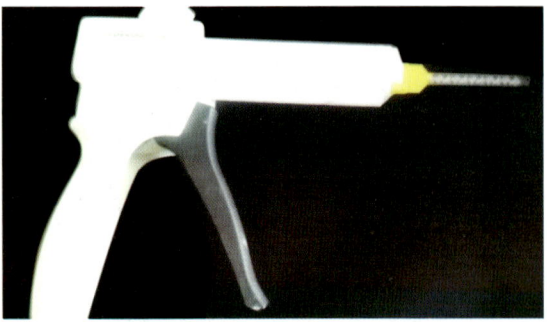

Fig. 10.29b: Automixing gun

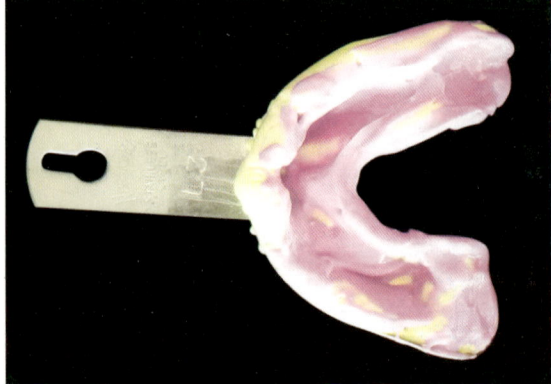

Fig. 10.30: Light body over putty impression

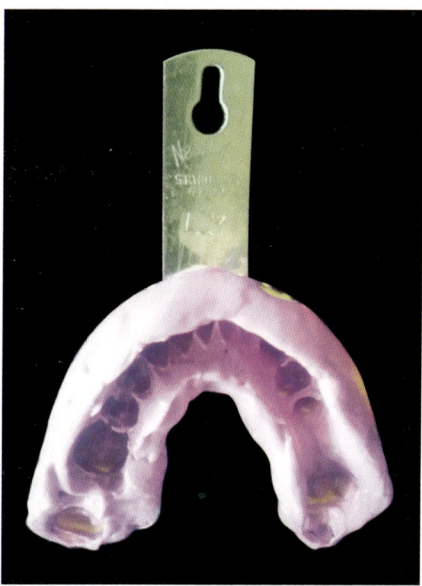

Fig. 10.31: Final putty wash impression

mouth so that the patient closes in maximum intercuspation without interference.

- Putty material is loaded on both sides of the triple tray and simultaneously the light body material injected onto prepared abutments and opposing teeth (Fig. 10.33).
- The tray is inserted in patient's mouth and patient asked to close in maximal intercuspation. The occlusion is verified by checking the contralateral side (Fig. 10.34).

Limitation of putty-wash technique

The putties were developed initially to reduce the shrinkage of condensation silicones; however, with addition silicones, the polymerization contraction and dimensional stability are excellent. The addition silicone

restorations in each arch and they record the prepared and adjacent teeth, opposing teeth and maximal intercuspation occlusion on bite.

The technique is advantageous as it eliminates the need for an articulator, minimizes deformation of mandible during opening and utilizes less material.

Procedure

- The triple tray of correct size (Fig. 10.32) is selected and verified for fit in patient's

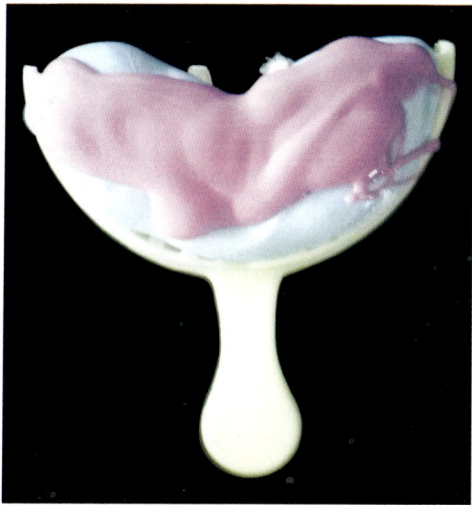

Fig. 10.33: Putty loaded in tray

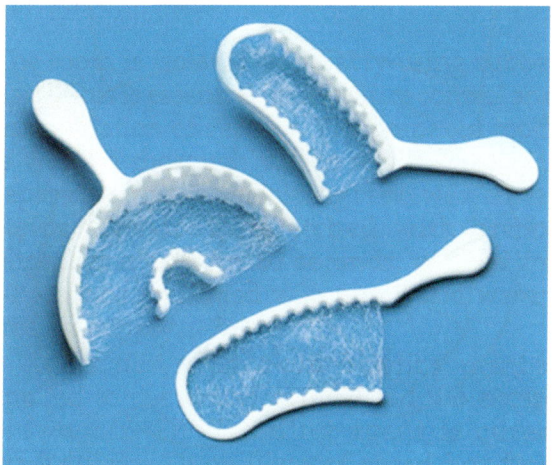

Fig. 10.32: Triple tray

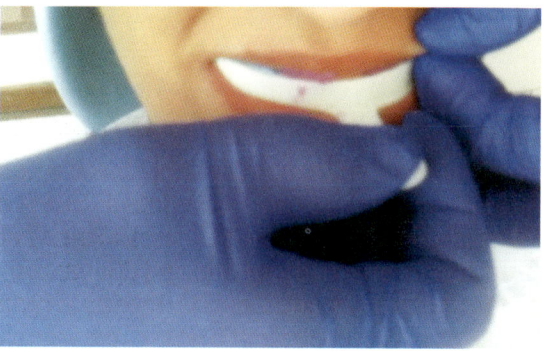

Fig. 10.34: Tray insertion in patient's oral cavity

putty-wash impressions are preferred because of their better handling features.

Summarily, there are three ways of recording a putty-wash impression:

- One-stage impression: Putty and wash are recorded simultaneously (also called twin mix or laminate technique)
- Two-stage impression: Putty is recorded first and after setting relined with a thin layer of wash.
- Two-stage impression creating space: A space is created for the wash. The space is created by:
  - Applying polythene spacer over the teeth before impression making with putty
  - Putty impression can be recorded before tooth preparation
  - Providing escape channels in the putty impression for the wash.

The main problem, which may lead to distortion, is recoil. Recoil works in the following way: Considerable forces are needed to seat putty impression, which can result either in outward flexion of the tray wall or the incorporation of residual stresses within the material. On removing the tray from the oral cavity, the tray walls rebound, which may lead to undersized (bucco-lingually) dies.

The putties of lower viscosity also produce similar distortions with plastic trays. Rigid metal trays can minimize such distortions and are recommended for putty-wash impressions. Such distortions may occur using two-stage impression technique also (Hydrostatic pressure generated during setting with wash in unspaced impression). It is established that the most convenient and reliable way of recording a putty-wash impression is to use the one stage technique with addition silicone putty in a rigid metal tray.

v. Evaluating the Impression

The final impression should be thoroughly checked before making the cast. The following features are of importance:

- There should be no tray show-through from any area of the impression; however, the stops used in the tray might show through the impression. Even minor show-through or visible thin layer of impression within the area to be restored is to be discarded.
- There should be no voids present, especially, within the area to be restored.
- The impression is reviewed thoroughly for tears and fractured margins.
- The impression material should fully cover the finish lines (minimum 0.5 mm beyond the finish line). And also, there should be no thin areas around finish line, because such unsupported areas distort under the weight of the stone.
- There should be no shiny smooth surfaces in the impression (moisture contamination at particular area may give rise to such surfaces).

The addition silicones release hydrogen after setting, which produce voids in the gypsum casts. To avoid these voids, hydrogen absorbers such as palladium black and polymer fillers are used. Alternatively, one can opt for either of the following:

- One hour delay in pouring (in case of Epoxy casts, the pouring is delayed for 12 hours since epoxy resin takes longer time for setting).
- Keep the impression in vacuum for five minutes
- Keep the impression in hot water, cool and then pour

Advances in elastomeric impression material

Vinly polyether silicone (VPES): Vinyl polyether silicone is hybrid of polyether and addition silicones.

The material combines the tear strength and dimensional stability of addition silicones and the wettability and flow of polyethers. It is available in multiple viscosities and with multiple setting times that enable its usage in every situation. It can be disinfected without distortion. The

Table 10.3: Elastomeric impression materials; commercial preparation and properties

Product (company)	Working time (minutes)	Time in oral cavity (min.)	Elastic recovery	Flexibility	Tear strength
Addition silicones: Light body					
Affinis (Coltene)	1.0	2.09	Very high	Low	Medium
Aquasil Ultra LV/XLV (Dentsply)	2.25–2.75	5.0	Very high	Medium	Very high
Exafast NDS (GC)	1.0–1.20	1.5	Very high	Medium	Low medium
Flexitime correct flow (Heraeus Kulzer)	2.5	5.0	Very high	Medium	Medium
1st Impression PVS:	1.25	2.25	High	Low	Medium
Fast Set (Den-Mat)	2.5	4.5	Very high	Low	Medium
1st Impression PVS: Regular Set (Den-Mat)					
Imprint II Garant (3M ESPE)	1.0	4.0	Very high	Low	Medium
Virtual: Fast Set (Ivoclar vivadent)	1.55	2.5	Very high	Low	Medium
Addition silicones: Heavy body					
Affinis: Coltene (Coltene/Whaledent)	1.0	2.5	Very high	Very low	Medium
Aquasil Ultra Heavy (Dentsply)	2.25–2.75	5.0	Very high	Low	High
Exafast NDS (GC America)	1.25	1.5	Very high	Low	High
Examix NDS (GC America)	2.0	4.0	Very high	Low	High
Exajet: Fast set (GC)	1.5	2.5	Very high	Low	Medium
Exajet: Regular set (GC)	2.0	3.0	Very high	Low	Medium
Flexitime (Heraeus Kulzer)	2.5	5.0	Very high	Very low	Medium
1st Impression PVS: Fast Set (Den-Mat)	1.25	2.25	Very high	Very low	Medium
1st Impression PVS: Regular Set (Den-Mat)	2.5	4.5	Very high	Very low	Medium
Imprint II Penta (3M ESPE)	2.0	4.0	Very high	Low	Very high
Virtual : Fast Set (Ivoclar Vivadent)	1.25	2.5	Very high	Low	Medium
Polyethers					
Impregum Garant Soft (3M ESPE)	2.0	3.5	High	Medium	Medium
Impregum Penta Soft (3M ESPE)	2.5	3.5	High	Medium	High

commercial preparation and properties of elastomeric impression materials are tabulated in Table 10.3.

Common errors: The various types of errors in rubber base impression material and the related causes are tabulated in Table 10.4.

Table 10.4: Types of errors and the causes (Elastomers)

Type of error	Causes
Distortion	• Inadequate ageing of the tray material • Lack of adhesion of the impression with the tray • Movement of tray during polymerization • Premature or improper removal from the mouth • Undue pressure during polymerization or during removal • Delay in seating the tray
Bubbles	• Air incorporated during mixing • Too rapid polymerization because of inadequate mixing • Premature gelation of syringe material preventing flow
Rough impression surface	• Improper mixing of the components • Incomplete polymerization caused by premature removal • Rapid polymerization might be due to high temperature
Rough cast surface	• Inadequate cleaning of impression • Excess water left in the impression • Premature removal of impression • Improper manipulation of stone plaster

3. Light Cure Impression Material

The light cure impression material contains elastomeric resin along with dimethacrylate, polyether methane and silicon dioxide as filler. The material is available in two viscosities. The light body is packed in syringes and the heavy body in tubes. The light body is applied first followed by heavy body. The impression is light cured with larger diameter probe. The material after setting shows better physical properties. Commercially available light cure impression materials are Genesis, Polyjel NF, etc.

Properties

• Highest resistance to tear
• Better dimensional stability
• Better flow
• Compatible with stone and die materials
• Can be electroplated
• Material should be stored away from direct light (light cures the material)

Advantages

• Control over working time
• Short curing time
• Better physical properties (excellent elasticity)
• Excellent tear resistance
• Highly biocompatible, can be cold disinfected with no loss of quality
• Dimensionally stable (impression can be poured even after two weeks)
• No by-products (production of gases, etc.)

Disadvantages

• Special tray (transparent tray) is required through which light can be passed
• Difficult to light cure at some areas
• Not fair in severe undercuts (material is rigid)
• Incomplete cure of the material can lead to distortion
• Costly

The properties of currently used impression materials are given in Table 10.5.

Copper Band Impressions

The copper band is used primarily for single tooth impression. It can also be used for

Table 10.5: Properties of impression materials

	Agar	Alginate	Polysulfide	Condensation silicone	Addition silicone	Polyether	Light cured
Availability	Preparation (boil, temper and store)	Powder and water	2 pastes	2 pastes	2 pastes	2 pastes	2 pastes
Handling (ease of use)	Technique sensitive	Good	Fair	Fair	Good	Good	Fair
Patient acceptance	Thermal shock because of heat	Pleasant	Unpleasant	Pleasant	Pleasant	Unpleasant	Pleasant
Ease of removal	Very easy	Very easy	Easy	Moderate	Moderate	Moderate to difficult	Moderate
Working time (minute)	7–15	2.5	5–7	3	2–4.5	2.5	5–7
Setting time (minute)	5	3.5	8–12	6–8	3–7	4.5	3–4
Dimensional stability	Pour after one hour	Immediate pour	Pour after one hour	Immediate pour	Pour after one week	Pour after one week	Pour after one week
Die material	Stone	Stone	Stone	Stone	Stone	Stone	Stone
Electroplating	No	No	Yes	Yes	Yes	Yes	Yes
Ease of disinfection	Poor	Poor	Fair	Excellent	Excellent	Fair	Fair

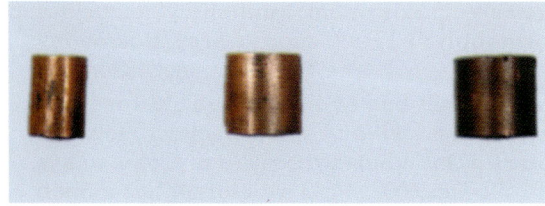

Fig. 10.35: Copper bands

multiple preparations when there are vague margins on one or two preparations that are not adequately replicated on the impression (Fig. 10.35).

The steps followed for copper band impressions are:

- Select copper band diameter by trial and error accordingly fitting the preparation.
- The selected copper band is annealed by heating over the flame and quenched in methylated spirit or alcohol.
- Mark approximate portion of finish line with a marker and cut the same with sharp scissors. The rough edges are smoothened with carborundum disc and stones.
- Evaluate the fit. The band should extend 1.0 mm beyond finish line and produce minimal tissue blanching.
- The band should have around 1.0 mm free space all around to accommodate for the impression material.
- A niche is given on top of the band, which will designate the buccal surface during making of the impression. The band is now ready for impression.
- Cover operator's fingers with Vaseline or petroleum jelly.
- Gently heat the green stick wax or compound over the Bunsen burner flame and compress the warm mass with lubricated fingers.
- Evaluate the viscosity and temperature, reheat or temper in a warm water bath if necessary.
- Push the band along with the material onto the preparation gently pressing with the fingers. (The buccal side of the band with niche should be carefully placed.)
- The impression material should be minimum 2.0 mm more than the coronal aspect of the preparation.
- The copper band is cooled with water.
- Remove the band from the preparation.
- Evaluate preparation side of the band. Relieve any excess by cutting with slow speed burs.
- The impression can be relieved to compensate for the light body rubber base impression.
- Instead of green stick wax or compound, the putty of the rubber base can also be used.
- In case the putty is used, the inner surface can be coated with adhesive as per instructions from the manufacturers.
- A couple of holes can be drilled through the band to decrease the hydrostatic pressure.
- The die can be prepared by pouring Type IV Gypsum and can be transferred to the original cast for adjustments of proximal contact and occlusion.

Disinfection of Impression

Various types of micro-organisms get entrapped within the impression, which if not disinfected, can refer to the casts in the laboratory. It has been established that micro-organisms such as *Staphylococcus aureus*, *Escherichia coli* and *Candida albicans* could survive on impression materials. It is essential to analyze disinfection procedures that should inactivate the micro-organisms without affecting the impression material. The different disinfectant agents have been and are being used to disinfect the impression (Fig. 10.36).

The disinfectant agent is a part in the impression material kit in some of the materials available. Generally, the impression can be disinfected by immersing in 2.5% sodium hypochlorite or 2.0% glutaraldehyde. The time of immersion should be brief

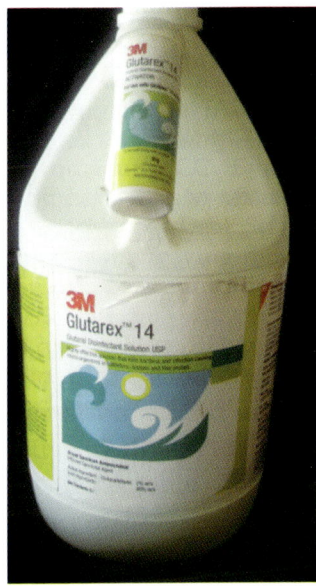

Fig. 10.36: Disinfectant agent

Table 10.6: Commonly used disinfectants	
Product name	**Composition**
Cidex	2.0% glutaraldehyde
Techno-sept	0.7% ampholytic soap and 4.0% propanol-2
Hibitane	0.5% chlorhexidine
Chloramine	5.0% sodium salt of p-toluidine
Benzalkon	1.0% benzalkonium chloride
Surface phenol derivatives	0.5% mix of 2-phenyl phenol and chloro-cresol
Hyposol	3.0% sodium hypochlorite

(between 3 and 7 minutes). Prolonged immersion may produce measurable distortions and certain chemicals used, may change the surface hardness of the material. Disinfection with 2.0% glutaraldehyde solution showed a slight expanding effect (0.03%) on the dimensional stability of rubber base impression material. The disinfectants increase the wettability of polysulfide and reduce the dimensional stability of hydrophilic silicones. The polyether impressions are adversely affected with disinfection by immersion. A chlorine compound using short immersion time (2–3 minutes) minimizes dimensional change with polyether impressions; alternatively, spraying only can disinfect the impression. The surfactants improve the wettability and simplify pouring of gypsum. However, addition of surfactants makes the preparation of electroformed dies more difficult, because the metalizing powder does not adhere well to the hydrophilic impressions. Recently, microwave energy has been used to disinfect the impressions.

The routinely used disinfectants are given in Table 10.6.

The UV light has also been used as disinfectant. The UV lights are effective especially against Candida organisms without producing dimensional change or surface roughness of the impression material. After disinfection, the impression should not be kept in air. Chlorine compounds or iodophors are preferred in alginate impressions keeping the exposure time less than 10 minutes. The chlorine compound is not compatible with zinc oxide impression and impression compound. Iodophors and glutaraldehyde are preferred.

Disadvantages of Disinfection

The following disadvantages are commonly encountered:
- Unpleasant odour of glutaraldehyde and chlorine solutions.
- Chlorine containing solutions may bleach certain materials.
- Iodine containing solution may stain the materials.
- Some individuals exhibit sensitivity to glutaraldehyde and/or iodine (hands should not be exposed to these solutions).

The protocol of disinfection is summarized as:
- The impression should be rinsed to remove saliva, blood and other debris.
- The patients are considered as potentially infectious.

- The impression is immersed in 2% glutaraldehyde solution for one hour.
- The protocol is effective in rubber base materials; however, alginate and zinc oxide eugenol impressions are immersed for shorter duration.

Bibliography

1. Abdelaziz KM, Combe EC and Hodges JS. The effect of disinfectants on the properties of dental gypsum: 1. Mechanical properties. J. Prosthodont: 2002;11:161–7.
2. Abdelaziz KM, Combe EC and Hodges JS. The Wetting of surface-treated silicone impression materials by Gypsum mixes containing dis-infectants and modifiers. J. Prosthodont.: 2005; 14:104–9.
3. Abdelaziz KM, Hassan AM and Hodges JS. Reproducibility of sterilized rubber impressions. Braz. Dent. J.: 2004;15:209–13.
4. Adhapure P, Bhandari J and Shinde J. Advances in soft tissue management: A review. Int. J. Basic and Appl. Med.Sci.: 2015;5:57–61.
5. Albaker AM. Gingival retraction: Techniques and materials: A review. Pakistan Oral and Dent. J.: 2010;30:545–51.
6. Al-Bakshi IA, Hussey D and Al-Omari MW. The dimensional accuracy of four impression techniques with the use of addition silicone impression materials. J. Clin. Dent.: 2007;18:29–33.
7. Almortadi N and Chadwick RG. Disinfection of dental impressions-compliance to accepted standards. Br. Dent. J.: 2010;209:607–11.
8. Ashley M, McCullagh A and Sweet C. Making a good impression (Dental Alginates). Dental Update: 2005;32:169–70.
9. Baba N Z., Goodacre C J and Jekki R: Gingival displacement for impression making in fixed prosthodontics. Dent Clinics North Am. (2014) 58, 45–68.
10. Balkenhol M, Kanehira M, Finger WJ and Wostmann B. Working time of elastomeric impression materials: Relevance of rheological tests. Am. J. Dent.: 2007;20:347–52.
11. Baumann MA. The influence of dental gloves on the setting of impression materials. BDJ. 1995;179: 130–5.
12. Beier US, Kranewitter R and Dumfahrt H. Quality of impressions after use of the Magic FoamCord gingival retraction system: A clinical study of 269 abutment teeth. Int. J. Prosthodont.: 2009;22: 143–7.
13. Bergman B. Disinfection of prosthodontic impression materials: a literature review. Int. J. Prosthodont.: 1989;2:537–42.
14. Bindra B and Heath JRI. Adhesion of elastomeric impression materials to tray. J. Oral Rehab.: 1997; 24:63–9.
15. Boening KW, Walter MH and Schuette U. Clinical significance of surface activation of silicone impression materials. J. Dent.: 1998;26:447–52.
16. Carrotte PV, Johnson A and Winstanley RB. The influence of the impression tray on the accuracy of impressions for crown and bridge work-an investigation and review. B.D.J.: 1998;185:580–5.
17. Chai J, Takahashi Y and Lautenschlager EP. Clinically relevant mechanical properties of elastomeric impression materials. Int. J. Prosthodont: 1998;11:219–23.
18. Chee WW and Donovan TE. Polyvinyl siloxane impression material: a review of properties and techniques. JPD: 1992;68;728–32.
19. Cloyd S and Puri S. Using the double cord packing technique of tissue retraction for making crown impressions. Dent. Today: 1999;18:54–9.
20. Craig RG, Urquiola NJ and Liu CC. Comparison of commercial elastomeric impression materials. Oper. Dent.: 1990;15:94–104.
21. Craig RG. A review of properties of rubber impression materials. J. Mich. Dent. Assoc.: 1977; 59:254–61.
22. Craig RG. Review of dental impression materials. Adv. Dent. Res.: 1988;2:51–64.
23. de Camargo LM, Chee WWL and Donovan TE. Inhibition of polymerization of polyvinyl siloxanes by medicaments used on gingival retraction cords. J. Prosthet. Dent.: 1993;70: 114–7.
24. Devan MM. Basic principles in impression making JPD: 2005;93:503–8.
25. Donovan TE and Chee WL. A review of contemporary impression materials and techniques. Dent. Clin. North Am.: 2004;48:445–70.
26. Endo T and Finger WJ. Dimensional accuracy of a new polyether impression material. Quint. Int.: 2006;37:47–51.
27. Falk A, Steyern PV, Fransson H and Thoren MM. Reliability of impression replica technique. Int. J. Prosthodont.: 2015;28:179–80.
28. Gelbard S, Aoskar Y, Zalkind M and Stern N. Effect of impression materials and techniques on

the marginal fit of metal castings. JPD: 1994;71: 1–6.

29. German MJ, Carrick TE and McCabe JF. Surface detail reproduction of elastomeric impression materials related to rheological properties. Dent. Mater.: 2008;24:951–6.

30. Gherlone EF, Maiorana C, Grassi RF, Ciancaglini, R. and Cattoni, F. The use of 980 nm diode and 1064 nm ND:YAG laser for gingival retraction in fixed prosthesis. J. Oral Laser Appli.:2004;4: 183–90.

31. Giordano R. Impression materials: basic properties. Gen. Dent.: 2000;48:510–6.

32. Hamalian TA, Nasr E and Chidiac JJ. Impression materials in fixed prosthodontics: influence of choice on clinical procedure. J. Prosthodont.: 2011; 20:153–60.

33. Herrera SP and Merchant VA. Dimensional stability of dental impressions after immersion disinfection. J. Am. Dent. Assoc.: 1986;113:419–22.

34. Ingraham R and Sochat R. Rotary gingival curettage: A technique for tooth preparation and management of the gingival sulcus for impression taking. Int. J. Periodontol. Restorative Dent.: 1981; 1:9–33.

35. Johnson GH, Lepe X, Aw TC. The effect of surface moisture on detail reproduction of elastomeric impressions. J. Prosthet. Dent.: 2003;90:354–64.

36. Kahn R, Donovan T and Chee W. Interaction of latex gloves and polyvinylsiloxane impression materials: a screening survey. Int. J. Prosthodont.: 1989;2:342–6.

37. Kanaparthy A and Kanaparthy R. Management of gingival tissue in restorative procedures. Eur. J. Pharma. and Med. Res.: 2015;2:73–8.

38. Khajuria RR, Sharma V, Vadavagi SV and Singh R. Advancements in tissue displacement: A review. Annals of Dental Specialty: 2014;2:100–3.

39. Laufer BZ, Baharav H, Ganor Y and Cardash H. The effect of marginal thickness on the distortion of different impression materials. J.P.D.: 1996;76:466–71.

40. Lee IK, Delong R, Pintado MR and Malik R. Evaluation of factors affecting the accuracy of impressions using quantitative surface analysis. Oper. Dent.: 1995;20:246–52.

41. Lepe X and Johnson GH. Accuracy of polyether and addition silicone after long term immersion disinfection JPD: 1997;78, 245–9.

42. Livaditis GJ. The matrix impression system for fixed prosthodontics. J. Prosthet. Dent.: 1998;79: 200–7.

43. Lowe R. Mastering the art of impression making. Inside Dent.: 2006;2:38–9.

44. Mandikos MN. Polyvinyl siloxane impression material: an update on clinical use. Aust. Dent. J.: 1998;43:428–34.

45. Martin N, Martin MV and Jedynakiewicz NM. The dimensional stability of dental impression materials following immersion in disinfecting solutions. Dent. Mater.: 2007;23:760–8.

46. Matis BA, Valadez D and Valadez E. The effect of the use of dental gloves on mixing vinyl polysiloxane putties. J. Prosthodont.: 1997;6:189–92.

47. Mazzanti G, Dankle C, Tita B, Vitali F and Signore A. Biological evaluation of a polyvinyl siloxane impression material. Dent. Mater.: 2005;21: 371–4.

48. McCabe JF and Brownman AJ. Rheological properties of dental impression materials. BDJ: 1981;151:179–83.

49. Messing JJ. Copper band technique. Br. Dent. J.: 1965;119:246–8.

50. Millar B. How to make a good impression (crown and bridge). BDJ: 2001;191:402–3.

51. Moon MG, Jarrett TA, Morlen RH and Fallo GJ. The effect of various base/core material on the setting of a polyvinyl siloxane material. JPD: 1996;76:608–12.

52. Nally FF and Storrs J. Hypersensitivity of dental impression materials. BDJ: 1973;134:244–6.

53. Nissan J, Rosner O, Bukhari MA, Ghelfan O and Pilo R. Effect of various putty-wash impression techniques on marginal fit of cast crowns. Int. J. Periodontics Restorative Dent.: 2013;33:e37–42.

54. Padbury Jr. A. and Wang, H.I. Interactions between the gingiva and the margin of restorations. J. Clin. Periodontot.:2003;30:379–85.

55. Perakis N, Belser VC and Magne P. Final impression: A review of material properties and description of current technique. Int. J. Periodont. and Restorative Dent.: 2004;24:109–17.

56. Peutzfeldt A and Asmussen E. Accuracy of alginate and elastomeric impression materials. Scand. J. Dent. Res.: 1989;97:375–9.

57. Poss S. An innovative tissue retraction material. Compend. Contin. Educ. Dent.: 2002;23:13–7.

58. Ray KC and Fuller ML. Isolation of Myco-bacterium from dental impression material. J. Prosthet. Dent.: 1963;13:390–6.

59. Re D, Angelis FD, Augusti G, Augusti D, Caputi S, Amario M and D'Arcangelo C. Mechanical

properties of elastomeric impression materials:An in vitro comparison. Int. J. Dent.:Art.ID428286, 2015;1–8.

60. Rowe AHR and Forrest JO. Dental impressions. The probability of contamination and a method of disinfection. Br. Dent. J.: 1978;145:184–6.

61. Rubel BS. Impression materials: a comparative review of impression materials most commonly used in restorative dentistry. Dent. Clin. North Am.: 2007;51:629–42.

62. Rudolph H, Rohi A, Walter MH, Luthardt RG and Quass S. Performance of fast-setting impression materials in the reproduction of subgingival tooth surfaces without soft tissue retraction. Int. J. Prosthodont.: 2014;27:366–75.

63. Samet N, Shohat M, Livny A and Weiss EI. A clinical evaluation of fixed partial denture impressions. J.P.D.: 2005;94:112–7.

64. Shiozawa M, Takahashi H and Iwasaki N. Effect of the space for wash materials on sulcus depth reproduction with addition silicone using two-step putty-wash technique. Dent. Mater. J.: 2013; 32:150–5.

65. Shogo M. Disinfection method for impression materials. Freedom from fear of hepatitis B and AIDS. JPD: 1986;56:451–4.

66. Singh K, Sahoos S, Prasad KD and Singh A. Effect of different impression techniques on the dimensional accuracy of impressions using various elastomeric impression materials: an in vitro study. J. Contemp. Dent. Pract.: 2012;13:98–106.

67. Stober T, Johnson GH and Schmitter M. Accuracy of the newly formulated fast-setting elastomeric impression material. J. Prosthet. Dent.: 2010;103: 228–39.

68. Sydiskis RJ and Gerhardt DE. Cytotoxicity of impression materials. JPD: 1993;69:431–5.

69. Thongthammachat S, Moore BK, Barco MT, Hovijitra S, Brown DT and Andres CJ. Dimensional accuracy of dental casts : influence of tray material, impression material and time. J. Prosthodont.: 2002;11:98–108.

70. Todd JA, Oesterie LJ, Newman SM and Shellhart WC. Dimensional changes of extended-pour alginate impression materials. Am. J. Orthod. Dentofacial Orthop.: 2013;143:s55–63.

71. Wassell RW, Barker D and Walls AWG. Crowns and other extracoronal restorations: Impressions materials and technique. Br. Dent. J.: 2002;192: 679–90.

11

Interim Restorations

When confronted with extensive and/or complex treatment plans, judicious sequencing is vital to both patient and the operator. Usually, permanent solution to patient's esthetics and functional concerns are not indicated at treatment onset; yet social interaction make these considerations a concern to the patient. The interim treatment enhances patient motivation, which frequently determines the acceptance and successful completion of the chosen treatment plan.

Interim or temporary treatment includes all those procedures that are carried out before the fabrication of final restoration to maintain optimal health of the oral tissues, occlusion and also the esthetics of the patient.

Interim or provisional restorations, many a times, may have to function for extended periods because of unforeseen events, such as laboratory delays, etc. The delay in placing the permanent restoration may be deliberate. The temporary restorations are prolonged, especially, in case of occlusal rehabilitation to acclimatize the same with the temporo-mandibular joint functioning and the periodontium. Whatever the intended period of temporary restoration, it should never be ill placed. Inadequate restorations may lead to unnecessary problems. Adequately placed restorations enhance the final outcome as well as psychological well-being of the patient.

Rationale for giving a temporary restoration:
- Preserves pulp vitality
- Ensures gingival health
- Prevention of passive tooth eruption and mesial drift
- Patient's comfort
- Esthetics
- Maintains occlusal function
- Psychological well-being

REQUIREMENTS OF A TEMPORARY RESTORATION

An optimum temporary restoration must satisfy many interrelated factors such as:

A. Biological
B. Mechanical
C. Esthetic
D. Convenience

A. Biological

a. *Pulp protection:* The temporary restoration should be non-irritating and non-toxic. A temporary restoration must seal and insulate the prepared tooth surface from the oral environment to prevent any irritation to the pulp.

b. *Protection of the periodontium:* It should have good marginal fit, proper contour and a smooth surface. It should not impinge upon the gingival tissues. All these features prevent plaque deposition and subsequently the gingival periodontal diseases.

c. *Preserving occlusal accuracy:* It should maintain proper contact with adjacent and opposing teeth to avoid extrusion and/or drifting of the teeth, preserving the occlusal accuracy and stability.

B. *Mechanical*

It should possess sufficient strength to withstand normal occlusal forces. It should protect teeth weakened by crown preparation and make them resistant to fracture; more so, the occlusal forces are dissipated normally with temporary restorations.

C. *Esthetic*

The appearance of a temporary restoration is important both for anterior and posterior teeth. Although, it may not be possible to duplicate the appearance of natural teeth, good texture, contour, color and translucency are essential qualities of a desirable temporary restoration. The restoration should not make the patient look abnormal at any stage (should not be conspicuous).

D. *Convenience*

The convenience of the operator and the patient should be taken care of while placing interim restorations.

a. *Chair side time:* It should be less time consuming.

b. *Manipulation:* The manipulation should be easy to manipulate; should have adequate working time and rapid setting time during insertion. The removal should also be easy at time of placing a permanent restoration.

c. *Good patient acceptance:* It should be well tolerated by the patient. It must be non-irritating, non-toxic and odorless.

d. *Cost factor:* It should be relatively inexpensive, or cost effective.

Limitations of Provisionalization

- Lack of inherent strength (the provisional restorations may fracture in long span coverage, especially in patients with bruxism or other parafunctional habits).
- Poor marginal adaptation.
- Color instability.
- Poor wear resistance.
- The restorations may drift, especially during heavy occlusal stresses.
- Odor emission (resins particularly auto-polymerizing types are porous and subsequently produce bad odor).
- Inadequate bonding characteristics.
- Poor tissue response to irritation.
- Time consuming.
- Increased cost factor.

MATERIALS USED FOR INTERIM RESTORATIONS

I. For Intracoronal Preparation

   i. Gutta-percha
  ii. Zinc oxide eugenol
 iii. Non-eugenol preparations
 iv. Zinc phosphate cement
  v. Polycarboxylate cement

II. For Extracoronal Preparation

a. Prefabricated crowns
   i. Polycarbonate crowns
  ii. Cellulose acetate crowns
 iii. Aluminium shell crowns
 iv. Stainless steel crowns
  v. Nickel chromium crowns
b. Custom made crowns
   i. Heat-cure acrylic crowns
  ii. Self-cure acrylic crowns

I. For Intracoronal Preparations

i. *Gutta-percha*

Gutta-percha is a form of rubber; chemical components of Gutta (hydrocarbon) along with albane/guttane groups. The ingredients such as zinc oxide, waxes, calcium hydroxide, magnesium hydroxide, etc. are added to achieve desirable working properties. Gutta-percha is supplied in three forms:

- Low heat (softens below 200°F)
- Medium heat (softens within 200–210°F)
- High heat (softens within 230–250°F)

Manipulation

The gutta-percha stick is softened over an alcohol lamp or Bunsen burner. Avoid overheating as it may burn leading to oxidation of its components and affecting its properties. The softened gutta-percha is inserted in the wet cavity in bulk and pressed gently. The wet burnisher of appropriate size can be used to condense the gutta-percha. Remove excess material immediately with a hot flat spatula or burnisher, trimming the margins. The occlusal surface is smoothened with warm instrument. The occlusion is adjusted and evaluated.

Physical properties

- Softens on heating and hardens on cooling
- Almost colorless (slight pink or gray hue)
- Odorless
- Slightly elastic and contracts during solidification
- Non-irritating to soft tissues
- Poor mechanical properties
- Ease of insertion and removal

Disadvantages

- Poor strength and abrasion resistance
- Excessive shrinkage (coefficient of thermal expansion is 198×10^{-6}); can be used for limited period only (say for a day or so).
- Disintegrates due to oxidation after some time
- Plastic flow is higher

ii. Zinc Oxide Eugenol Cement

The zinc oxide eugenol cement is the most accepted and widely used temporary restorative material. The powder consists of 70% zinc oxide and 25% glass or silica and the liquid consists of eugenol (Fig. 11.1).

Zinc oxide eugenol offers better biocompatibility than other dental cements. It is a good sealer and insulator for dental pulp. It has an antiseptic effect on micro-organisms remaining in dentin and also act as sedative and anti-inflammatory over the pulp. The mixed/set cement has natural pH of 7.0. The strength of zinc oxide eugenol is not sufficient to resist forces of mastication. The cement lacks resistance to wear and is soluble in oral fluids.

Basically, two types of zinc oxide eugenol cements are available.

Type I: ZOE used as a base or temporary restorations

Type II: ZOE used as cavity liner and for cementation

Earlier, cements containing equal amounts of zinc oxide (100%) and eugenol (100%) were easy to mix and place in the cavity; however, it was hydrolytically unstable and showed poor strength. The setting reaction was slow, which was advantageous since large quantity of material could be mixed at the beginning of the day and stored.

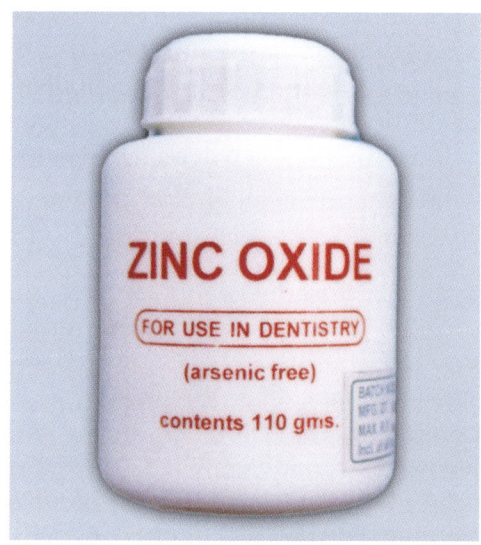

Fig. 11.1: Zinc oxide powder

The cement was later modified to improve upon the working, handling and setting characteristics. Improved version of the cement was achieved by two ways:

   i. Partial substitution of eugenol by ortho-ethoxybenzoic acid (EBA)

  ii. Addition of finer quality of aluminium oxide or resin polymer to the powder component

i. *EBA (ortho-ethoxybenzoic acid) modified cement:* Ethoxybenzoic acid (EBA) has been tried to improve upon the physical properties of zinc oxide eugenol. EBA chelates with zinc and forms an ionic complex, zinc benzoate. Certain fillers are added to the powder such as quartz, alumina, etc. to reduce the solubility and disintegration of the cement. The powder consists of 70% zinc oxide and 30% alumina or quartz. The liquid consists of EBA 62.5% and eugenol 37.5%.

Addition of EBA leads to improved properties such as:

- Large amount of powder can be incorporated in the liquid so as to obtain better consistency of the mix cement.
- Increases compressive, tensile and shear strength (close to zinc phosphate).
- Decreases the setting time; however, if the concentration of EBA is more than 70%, the setting time is sharply increased.
- Density is one and half times more than the conventional zinc oxide eugenol cement.
- Coefficient of thermal expansion increases.
- Solubility and disintegration also increases.
- No adverse effect on pulp.

ii. *Resin modified zinc oxide eugenol cement:* The resin (polymeric) component like polymethyl methacrylate is added to the conventional zinc oxide powder.

20% polymethyl methacryalte is usually added to zinc oxide powder. The liquid is eugenol (85%) along with olive oil and accelerators like zinc stearate and zinc acetate (15%).

The addition of resin improves the strength, homogenicity and smoothness and decreases flow, brittleness and solubility of the cement. Zinc stearate and zinc acetate act as accelerator and improve strength of the cement. Olive oil acts as plasticizer and masks the irritating effect of eugenol.

Vanillate esters have also been added to have high strength, low solubility and low disintegration values. Some zinc oxide cements contain antibiotics and steroids as anti-inflammatory agents. Barium sulphate added for radiopacity; though usually not preferred.

Manipulation: The conventional zinc oxide eugenol cement is available in powder and liquid form. Mixing is carried out on a clean glass slab or disposable mixing pad using stainless steel spatula. The required amount of powder and liquid is dispensed on the slab. The powder in bulk is incorporated in the liquid and thoroughly spatulated.

Smaller amount of powder, if required, can be added and subsequently spatulated. The correct consistency is achieved when the mix is putty like and can be picked with fingers without sticking. The clean plastic instruments are used to fill the cavity. A moist cotton pellet is patted over the surface to enhance setting. The humid environment hastens the setting process. The anhydrous zinc oxide does not react with eugenol (water is an essential feature in setting reaction). Following features influence the rate of setting.

- A drop of water accelerates the setting reaction but excessive water tends to decrease the same. Humidity fastens the reaction.
- Additives such as zinc stearate, zinc acetate, resins alcohols, etc. act as accelerators.
- Within limits, greater the zinc oxide to eugenol, faster is the setting.
- Higher the temperature, shorter the setting time.
- Smaller the particle size of zinc oxide, shorter the setting time.

Clinical benefits of eugenol

Eugenol exerts many beneficial effects, such as:

- Eugenol is bactericidal at relatively higher concentration. At low concentration, eugenol acts like local anesthetic; helps in dissolution of inflammation. It also inhibits neurogenic activities.
- Higher dose of eugenol is toxic to pulp; cause tissue damage and may exert neurotoxic effect.
- Marginal adaptability (zinc oxide eugenol cement) is excellent; prevents leakage and subsequent growth of bacteria.

iii. *Non-eugenol Preparations*

The powder of non-eugenol preparations contains zinc oxide, zinc sulphate, calcium sulphate, glycol acetate, polyvinyl acetate, polyvinyl chloride acetate and other pigments in traces. The setting reaction is initiated by saliva or water. Cavit is the most commonly used non-eugenol cement preparation (Fig. 11.2). The properties of cavit are:

- Shows higher linear expansion (marginal adaptability is improved).
- Non-satisfactory for luting purposes (film thickness is 91μ).
- The strength and the pH of the material is comparable to conventional zinc oxide eugenol.
- When inserted into dry cavities, it creates negative pressure causing aspiration of odontoblasts leading to pain.

iv. *Zinc Phosphate Cement*

Zinc phosphate cement is widely used as temporary restorative material and also as luting agent (Fig. 11.3). The cement is of two types depending upon the particle size, having the same composition.

Type I: (luting cement) Fine grain powder particles (film thickness 25 μ).

Type II: (temporary cement) Medium-sized powder particles.

The powder consists of zinc oxide along with magnesium oxide, bismuth trioxide, barium sulphate etc.; whereas the liquid is primarily 37% phosphoric acid and water along with traces of aluminium and zinc.

The setting reaction is basically the acid–base reaction. The factors, which control the setting rate, are:

- Composition of liquid (percentage of water and buffering salts).
- Particle size of the powder (smaller the particle size, faster is the reaction).
- Decreasing the powder/liquid ratio can increase setting time.
- Rate at which the powder is incorporated in the liquid. If all the powder is added at once, the reaction is very rapid.
- Temperature during mixing affects the setting reaction. Decreasing the temperature by cooling the glass slab increases the setting time.

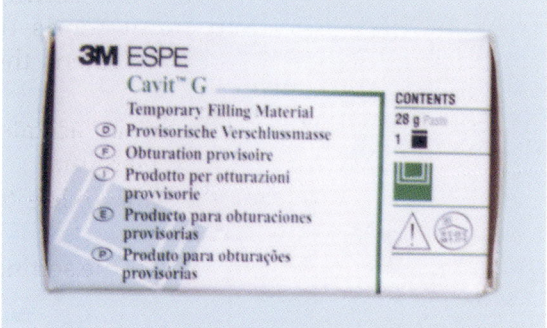

Fig. 11.2: Cavit (Non-eugenol preparation)

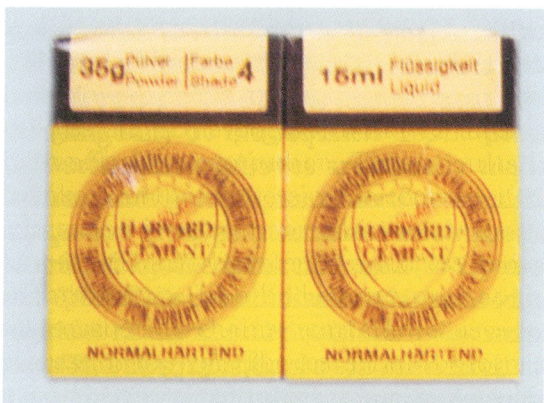

Fig. 11.3: Zinc phosphate cement

- The addition of water decreases the setting time and loss of water increases the setting time.

Manipulation: The reaction after mixing the powder and liquid is highly exothermic. It is necessary to dissipate the heat, otherwise reaction will be too rapid. A properly cooled glass slab is to be used for this purpose. The temperature of the glass slab should not be lowered around dew point otherwise water droplets will form and contaminate the mix. A cool slab allows incorporation of more powder leading to better physical properties. The commonly used powder/liquid ratio is 2.5: 1 for temporary restorations. The liquid bottle should be stored in a normal environment. Exposure to air leads to change in water/acid ratio, which affects the subsequent setting and physical properties of the set cement. The bottle should not be kept in refrigerator; otherwise the condensed water may affect the physical properties. Repeated opening of the liquid bottle especially for a longer period should be avoided. Usually, the last one-fifth of the liquid is discarded. The liquid should not be kept over the glass slab for a longer duration to avoid contamination.

The mixing is carried out with long narrow bladed stainless steel spatula on a cool glass slab. The cement is mixed with the spatula held flat on the surface of the slab and moving in a rotary motion. The mixing should always be accomplished in small increments so as to achieve proper consistency. The mixing is usually completed in 60 seconds in normal environment.

v. *Polycarboxylate Cement*

The polycarboxylate cement is an improved quality of zinc phosphate cement. The powder basically is that of zinc phosphate cement with minor addition of stannous fluoride. The liquid is an aqueous solution of polyacrylic acid (Fig. 11.4). The polyacrylic acid helps in adhesion; whereas stannous fluoride imparts anticariogenic properties.

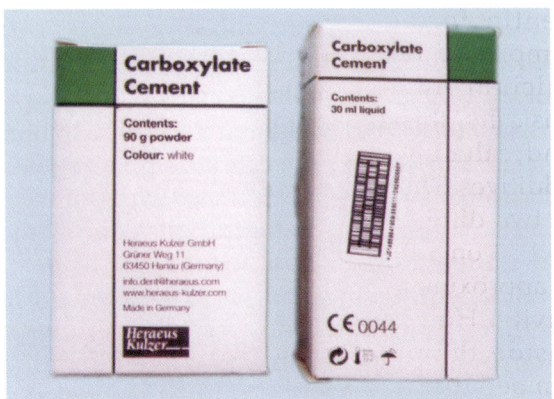

Fig. 11.4: Polycarboxylate cement

Manipulation

The setting reaction involves acid–base phenomenon. The recommended powder/liquid ratio is 1:1 for restorative purposes. The liquid of the cement should not be stored in refrigerator because the liquid tends to get thickened (gel formation).

Mixing is carried out on a glass slab or a non-absorbent paper pad. The cool glass slab is preferred as it allows extension of the working time. The exposure of the liquid to air is avoided since it may lead to loss of water, subsequently increasing the viscosity of the liquid.

Powder is incorporated into the liquid in two or three large increments using rapid spatulation. The mix should be completed in 30 seconds to allow maximum length of working time. The consistency of the cement is viscous and will flow back under its own weight when drawn with a spatula. The mechanical/physical properties are comparable to zinc phosphate cement having advantage of biological compatibility, adhesion and less irritating to underlying tissues.

vi. *Calcium Hydroxide Paste*

Calcium hydroxide with its improved qualities is being preferred as temporary restoration. The higher pH value is useful for killing the bacteria at the site and inducing secondary dentin formation. The commonly used temporary restorative material containing calcium hydroxide is Dycal (Fig. 11.5). Basically, this is a combination of zinc oxide and calcium hydroxide along with other additives. The base and the catalyst (available in two different tubes) are mixed in the ratio of 1 : 1 on a disposable pad. The setting time is approximately one minute outside the oral cavity. However, it decreases substantially inside the oral cavity because of higher temperature and humidity.

Light cure calcium hydroxide has also been used as temporary restorations (Fig. 11.6). The material exhibits better physical properties like better compressive strength and less solubility in oral fluids. The calcium hydroxide preparation is preferred as interim restoration where composite is to be used as final restoration. The base of calcium hydroxide is compatible with composites. Calcium hydroxide base is also preferred in rampant caries, which slows down the progress of caries before final restoration.

The light cure materials used for temporization mostly exhibit volumetric changes on solidification. These materials

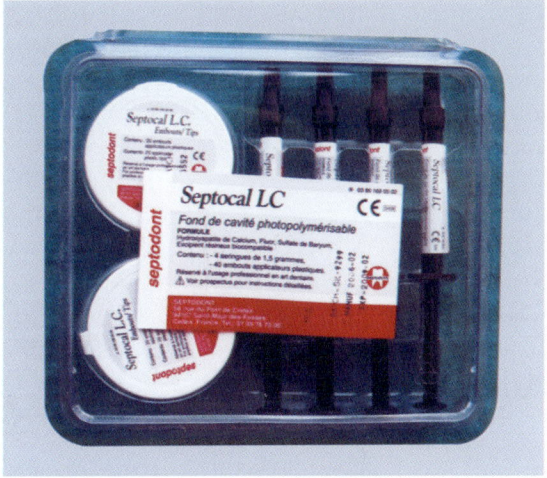

Fig. 11.6: Light cure calcium hydroxide (Septocal LC)

shrink and cause marginal discrepancy. Also, the resins employed are exothermic and are not entirely biocompatible.

Different types of resins have been tried. Epimine resins produce considerably less exothermic heat during polymerization. It produces better marginal adaptation when compared to other resins. However, it is not commonly used because it is expensive, has poor resistance to abrasion and discolor with time. Urethane dimethacrylate resin satisfies most of the requisites and is currently being used.

II. For Extracoronal preparations

The provisional restorations for extracoronal preparations are either prefabricated or can be fabricated in the clinic/laboratory.

a. Prefabricated Crowns

Various types of prefabricated crowns are being used as provisional restorations, such as:

i. Polycarbonate crowns: The polycarbonate crowns are manufactured in a single medium color; the variety of shades are not available. The single shade is, however, resistant to discoloration as compared to custom resin crowns. The crowns are mostly used for

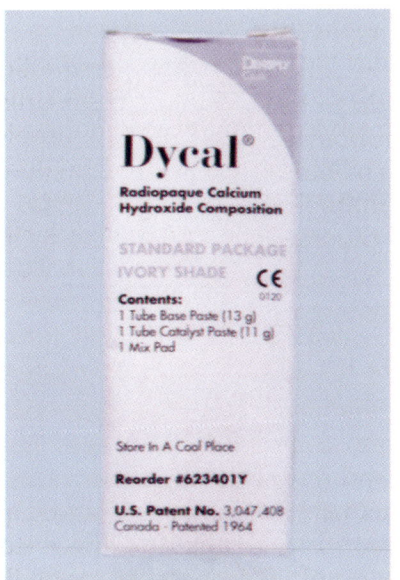

Fig. 11.5: Calcium hydroxide (Dycal)

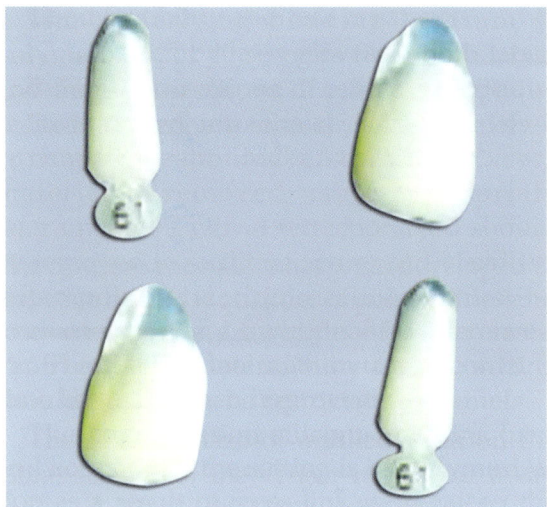

Fig. 11.7: Polycarbonate crowns

anterior teeth, providing reasonable esthetics (Fig. 11.7). A wide range of anterior polycarbonate crowns are available; however, the variety of posterior crowns is limited. Although, these are available in a single shade, this can be modified to a limited extent by the shade of the underlying luting cement.

ii. *Cellulose acetate crowns:* Cellulose acetate is a thin transparent material available in all tooth shapes and sizes (Fig. 11.8). The requisite shade is provided by the auto-polymerising resin used under these crowns. After polymerization, the cellulose acetate is peeled off and discarded. The additional resin may be reinforced, if need be (usually required for establishing proximal contacts).

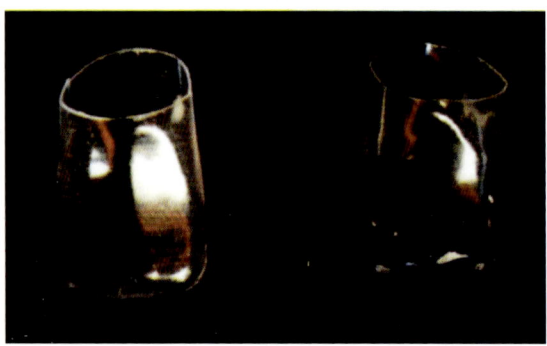

Fig. 11.8: Cellulose crowns

Procedure for fabrication

- Measure the incisal-cervical and mesio-distal width of the crown space with a Boley gauge or dividers prior to crown preparation. (In case of post-core or other situations, size of adjacent tooth is taken.) If the measurements do not exactly coincide with the available crown, the larger crown is selected (smaller crown may result in poor morphology).
- The crown can be trimmed to coincide with the margins.
- Try the crown on the prepared tooth. When properly aligned without gingival tissue impingement, it is ready to be lined with resin.
- Apply a thin coat of petrolatum onto the prepared tooth and adjacent gingival tissues. The auto-polymerizing resin is mixed and filled in the crown. When the resin just looses its gloss, the crown is pushed and adjusted over the tooth.
- Marginal excess should be finished immediately after placement; if delayed, the doughy resin will tend to pull away from the margin.
- Loosen the crown and reinsert it. Repeat the procedure two to three times while the resin is in rubbery stage.
- Remove the cellulose acetate crown cover before the resin has fully polymerized and place the fabricated resin crown in warm water.
- When the resin has fully set, the crown so prepared is finished with carborundum and fine grit garnet disks and stones.
- Try the crown on the patient and check for any occlusal disharmony. Adjust the lingual surface to give the desired occlusal contacts.
- Polish and cement this provisional crown.

iii. *Aluminium shell crowns:* The aluminium shell crowns are mainly used for posterior teeth (Fig. 11.9). A shell of suitable diameter is selected and festooned to adapt to the preparation. A luting cement is applied inside

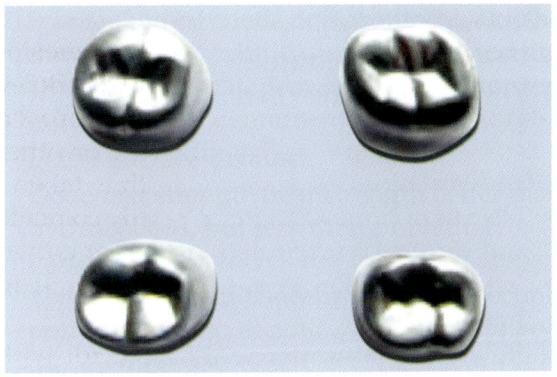

Fig. 11.9: Aluminium crowns

the shell and the same is placed over the prepared tooth. Aluminium shells can adapt easily to the patient's occlusion; however, they lack the rigidity required for acceptable marginal strength and the proximal contacts.

iv. Stainless steel crowns: The stainless steel crowns are used mainly for the deciduous and young permanent posterior teeth (Fig. 11.10). The thin stainless steel is effectively malleable and get conform to the occlusion. The cervical bands can be slightly constricted to favour gingival health.

v. Nickel chromium crowns: Nickel chromium crowns are mainly used in primary teeth; however, these have been tried in adult teeth

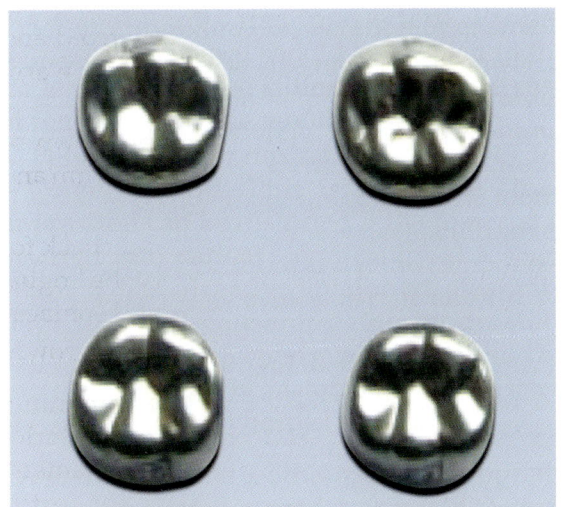

Fig. 11.10: Stainless steel crowns

also. The crowns are trimmed and adapted with contouring pliers to fit the underlying tooth.

Selection of the size of the crowns is critical. Care has to be taken not to extend it apical to the finish line of the prepared tooth, as it will impinge gingival tissues. The crown is fitted without using any luting agent.

b. Custom Made Crowns

The custom made crowns are of following types:

i. Heat-cure acrylic crowns

Heat-cure acrylic is commonly employed material for fabrication of temporary crown. The crown is fabricated on the diagnostic cast (die), finished and tried clinically on the prepared tooth. Minor adjustments of the crown, if required, can be carried out in the oral cavity.

Procedure
- The tooth is prepared clinically for the specific crown. The rubber base impression is taken and the cast prepared.
- Alternatively, the tooth is prepared on the diagnostic cast fabricated before tooth preparation (The preparation should be more conservative than the eventual tooth preparation and should have supragingival margins).
- Coat the prepared tooth with separating medium.
- The wax up cover simulating crown morphology is fabricated on articulated casts.
- The wax is removed by boiling and heat-cure resin is applied on the lost-wax surface. The resin is cured in boiling water, cooled and the restoration is removed.
- Smooth and polish the temporary restoration.
- Try the temporary restoration onto the prepared tooth.
- Adjust the occlusion (crown may be relined by self-cure resin, if need be).

- Confirm the marginal fit and occlusion, refinish, polish and cement the restoration.

Advantages
- The chair side time is reduced. Most of the procedures have been completed before the patient's visit.
- Less heat is generated in the oral cavity. The self-cure resin used clinically is comparatively small.
- Contact between monomer and the soft tissues is minimal, avoiding allergic reactions.

Disadvantages
- Cost factor (extra laboratory expenses).
- Time consuming, especially in duplicating process.

ii. *Self-cure acrylic crowns:* The provisional crown can also be fabricated using self-cure acrylic resin, eliminating the need for laboratory procedures required with heat-cure resin.

Procedure
- Rubber base impression of the tooth is taken prior to its preparation.
- The borders and inter-proximal extensions of the impression are trimmed and the impression is stored.
- The tooth is prepared for a specific crown; cast is prepared after taking the impression with rubber base impression material.
- A mix of self-cure acrylic resin is placed in the section of the impression corresponding to the crown preparations.
- The tooth preparation on the die (cast) is lubricated and pushed into the impression.
- The die/cast is taken out after the resin sets in the impression.
- The resin restoration is then removed from the impression, finished, polished and tried in the oral cavity.
- The occlusion is adjusted, if need be.
- The final interim restoration is cemented.

Advantages
- Cost factor is reduced.
- Do not require extensive laboratory technique.

Disadvantages
- Heat of polymerization may damage pulp/ soft tissues, if fabricated in oral cavity.
- Allergic reaction to the monomer in some patients.
- Inherently poor marginal fit.

Cementation of Acrylic Crowns

For cementation of temporary acrylic crowns, zinc oxide eugenol is not used as cementing medium; however, non-eugenol cements based on the liquid containing ortho-ethoxy-benzoic acid, ortho-methoxybenzoic acid, etc. are preferred. One of the reasons for the use of the eugenol-free cement is that the presence of free or leached eugenol has a softening effect on the resin. The effects of both eugenol and non-eugenol preparations on pulp and gingival tissues are the same. Glass-ionomer cement is the preferred choice to be used as cementing medium; alternatively, these can be cemented with self-cure resins.

Bibliography

1. Balkenhol M, Knapp M, Ferger P, Heun U and Wostmann B. Correlation between polymerization shrinkage and marginal fit of temporary crowns. Dent. Mater.: 2008;24:1575–84.
2. Banihashemrad SA, Mogaddas MJ, Mokhtari MR, Farazi F, Garajjan A and Mehrara R. Clinical evaluation of periodontal parameters in correct marginal dental restorations. Int. J. Stomatol. Res.: 2012;1:31–4.
3. Behrand DA. Temporary protective restorations in crown and bridge work. Aust. Dent. J.: 1967;12: 411–6.
4. Boskman L and Tousignant G. Temporization simplified. Oral Health: 2011;40–50.
5. Cardoso M, Torres MF, Rego MR dM and Santiago LC. Influence of application site of provisional cement on the marginal adaptation of provisional crowns. J. Appl. Oral Sci.: 2008;16: 214–8.

6. Carvalho CN, de Oliveria B and Loguercio AD. Effect of zinc oxide eugenol (ZOE) temporary restoration on resin-dentin bond strength using different adhesive strategies. J. Esthet. Restor. Dent.: 2007;19:144–53.

7. Castelnuovo J and Tjan AH. Temperature rise in pulpal chamber during fabrication of provisional resinous crowns. J. Prosth. Dent.: 1997;78:441–6.

8. Dumbrigue HB. Composite indirect-direct method for fabricating multiple-unit provisional restorations. J. Prosthet. Dent.: 2003;89:86–8.

9. Edwards DE. Temporary crowns materials and techniques. Contemp. Dent. Asst.: 2007;34–9.

10. Fox CW, Abrams BL and Doukoudakis A. Provisional restorations for altered occlusion. J. Prosth. Dent.: 1984;52:567–72.

11. Gauthier MA, Stangel I, Ellis TH and Zhu XX. Oxygen inhibition in dental resins. J. Dent. Res.: 2005;84:725–9.

12. Gilson TD and Myers GE. Clinical studies of Dental cements II. Further investigation of zinc oxide eugenol cements for temporary restorations. J.Dent.Res.: 1972;48:366–7.

13. Goldstein MB. Long-term composite provisionalization: the conversion. Dent. Today: 2008;27, 80:82–3.

14. Gratton DG and Aquilina SA. Interim restorations. Dent. Clin. North Am.: 2004;48:487–97.

15. Haselton DR, Diaz Arnold AM and Vargas MA. Flexural strength of provisional crown and fixed partial dentures. J. Prosth. Dent.: 2002;87:225–8.

16. Haselton DR, Diaz Arnold AM and Vargas MA. Color stability of provisional crown and fixed partial denture resins. J. Prosth. Dent.: 2005;93: 70–5.

17. Hirsh LS and Marion LR. Esthetic provisionalization for a combined porcelain veneer and anterior single crown case. Compend. Contin. Educ. Dent.: 2011;32:38–42.

18. Le TM. An analysis of direct versus indirect provisionalization. Dent. Today: 2006;25, 136:138–41.

19. Lui JL, Setcos JC and Phillips RW. Temporary restorations: a review. Oper. Dent.: 1986;11:103–10.

20. Malone M. Smile design and advanced provisional fabrication. Gen. Dent.: 2008;56:238–42.

21. Mancuso A. Provisionalization of the anterior aesthetic case. Dent. Today: 2000;19:88–9.

22. Marashi J. Temporization: freehand artistry defining clinical success. Dent. Today: 1996;24: 134–6.

23. Markowitz K, Moyniham M, Liu M and Kim S. Biological properties of eugenol and zinc oxide eugenol. O Surg., O Med., O. Path.: 1992;73:729–37.

24. Mitrani R, Phillips K and Escudero F. Provisional restoration of teeth prepared for porcelain laminate veneers: an alternative technique. Pract. Proced. Aesthet. Dent.: 2003;15:441–5.

25. Nejatidanesh F, Lotfi HR and Savabi O. Marginal accuracy of interim restorations fabricated from four interim autopolymerizing resins. J. Prosth. Dent.: 2006;95:364–7.

26. Osman YI and Owen CP. Flexural strength of provisional restorative materials. J. Prosth. Dent.: 1993;70:94–6.

27. Rakhshan V. Marginal integrity of provisional resin restoration materials: A review of the literature. Saudi J. Dent. Res.: 2014;30:1–8.

28. Regish KM, Sharma D and Prithviraj DR. Techniques of fabrication of provisional restoration: an overview. Int. J. Dent.:Art. ID134659, 2011;1–5.

29. Robert DB. Flexible casts used in making indirect interim restorations. J. Prosth. Dent.: 1992;68: 372–4.

30. Schwedhelm Er. Direct technique for the fabrication of acrylic provisional restorations. J. Contemp. Dent. Pract.: 2006;7:157–73.

31. Slutzky H, Weiss EI, Lewinstein I, Slutzky S and Matalon S. Surface antibacterial properties of resin and resin modified dental cements.: Quint. Int.: 2007;38:55–61.

32. Slutzky H, Slutzky-Goldberg I, Weiss EI and Matalon S. Antibacterial properties of temporary filling materials. J. Endod.:2006;32:214–7.

33. Small BW. Indirect provisional restorations. Gen. Dent.: 1999;47:140–2.

34. Sneed WD and Knight JS. Simple technique to fabricate provisional restorations for porcelain veneers. J. Esthet. Restor. Dent.: 2001;13:115–9.

35. Spear F. An interdisciplinary approach to the use of long-term temporary restorations. J. Am. Dent. Assoc.: 2009;140:1418–24.

36. Strassler HE. In-office provisional restorative materials for fixed prosthodontics: part 1—polymeric resin provisional materials. Inside Dent.: 2009;5:70–4.

37. Strupp WC. Provisional materials. Compendium: 2010;31:166–9.

38. Wang RL, Moore BK, Goodacre CJ, Swartz ML and Andres CJ. A comparison of resins for fabricating provisional fixed restorations. Int. J. Prosthodont.: 1989;2:173–84.

39. Waerhang J. Temporary restorations: advantages and disadvantages. Dent. Clin. North Am.: 1980; 24:305–16.

40. Wassell W, St. George S, Ingledew RP and Steel JG. Crowns and other extracoronal restorations: Provisional restorations. Br. Dent. J.: 2002;192: 619–30.

41. Weaver RG, Johnson BE, Cvar JF and McCune RJ. Clinical evaluation of intermediary restorations. J. Dent. Children.: 1972;39:189–93.

42. Youdelis RA and Fancher R. Provisional restorations: an integrated approach to periodontics and restorative dentistry. Dent. Clin. North Am.: 1980;24:285–303.

43. Young DHM, Smith CT and Morton D. Comparative in vitro evaluation of two provisional restorative materials. J. Prosth. Dent.: 2001;85:129–32.

12

Luting Agents

The extensive loss of tooth structure, may be because of endodontic procedures, repeated re-treatments and/or fracture of cusps, etc. warrant the use of indirect restorations. These restorations are the operator's choice whenever occlusal modifications are required. Indirect restorations are supposed to be luted to the prepared tooth surface by different materials. Over the years, the advancement of these materials has influenced the success of indirect restorations.

Literally, the word 'luting' is defined as the use of a moldable substance to seal joints and cement two substances together. Luting space is the space between two surfaces to be filled with an adhesive film. Adhesion, on the other hand, can be defined as coupling of similar or dissimilar substrates by a special adhesive. An adhesive is non-metallic substance, which is able to connect surfaces by adhesion and cohesion. One important factor for adhesion is wettability of the substrate. The measure for wettability is the contact angle (distribution of any liquid on the bonded substrate measured by the tangent to the surface). The more thc free surface energy, the smaller the contact angle and better wettability for bonding agents. The saliva, however, decreases the free surface energy and consequently, lowers the wettability. The advantages of luting process in dentistry are

relatively low thermal and mechanical stresses affecting the bonded substrates.

In spite of the best care and precision, it has been established that the cast restorations leave a gap of about 50–100 μ sufficient for microleakage and subsequently the secondary caries. More so, the gap may facilitate sliding of restoration within the cavity, disturbing the hydrodynamism in dentinal tubules, subsequently enhancing the sensitivity and other complications. It is established that the presence of any material between two surfaces leads to increase in friction by increasing the surface area in contact. This friction prevents the movement/sliding of restoration in the prepared cavity. The luting agents are utilized to achieve the requisite friction.

The preparation/cutting depth for the cast restoration is preferred in such a way so as to have adequate amount of remaining dentin, which will act as a base and insulator. In case, the remaining thickness of dentin is less than 2.0 mm, then it is substituted with a base or lining cements. Practically, dentin is the best insulator as compared to any cement material of equivalent thickness.

Base is the material or combination of materials, which is used as substitute for lost dentin; the liner, which synchronises the base (the material may or may not be the same) is used for protection against chemical, thermal, mechanical and electrical stimuli as well as from bacteria and toxins.

The base is not indicated in many occasions (presence of 2.0 mm of remaining dentin). Luting agent, however, is the necessity of every cast restoration. Base is needed for protection; whereas luting agent is required for seating and sealing of the restoration.

The usual phenomenon for luting in dentistry is micro-mechanical attachment involving intermolecular bonds. However, with the advent of bonding agents and adhesive luting agents, this concept is changed. The luting agent interlocks between the irregularities of the surfaces, obstructing the mobility between the bonded substrates.

The choice of cement depends on the functional and biological demands of the particular clinical situation. The mechanical and biological properties of various luting agents differ from each other. In the oral environment, luting cements should withstand masticatory and parafunctional stresses, maintaining their integrity while stresses are being transferred from indirect restorations to tooth structure. These stresses, however, vary in different clinical situations. Stronger luting agents are required where greater stresses are anticipated.

Requirements of a Luting Agent

The clinical requirements of a luting agent are:

1. *Strength:* An ideal luting agent should have sufficient strength to resist fracture and also long-term fatigue stresses. The luting agent is to bear functional forces along with the indirect restoration.

   The minimum compressive strength of 70 MPa is considered optimum for luting agents. Generally, the luting agents have sufficient compressive strength; however, the tensile strength is poor (oblique forces may destabilize the restoration). The researchers have tried to improve the properties of luting agent by modifying their composition. Addition of phytic acid

to zinc phosphate, amino acid monomer to glass-ionomer and resin fibers to resin cements could improve mechanical properties. The luting agents, which exhibit high creep, do not perform well. Clinically, glass-ionomers have higher creep values than zinc phosphate cements. Composites also have similar creep values. Change in water/powder ratio and the manipulation technique may affect the mechanical properties; however, adhesive resins are little affected by these features. The filled resin luting agents generally exhibit higher values (compressive strength and other mechanical properties such as modulus of elasticity, fracture toughness, etc.) than traditional unfilled resins.

2. *Wetting:* After the preparation, the tooth leaves a rough surface covered with debris. The tooth surface and the restoration should be thoroughly cleaned so as to enable the cement to wet both the surfaces. The wetting helps the cement flow into irregularities on both the surfaces sealing the gaps between the restorations and the tooth surfaces.

3. *Flow:* The luting agent should have sufficient flow so as to fill the interfaces between the tooth and the restoration. Clinically, the materials can be mixed at lower powder/liquid ratio to enhance flow. Seating the restoration under dynamic load (patient is instructed to close firmly and keep pressed); this results in superior flow of the luting agent and complete seating of the restoration.

4. *Film thickness:* The minimum film thickness required for effective luting is less than 25 μ. To achieve adequate film thickness, the particles of luting cement should be 5–10 μ in diameter. The film thickness, clinically achieved, varies from 20 to 100 μ. The film thickness of the material depends upon viscosity of mixture and also availability of space for displacement of cement.

The type of luting agent affects film thickness; however, the type of restoration is not significant. The mixing technique has also been shown to influence film thickness. The higher viscosity of the luting agent may elevate or tilt the restoration. The resin cements, because of their higher viscosity, may lead to tilting of castings.

Film thickness is also influenced by manipulative variables such as mixing temperature and powder/liquid ratio. As film thickness increases, the tensile bond strength of cements to cast alloy decreases; however, polycarboxylate cements have shown opposite results.

5. *Overhang control:* All luting cements leave some form of overhang after seating of the indirect restorations. The working time and easy removal of the cement are pre-requisite of an ideal luting agent. The criteria of time as regard removal of the overhang are very important. The 'cleaning' of set zinc phosphate and polycarboxylate cements is comparatively easier than glass-ionomers, composites and dual-cure cements. In such cases, the 'cleaning' is carried out before the cement is set completely, i.e. partly set cements. Once the 'extra' cement is cleaned from all the sides, the patient is again asked to press the restoration. The pressing of restoration will fill the gaps between the tooth and restoration, if any. Once the cement is set, the probe should not be touched at the margins. Use of probe will remove the set cement, subsequently leaving the gap for caries and sensitivity. The low viscosity luting agents can only be used under easily accessible margins. Earlier, the luting agents, which change colour after setting were considered effective; however, recent studies opined that such color may jeopardize the esthetics.

6. *Wear of luting cement:* It is established that marginal gaps and recurrent caries are definite factors for failures in indirect restorations. In case of ceramic/composite inlays and crowns, because of increased restoration–tooth gap, the concern of wear of luting agents is gaining importance. The wear resistance of almost all cements is less than that of resin cements. It is postulated that luting agent wear might be self-limiting because of simultaneous wear of enamel margins.

The quantitative/three-dimensional measure of wear within the luting space is carried out using advance computer technology and optical scanning methods. The wear at the margins is a cause of concern to the operator, since it may lead to recurrent caries after passage of time.

7. *Dissolution in oral fluids:* The dissolution of luting agents in oral fluids is significant as all margins are accessible to saliva. An ideal luting agent should be impervious to oral fluids and resist dissolution. With the exception of cast gold restorations, where the beveling may minimize the salivary contact with the margins, all other restorations are susceptible to salivary contact. The cement dissolution has been shown to be independent of the marginal width as explained by Fick's law of diffusion (Fick's law states that the flux of a component of concentration across the membrane of a unit area, in a predefined plane, is proportional to the concentration differential across the plane). Modifying the powder/liquid ratio certainly has a dramatic effect on solubility. The polycarboxylate cements being thixotropic (semisolid when left standing and fluid when subjected to stresses), if mixed in higher liquid/powder ratio, show increased solubility. The dissolution of resin cement is minimum, followed by glass-ionomer cements, polycarboxylate cements and zinc phosphate cement.

The combined effect of wear and dissolution of the luting cement is significant clinically.

8. *Biocompatibility:* An ideal luting agent should have a little or no interaction with body tissues and fluids. It should be non-toxic and should have low allergic potential. The zinc phosphate and glass-ionomer cements are of concern because these can initiate pulpal irritation. However, glass-ionomer cement has been shown to reduce demineralization around crowns despite reduced solubility as compared to zinc phosphate cement. Glass-ionomers also increase the fluoride concentration in the saliva. Many luting agents do possess antimicrobial properties, but their effect diminishes with time. Antimicrobial agents have been added into luting agents but their clinical significance remains doubtful.

9. *Microleakage and modulus of elasticity:* Microleakage of bacteria and their products around dental restorations may lead to pulpal reactions and also affect the prognosis of the restoration. The non-adhesive resins have higher microleakage compared with traditional cements; whereas adhesive resin systems have less microleakage. The configuration of marginal gaps, which favours penetration of bacterial toxins, etc. has not been specified. A few authors could not observe any significant correlation between marginal gaps and micro-leakage. The degree of microleakage is invariably higher with preparation margins in dentin than in enamel.

Modulus of elasticity relates to cement deformation and marginal gap formation. The cement with higher modulus of elasticity is important to prevent microleakage. The modulus of elasticity value for luting agents should be between dentin and indirect restorative material. The modulus of elasticity for dentin, casting alloys and all ceramic materials is 18–30 GPa, 90–220 GPa and 55–230 GPa respectively. A high modulus of elasticity is important, especially at high masticatory stress areas or long span prosthesis. Zinc phosphate cement has highest modulus of elasticity and resin-modified glass-ionomer being the least. The resin modified glass-ionomers should be limited to low stress bearing areas or single restoration.

10. *Radiopacity:* Radiopacity of the luting agents is helpful in diagnosis of recurrent decay, detection of open gingival margins and the excess material. The luting agent should be more radiopaque than dentin. It is difficult to detect a cement line radiographically if the material is not significantly more radiopaque than dentin. In case of inaccessible areas and where marginal fit is not ideal, optimal radiopacity helps ensure complete removal of excess material and also distinguishes marginal gap cements from recurrent decay.

Radiopacity depends upon the type and proportion of filler particles. The auto-polymerizing resins are less radiopaque than dentin. The other cements are radiopaque as required.

11. *Clinical performance:* Various factors affect the clinical performance of luting cements. The correlation between labora-tory measurements of the properties and clinical performance has not been established. A few authors observed no significant difference in clinical success between restorations cemented with zinc phosphate and those cemented with a reinforced zinc oxide eugenol. Glass-ionomer cements are more effective for base metals; resin cements have shown promising results with composite/ceramic restorations.

The clinical performance of the luting agents vary with the choice of material, type of restoration, stresses onto the restoration and the oral environment.

TYPES OF LUTING AGENTS

1. Zinc Phosphate Cement

Zinc phosphate cement is the most commonly used luting agent (Fig. 12.1), for luting of metal inlays, onlays and crowns. ADA specification no. 8 designates zinc phosphate cement as of two types:

Type I—for cementation of indirect restorations.

Type II—for all other uses.

This cement does not chemically bond to any surface and provides seal by mechanical retention only. The taper, length and surface area of tooth is critical for successful restoration.

The compressive strength (80–110 Mpa), tensile strength (5–7 Mpa), modulus of elasticity (136 Mpa) can resist masticatory forces. The 25 μ film thickness makes it the material of choice for luting purpose.

However, zinc phosphate cement reveals higher dissolution at almost all pH levels and also gets abraded with toothbrush or other mechanical means of cleaning. The buccal, lingual and occlusal surfaces are more prone to such types of erosion/abrasion.

Advantages

- Adequate film thickness (25 μ)
- Excellent flow
- Dimensionally stable, no expansion/ shrinkage
- Cost effective

Disadvantages

- Solubility in oral fluids
- Poor tensile strength
- Easily gets abraded
- No chemical bond
- Potential for pulpal irritation

2. Polycarboxylate Cement

Polycarboxylate cement exhibits chemical adhesion to the tooth structure through interaction of carboxylic acid groups of the cement with calcium of the dentin (Fig. 12.2).

Despite the adhesion of the cement to tooth structure, the retention potential of polycarboxylate cement and zinc phosphate cement is the same. The difference is in the mode of failure. In zinc phosphate cement, the failure occurs at cement–tooth interface; whereas in case of polycarboxylate, it occurs at cement–metal interface.

The cement does not bond to the metal in normal conditions. The dirty surface of the metal on the cavity side of casting is removed in order to improve the wettability. The surface can be air abraded and the casting should be thoroughly washed with water.

As the cement provides adhesion to tooth structure, a clean cavity surface is necessary in order to attain intimate contact and interaction between cement and the tooth. 10% polyacrylic acid solution is applied for 10 to 15 seconds, followed by rinsing with water to achieve the adhesion.

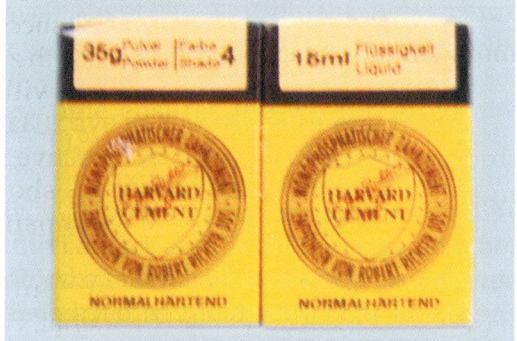

Fig. 12.1: Zinc phosphate cement

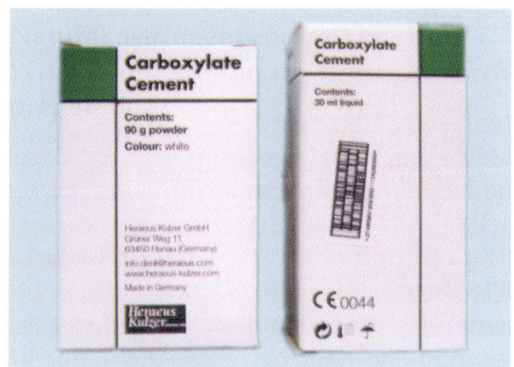

Fig. 12.2: Polycarboxylate cement

It has a low compressive strength (55 Mpa), higher tensile strength (8–12 Mpa) and greater plastic deformation than zinc phosphate cement. The 22–28 μ film thickness is appropriate for luting indirect restorations.

Polycarboxylate cement has been reported to be biocompatible with dental pulp and is best suited for cementation of single metal units in low stress areas. However, it is soluble in oral fluids.

Advantages

- Better tensile strength
- Excellent flow
- Adequate film thickness (22–28 μ)
- Biocompatible with pulp
- Provides chemical adhesion with tooth structure

Disadvantages

- Highly viscous (operator may add more liquid to get appropriate viscosity)
- Thixotropic properties
- Less wear resistant

3. Glass-Ionomer Cement

Glass-ionomer cements adhere to tooth structure by forming a bond by chelation of carboxyl groups with calcium of dentin (Figs 12.3 and 12.4).

The compressive strength (90–230 Mpa) is higher than zinc phosphate and polycarboxylate cements. The lower modulus of elasticity (20 GPa) makes it susceptible to deformation in areas of high masticatory stresses. The film thickness (25–30 μ) is appropriate for luting purposes.

The initial low pH during setting was thought to be a cause of sensitivity; however, it was established that pH remains low for short duration and becomes normal within one hour.

Advantages

- Exhibits cariostatic activity because of fluoride release (preferred where caries susceptibility is higher).

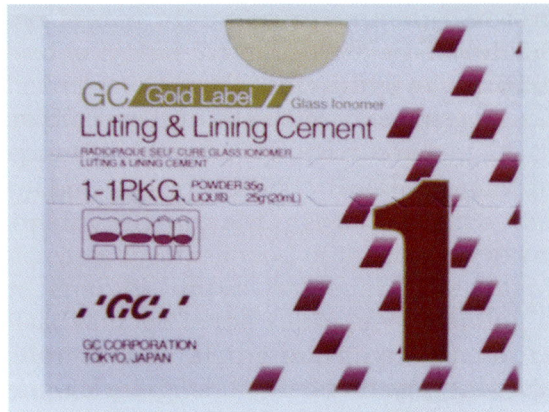

Fig. 12.3: Glass ionomer (luting and lining)

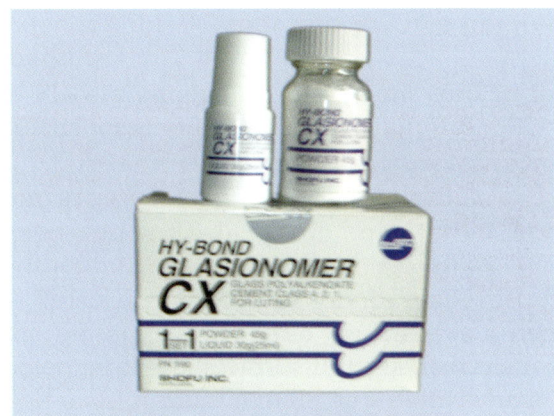

Fig. 12.4: Hy-bond glass ionomer

- The coefficient of thermal expansion is almost equivalent to that of tooth (no problem of expansion/shrinkage).
- Physical properties such as strength, flow and dissolution in oral fluids are better than other cements.
- Bonding to tooth structure.

Disadvantages

- It may lead to tooth sensitivity.
- Over hydration of tooth.

The modified form of glass-ionomer cements (resin reinforced glass-ionomer cement) has also been used as luting agent (Figs 12.5 and 12.6). They exhibit properties of glass ionomer cement coupled with better film thickness and strength. These systems

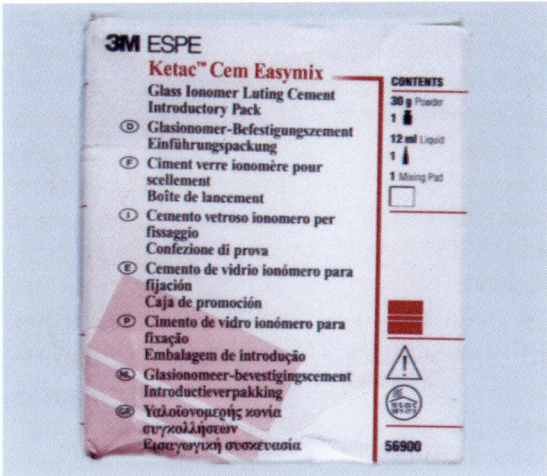

Fig. 12.5: Ketac-Cem Easymix

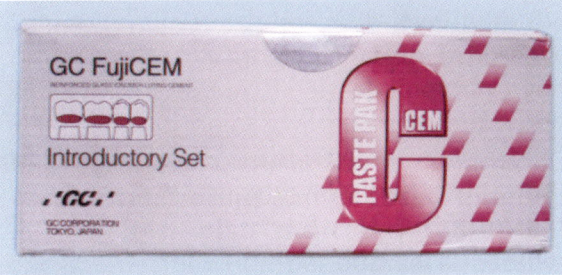

Fig. 12.6: GC FujiCEM

exhibit dual setting process consisting of photo-polymerization and an acid–base reaction. The final set material has glass particles in a matrix consisting of two networks, one derived from the resin and other from glass ionomer type reaction. The resin reinforcement produces higher bond strength to dental tissues and enhanced mechanical strength. The capsulated luting cement, Ketac-Cem has shown better strength. The resin-modified cements exhibit improved bonding and better marginal adaptation even after 24 hours of water storage. The possible reasons for improvement are:

• Hygroscopic expansion of the luting cement
• Reduced setting stress due to water absorption
• Improved bonding ability or setting during water storage

However, because of expansion of these cements, these should be used with caution in post and core restorations. All-ceramic crowns can also fracture because of expansion. The commonly used powder/liquid luting agents are summarized in Table 12.1.

4. Resin Cements

Resin luting cements have been in existence since long. The early formulations were chemically cured. Because of high polymerization shrinkage, tendency for pulpal irritation, microleakage and poor handling qualities, these luting agents are recently used.

The light activated resin cements are widely used as luting agents (Fig. 12.7). The chemically activated or auto-polymerizing systems (Panavia, C & B Metabond) are suited for luting of metal restorations. The polymerization of Panavia is strongly retarded by oxygen, which facilitates removal of excess resin (overhang removal is easy, prior to complete polymerization). Dual cure cements are also tried as luting agents. Dual cure cements were evolved to achieve complete cure in areas where the cure due to light polymerization is not complete like the lowermost layer of cement in porcelain inlays. The chemical activation is very slow, which provides extended working time. Until the cement is exposed to curing light, the operator has ample time for manipulation. Less micro-hardness of dual-cured luting cements have been reported, especially within first twenty-four hours when light curing was omitted; therefore, not used in metal restorations. The dual-cure cements are favourable for luting tooth colored restorations because they provide extended working time and controlled polymerization.

Resin cements, produced in dual-polymerized formulations are indicated for restorations having inaccessible margins, where initial light may not be reaching all parts of the restoration and the auto-curing is to complete the process. In case, the cement is

Table 12.1: Description of commonly used (powder/liquid) luting agents

Product name	Manufacturer	Composition	Film thickness (μ)	Setting time (minutes)
Fynal (Reinforced ZOE)	Dentsply/Caulk	Powder = zinc oxide; polymer Liquid = eugenol; acetic acid	30	5
Harvard cement (zinc-phosphate cement)	Richter & Hoffmann, Berlin, Germany	Powder-zinc oxide, magnesium oxide Liquid-phosphoric acid	25	6
Hy-Bond-ZP (zinc phosphate)	Shofu, Kyoto, Japan	Powder = zinc oxide; magnesium oxide; zinc fluoride; strontium fluoride; tannic acid Liquid = phosphoric acid; aluminium phosphate	21	8
Tenacin (zinc phosphate)	Dentsply/Caulk	Powder = zinc oxide; magnesium oxide Liquid = phosphoric acid; aluminium trihydrate	20	8
Bondalcap C (polycarboxylate)	Ivoclar/Vivadent	Powder = zinc oxide, magnesium oxide Liquid = polyacrylic acid	22	5
Durelon (polycarboxylate)	ESPE, Seefeld, Germany	Powder = zinc oxide; tin fluoride Liquid = polyacrylic acid	22	6–8
Hy-Bond-PC (polycarboxylate)	Shofu, Kyoto, Japan	Powder = zinc oxide; magnesium oxide; strontium fluoride; tannic acid Liquid = Polyacrylic acid; tricarboxylic acid	23	6–8
Liv Carbo (polycarboxylate)	GC America	Powder = zinc oxide; magnesium oxide; sodium fluoride Liquid = Polyacrylic acid	22	5
Poly Carb Water Set (polycarboxylate)	Pulpdent	Powder = zinc oxide; polyacrylic acid Liquid = water	22	7–8
Tylon-Plus (polycarboxylate) Water settable	Dentsply/Caulk	Powder = zinc oxide; polycarboxylic acid; stannous fluoride Liquid = water	22	6–7
Fuji I (glass ionomer)	GC Tokyo, Japan	Powder = fluoro-alumino-silicate glass Liquid = polyacrylic acid	22	6–8
Glass Lute (glass ionomer)	Pulpdent	Powder = fluoro-alumino-silicate glass Liquid = polyacrylic acid	25	6–7
Vivaglass Cem (glass ionomer)	Ivoclar/Vivadent	Powder = aluminium fluorosilicate glass; ytterbium trifluoride Liquid = polyacrylic acid, tartaric acid	25	5–7
Fuji Cem (resin modified glass ionomer)	GC, Tokyo, Japan	Paste A:fluoro-alumino-silicate, hydroxymethyl methacrylate, Paste B : polyacrylic acid, water, silica	18	6–8
Fuji Plus (resin modified glass ionomer)	GC, Tokyo, Japan	Powder = fluoro-alumino-silicate Liquid = Copolymer of acrylic and maleic acid	30	6–8

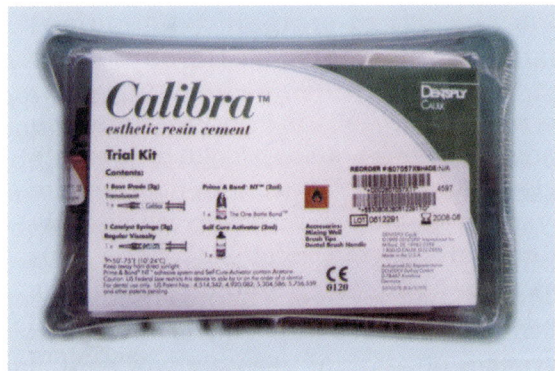

Fig. 12.7: Calibra-resin luting cement

not adequately polymerized, the clinical performance of the restoration is affected.

The dual-cure resins contain a new dimethacrylate polymer that modifies the rheology of the material facilitating easy removal of the excess material. However, these cements show significant decrease in their mechanical properties, especially the flexural strength.

Rely X™ Unicem (3M ESPE), a dual-cure resin cement is available in capsulated form (Fig. 12.8). The manufacturer claims that the cement is hydrophobic during setting, which enhances the dimensional stability of the cement. The handling and manipulation is simple. The initial set cement can be easily chipped off using an explorer. The cement possesses features like fluoride release, dual setting, shades for ceramic restorations and the potential for less postoperative sensitivity.

Another resin cement, Appeal™ (Vivadent NY), is a dual-cure cement with unique characteristics. The uniqueness of this system is the 'value based' shade system. The shades vary from '0' (translucent) to '7' (dark). The system is preferred for anterior applications. The anterior formulations are amine free to prevent the colour changes associated with previous formulations using amines for polymerization. In posterior applications, the dual-cure mode is used to ensure complete polymerization. Nexus™ 2 (Kerr), a dual-cure cement, is also available in four different shades, viz. clear, white, white opaque and yellow. Brown shade has also been introduced.

For resin cements, the pre-treatment of tooth with acid, primer/bonding is essential because it influences the condition of the dentin smear layer. An incomplete penetration of the smear layer with bonding agent or cement weakens the resulting bond. It is also assumed that the inter-diffusion of the smear layer with resin monomer may reinforce the bond; therefore, etching of the dentin may deteriorate the bond and should be avoided.

For veneers or translucent crowns, auto-cure or dual-cure resin cements should be avoided. Certain substances like para-toluidine necessary for chemical cure causes a measurable color change over a period of time. In such cases, light-cure cements are preferred. The higher filler composites can also be used as luting agents improving the abrasion resistance. When energy is applied to the composites, the consistency of the composite is changed to thinner viscosity resulting in easy control of the overhang.

The commonly used resin luting agents are summarized in Table 12.2.

Advantages
- Low film thickness
- Better compressive and tensile strength
- Lowest solubility
- Compatible with esthetic restorations
- Controlled working time
- Achieves appropriate bond strength

Disadvantages
- Postoperative sensitivity.
- Procedure is technique sensitive.

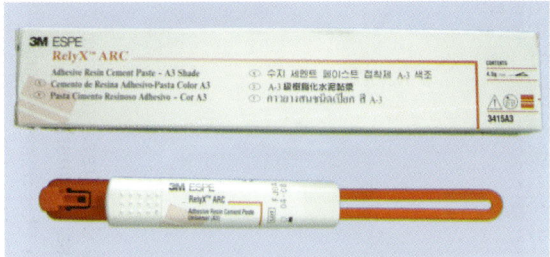

Fig. 12.8: Rely X-adhesive resin cement

Table 12.2: Description of commonly used resin luting agents

Product name	Manufacturer	Filler content (particle size)	Curing mode	Setting time (minutes)	Film thickness (μ)
C&B luting Composite	Bisco	46% (5 µm)	Self	6–7	30
C&B-Metabond	Parkell	Unfilled	Self	10	27
Cement-It!	Jeneric/Pentron	68% (1 µm)	Self	4	40
Choice porcelain Veneer system	Bisco	80% (6 µm)	Dual	7	60–70
Dicor MGC	Dentsply/Caulk	74% (2–4 µm)	Dual	11	
Dual cement	Ivoclar-Vivadent	61% (Microfill)	Dual	14–20	
Duo cement	Coltene/Whaledent	71% (0.5 µm)	Dual	8	
Duo-link	Bisco	67% (1 µm)	Dual	8	70–80
EnForce	Dentsply/Caulk	66% (1 µm)	Light/dual	6	60–70
FLC vision	Mirage dental system	71% (4 µm)	Light/dual	8	60–70
Flexi-flow	Essential dental system	63% (8 µm)	Self	5	40–45
Imperva dual resin cement	Shofu, Kotyo, Japana	77% (3 µm)	Dual	7.5	60–70
Lute-It!	Jeneric/Pentron	65% (0.8 µm)	Light/dual	4.5	45–50
Nexus	Kerr	68% (0.6 µm)	Light/dual	10	
Opal luting composite	3M ESPE, seefeld, Germany	82% (1.4 µm)	Light/dual	6	
Panavia	J. Morita	75% (N/a)	Self	1	44
Panavia 21	J. Morita	77% (N/a)	Self	1	45
Permalute	Ultradent products	70% (1.5 µm)	Dual	6–8	
Scotchbond resin cement	3M ESPE, seefeld, Germany	78% (1.4 µm)	Dual	6	70–80
Twinlook	Heraeus Kulzer	73% (0.7 µm)	Dual	4.5	60–70
Variolink II	Ivoclar-Vivadent	73% (1.0 µm)	Light/dual	15	80
RelyX ARC (Resin cement)	3M ESPE, seefeld, Germany	Bis-GMA, TEGDMA, silica and zirconium glass		6–8	45
Panavia F (Resin cement)	Kuraray, Osaka, Japan	BPEDMA, MDP, DMA, barium, boron and silicium glass, NaF		6–8	40
RelyX unicem (Self-adhesive resin cement)	3M ESPE, seefeld, Germany	Phosphoric acid methacrylates, dimethacrylates, inorganic fillers, fumed silica, initiators		6–8	50

Clinical Aspects of Cementation

The clinical aspect of cementation is important as many factors play part in successful cementation of the restorations. The cementation procedure is divided into two:

a. Seating
b. Retention

a. Seating

The discrepancies in the prepared tooth and the castings coupled with cementing pressure may lead to rebound of restoration. These discrepancies are to be compensated for proper seating of the restoration. The discrepancies can be minimized by coating the die with die-spacer, and/or relieving the die or etching the casting.

In seating the restoration, the features of luting cement, which play important role are:

- Rheology of cement
- Working time
- Film thickness
- Geometry of gap

The failure usually occurs at cement–tooth interface. The flow of cement is the key factor for successfully cementing the restorations. To achieve sufficient cement flow, the seating of restorations should be fast (within a few seconds) while the cement is sufficiently fluid.

The flow of zinc phosphate, polycarboxylate and ethoxybenzoic acid cements is sufficient under moderate pressure. The resin cements are less satisfactory in this respect.

The zinc oxide eugenol cement generates the lowest hydraulic pressure during seating, followed by polycarboxylate cement. Zinc phosphate cement exhibited the greatest hydraulic pressure. The seating force should be maintained at least for three minutes without any interruption while the cement is setting (Figs 12.9a and b).

Working time should be adequate so that the hydraulic action takes place before setting of cement. Mixing on a cool glass slab solves the problem to some extent.

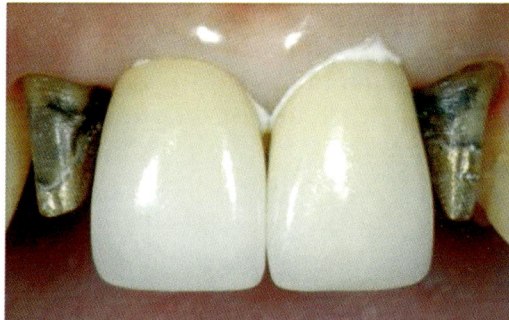

Fig. 12.9a: Excess cement at the margins

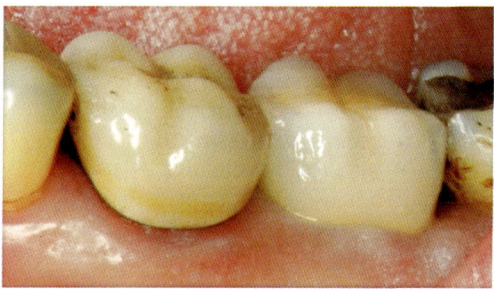

Fig. 12.9b: Excess cement removed from the margins

The excess of cement is to be removed. To achieve easy removal and minimizing the hydraulic pressure, a sort of path is created, which is known as 'venting'. It is confirmed that venting is a satisfactory method of achieving minimal film thickness under cast restorations; it also minimizes the hydraulic pressure.

b. Retention

It is established that almost all luting cements are fair in compressive strength and poor in tensile strength. The luting agents do not help in retention directly; however, better tensile strength of the cement may aid in retention.

The retention of the restoration mainly depends upon the following:

- The geometrical design of the tooth preparation, which in turn influences the stress distribution.
- Bonding efficiency of the luting cement to both the tooth and the restoration.
- Durability of the cement (resistance to mechanical breakdown and dissolution).

It is recommended that the cement with a high tensile strength be used to cement crowns and long span bridges since shear stresses in marginal area can exceed the strength of low strength cement.

Viscoelastic behaviour might be of more value than brittle characteristics. Dentin exhibits viscoelastic behaviour with a significant plastic deformation during fracture, which appears to be greater than that for the zinc phosphate and glass-ionomer cement. And also the modulus of elasticity of dentin in compression is slightly greater than that of zinc phosphate cements. Bonding between these materials influences the stress transfer between the cement, restoration and the tooth substance.

Bibliography

1. Aksornmuang J, Nakajima M, Foxton RM and Tagami J. Mechanical properties and bond strength of dual-cure resin composites to root canal dentin. Dent. Mater.: 2007;23:226–34.

2. Attar N, Tam LE and McComb D. Mechanical and physical properties of contemporary dental luting agents. J. Prosth. Dent: 2003;89:127–34.

3. Ayad MF, Rosenstiel SF and Salama M. Influence of tooth surface roughness and type of cement on retention of complete cast crowns. J. Prosth. Dent: 1997;77:116–21.

4. Balbosh A and Kern A. Effect of the surface treatment on retention of glass-fiber endodontic posts. J. Prosthet. Dent.: 2006;95:218–23.

5. Balbosh A, Ludwig K and Kern M. Comparison of titanium dowel retention using four different luting agents. J. Prosth. Dent: 2005;94:227–33.

6. Blatz MB, Sadan A and Kern M. Resin-ceramic bonding: a review of the literature. J. Prosth. Dent: 2003;89:268–74.

7. Borba M, Cesar PF and Griggs JA. Adaptation of fixed partial dentures. Dent. Mater.: 2011;27, 1119–26.

8. Bouillaguet S, Troesch S, Wataha JC, Krejci I, Meyer JM and Pashley DH. Microtensile bond strength between adhesive cements and root canal dentin. Dent. Mater.: 2003;19:199–205.

9. Braga RR, Cesar PF and Gonzaga CC. Mechanical properties of resin cements with different activation modes. J. Oral Rehabil.: 2002;29:257–62.

10. Cal E, Turkun LS, Torkun M, Toman M and Toksavul S. Effect of an antibacterial adhesive on the bond strength of three different luting resin composites. J. Dent.: 2006;34:372–38.

11. Chang J, Da Silva JD, Sakai M, Kristiansen J and Ishikawa-Nagai S. The optical effect of composite luting cement on all ceramic crowns. J. Dent.: 2009;37:937–43.

12. Cheung G J K and Botelho M G: Zirconia surface treatment for resin bonding. J Adhes Dent. (2015) 17, 551–8.

13. Cohen BI, Pagnillo MK, Newman I, Musikant BL and Duetsch AS. Retention of four endodontic posts cemented with composite resin. Gen. Dent.: 2000;48:320–4.

14. D'Arcangelo C, Cinelli M, De Angelis F and D'Amario M. The effect of resin cement film thickness on the pull-out strength of a fiber-reinforced post system. J. Prosthet. Dent.: 2007;98: 193–8.

15. Davidson CL, Van Zeghbroeck L and Freizer AJ. Destructive stresses in adhesive luting cements. JDR: 1991;70:880–2.

16. de la Macorra JC and Pradies G. Conventional and adhesive luting cements. Clin. Oral Invest.: 2002;6: 198–204.

17. De munck J, Van Landuy K, Peumans M, Poltevin A, Lambrechts P and Braem M. A critical review of the durability of adhesion to tooth tissue: methods and results. J. Dent. Res.: 2005;84:118–32.

18. Denike R and Ewoldsen N. Luting agents: critical appraisal. J. Esthet. Restorative Dent.: 2002;14:57–61.

19. Derand P and Derand T2000. Bond strength of luting cements to zirconium oxide ceramics. Int. J. Prosthodont.: 1991;13:131–5.

20. Desinova LA, Maev RG and Leontijev VK. Study of the adhesion between dental cement and dentin using a non-destructive acoustic microscopy approach. Dent. Mater.: 2009;25:557–65.

21. Duke ES. New technology directions in resin cements. Compendium.: 2003;24:606–8.

22. Eisenburger M, Addy M and Robbach A. Acidic solubility of luting cements. J. Dent.: 2003;31:137–42.

23. El-Badrawy WA and El-Mowafy OM. Chemical versus dual curing of resin inlay cements. J. Prosth. Dent: 1995;73:515–24.

24. el-Mowafy OM. The use of resin cements in restorative dentistry to overcome retention problems. J. Can. Dent. Assoc.: 2001;67:97–102.

25. Fleming GJP and Addison O. Adhesive cementation and the strengthening of all-ceramic dental restoration. J. Adhes. Sci. Tech.: 2009;23: 945–59.

26. Frankenberger R, Lohbauer U, Taschner M, Petschelt A and Nikolaenko SA. Adhesive luting revisited: influence of adhesive, temporary cement, cavity cleaning, and curing mode on internal dentin bond strength. J. Adhes. Dent.: 2007;9:269–73.

27. Frazier KB and Sarrett DC. Wear resistance of dual cured resin luting agents. Am. J. Dent.: 1995; 8:161–4.

28. Furukawa K, Inai N and Tagami J. The effect of luting resin bond to dentin on the strength of dentin supported by indirect resin composite. Dent. Mater.: 2002;18:136–42.

29. Galhano GA, Marques de Melo R, Pavanelli CA, Baldissara P, Scotti R, Valandro LF and Bottino MA. Adhesive cementation of zirconia posts to root dentin: evaluation of the mechanical cycling effect. Braz. Oral Res.: 2008;22:264–9.

30. Gemalmaz D, Ozcan M, Yoruc AB and Alkurn HN. Marginal adaptation of a sintered ceramic inlay system before and after cementation. J. Oral Rehab.: 1997;24:646–51.

31. Goodacre CJ, Campagni WV and Aquilino SA. Tooth preparations for complete crowns: An art form based on scientific principles. J. Prosthet. Dent.: 2001;85:363–76.

32. Goracci C, Sadek FT, Fabianelli A, Tay FR and Ferrari M. Evaluation of the adhesion of fiber posts to intraradicular dentin. Oper. Dent.: 2005; 390:627–35.

33. Gorodovsky S and Zidan O. Retentive strength, disintegration and marginal quality of luting cements. JPD: 1992;68:269–74.

34. Gu XH and Kern M. Marginal discrepancy and leakage in all- ceramic crowns : influence of luting agents and ageing conditions. Int. J. Prosthodont.: 2003;16:109–16.

35. Habib B, Fraunhofer JA and Driscoll CF. Comparison of two luting agents used for the retention of cast dowel and cores. J. Prosthodont.: 2005;14:164–9.

36. Hikita K, Van Meerbek B, De Munck J, Ikeda T, Van Landuyt K, Maida T, Lambrechts P and Peumans M. Bonding effectiveness of adhesive luting agents to enamel and dentin. Dental Mater.: 2007;23:71–80.

37. Hill EE and Lott J. A clinically focused discussion of luting materials. Aust. Dent. J.: 2011;56:67–76.

38. Hill EE. Dental cements for definitive luting: a review and practical clinical considerations. Dent. Clin. N. Am.: 2007;51:643–58.

39. Huber L, Cattani-Lorente M, Shaw L, Krejci I and Bouillaguet S. Push-out bond strength of endodontic posts bonded with different resin-based luting cements. Am. J. Dent.: 2007;20;167–72.

40. Irie M and Suzuki M. Current luting cements: marginal gap formation of composite inlay and their mechanical properties. Dent. Mater.: 2001; 17– 347.

41. Irie M, Suzuki K and Watts DC. Marginal and flexural integrity of three classes of luting cement, with early finishing and water storage. Dent. Mater.: 2004;20:3–11.

42. Jivraj SA, Kim TH and Donovan TE. Selection of luting agents. Part I. J. Calif. Dent. Assoc.: 2006;34: 149–60.

43. Kim TH, Jivraj SA and Donovan TE. Selection of luting agents, part 2. J. Calif. Dent. Assoc.: 2006;34: 161–6.

44. Kramer N, Lohbauer U and Frankenberger R. Adhesive luting of indirect restorations. Am. J. Dent.: 2000;13:60–76.

45. Kumbuloglu O, Lassila VJ, Vallittu PK. A study of the physical and chemical properties of four resin composite luting cements. Int. J. Prosthodont.: 2004;17:357–63.

46. Li ZC and White SN. Mechanical properties of dental luting cements. J. Prosth. Dent.: 1999; 81:597–609.

47. Malkoc MA, Sevimay M, Tatar I and Celik HH. Micro-CT detection and characterization of porosity in luting cements. J. Prosthodont.: 2015; 24:553–61.

48. Marchan S, Coldero L, Whiting R and Barclay S. In vitro evaluation of the retention of zirconia-based ceramic posts luted with glass ionomer and resin cements. Braz. Dent. J.: 2005;16:213–7.

49. Marcondes M, Souza N, Manfroi FB, Burnett LH and Spohr AM: Clinical evaluation of Indirect composite resin restorations cemented with different resin cements. J Adhes Dent. 2016:18;59–67.

50. McComb D. Adhesive luting cements—class, criteria and usage. Compend Cont. Educ. Dent.: 1996;17:759–62.

51. Milutinovic-Nikolic AD, Medi VB and Vukovic ZM. Porosity of different dental luting cements. Dent. Mater.: 2007;23:674–8.

52. Monticelli F, Toledano M, Tay FR, Sadek FT, Goraci C and Ferrari M. A simple etching technique for improving the retention fiber posts to resin composites. J. Endod.: 2006;32:44–7.

53. Munck JD, Vargas M, Landuyt KV, Hikita K, Lambrechts P and Meerbeck BV. Bonding of an auto-adhesive luting material to enamel and dentin. Dent. Mater.: 2004;20:963–71.

54. Oilo G and Euje DM. Film thickness of dental luting cements. Dent. Mater. 1986;2:85–89.

55. Olivera AB and Saito T. The effect of die spacer on retention and fitting of complete cast crowns. J. Prosthodont.: 2006;15:243–249.

56. O'Rourke B, Walls AW and Wassell RW. Radiographic detection of overhangs formed by resin composite luting agents. J. Dent.: 1995; 23:353–7.

57. Ozcan M and Bernasconi M: Adhesion of Zirconia used for dental restorations: A systematic review and meta analysis. J Adhes Dent. 2015;17:7–26.

58. Pameijer A. A review of luting agents. Int. J. Dent.:1–7, Article ID 752861; 2012.

59. Pegoraro TA, Da Silva NRFA and Carvalho RM. Cements for use in esthetic dentistry. Dent. Clin. N. Am.: 2007;51:453–71.

60. Perdiago J, Geraldeli S and Lee IK. Push-out bond strengths of tooth-coloured posts bonded with different adhesive systems. Am. J. Dent.: 2004;17: 422–6.

61. Perdiago J, Gomes G and Lee IK. The effect of silane on the bonding strength of the fiber posts. Dent. Mater.: 2006;22:752–8.

62. Piwowarczyk A and Lauer HC. Mechanical properties of luting cements after water storage. Oper. Dent.: 2003;28:535.

63. Piwowarczyk A, Lauer HC and Sorenson JA. Microleakage of various cementing agents for full cast crowns. Dent. Mater.: 2005;21:445.

64. Polat ZS, Tacir IH, Eskimez S and Celik MY. Retentive form of three fiber-reinforced resin composite posts and a zirconia post cemented with two adhesive luting agents: in vitro study. Dent. Mater. J.: 2007;26:672–6.

65. Proussaefs P. Crowns cemented on crown preparations lacking geometric resistance form. Part II: Effect of cement. J. Prosth. Dent: 2004; 13:36.

66. Qualtrough AJ, Chandler NP and Purton DG. A comparison of the retention of tooth-colored posts. Quint. Int.: 2003;34:199–201.

67. Radovic I, Monticelli F and Goracci C. Self-adhesive resin cements: a literature review. J. Adhes. Dent.: 2008;10:251–8.

68. Ramaraju S and Alla RK, Alluri VR and Raju MAKV. A review of conventional and contemporary luting agents used in dentistry. Am. J. Mater. Sci. and Engg.: 2014;2:28–35.

69. Rezende EC, Gomes GM, Szesz AL, Bueno CD, Reis A and Loguercio AD: Effects of dentin moisture on cementation of fibre posts to root canals. 2016;18:29–34.

70. Rosenstiel SF, Land MF and Crispin BJ. Dental luting agents: a review of the current literature. J. Prosth. Dent: 1998;80:280–301.

71. Rosentritt M, Behr M, Lang R and Handel G. Influence of cement type on the marginal adaptation of all ceramic MOD inlays. Dent. Mater.: 2004;20:463.

72. Seo D, Yi Y and Roh B. The effect of preparation designs on the marginal and internal gaps in Cerec 3 partial ceramic crowns. J. Dent.: 2009;37: 374–82.

73. Soares CJ, Soares PV, Pereira JC and Fonseca RB. Surface treatment protocols in the cementation process of ceramic and laboratory-processed composite restorations: A literature review. J. Esthet. and Rest. Dent.: 2005;17:224–35.

74. Staxrud F and Dahl J E: Silanising agents promote resin-composite repair. International Dent J. 2016; 65:311–5.

75. Sumer E and Deger Y. Contemporary permanent luting agents used in dentistry: A literature review. Int. Dent. Res.: 2011;1:26–31.

76. Weiser F and Behr M. Self-adhesive resin cements: a clinical review. J. Prosthodont.: 2015;24:100–8.

77. White SN and Yu Z. Film thickness of new adhesive luting agents. J. Prosthet. Dent.: 1992;67: 782–5.

13

Failures of Indirect Restorations

The most difficult task in our profession is to define failure. Different philosophers and various authors have defined failures in their own ways and whims. Usually, patient's dissatisfaction is considered as failure, though satisfaction/dissatisfaction is individual's perception. The variation in judgement amongst operators and also the patients is a common feature. If one person is not satisfied over placement of margins or color, etc.; the other may accept the same happily. Such variations in judgement are expected and make way for further improvement; otherwise, the restoration (inlay, onlay, crown or bridge) cannot be standardized. The level of acceptability always varies between the operator and the patient. Failures can also be categorized as 'established failure' and 'potential failure'. In case, both operator and the patient accept, the failure is designated as 'established' and in case one (either operator or the patient) do not accept, it is designated as 'potential'. Failures may occur even after appropriately performed restorative procedures. These are related with the complication encountered during and after fabrication of the restoration. A complication has been defined as 'a secondary disease or condition developing in the course of a primary disease or condition'. The knowledge regarding the clinical complications during restorative procedures enhances the clinician's ability to develop the most appropriate treatment plan and convey the patient as regard the possible complications and outcome of the treatment.

The causes of failures and the adequate remedies in indirect restorations are as follows:

1. Discomfort

Patient's discomfort should be taken seriously and attend immediately, otherwise the underlying cause for the discomfort may lead to unmanageable complications. The causes leading to discomfort can be:

a. *Traumatic functional occlusion:* The premature contact of high marginal ridge, cusp tip, incline planes or any other object during functional occlusion leads to discomfort to the patient (Fig. 13.1). The mobile and extruded teeth because of loss of periodontal support also creates discomfort. The premature areas can be corrected after carefully examining the wax records or articulating paper marks. Small stones are used to grind off the prematurities. The extruded teeth should be enveloped by taking more number of abutments in case of bridge; in case of single crown, it is preferably united with the adjacent healthy tooth. Care should be

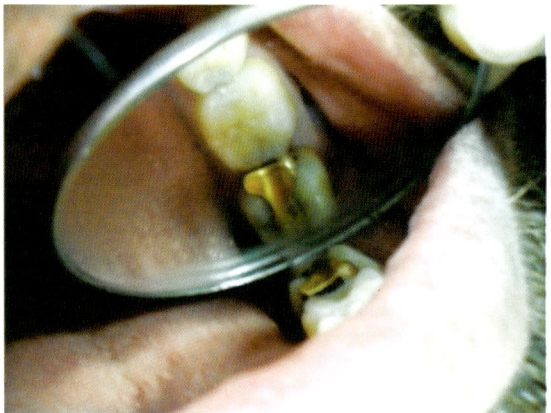
Fig. 13.1: Premature contact in inlay

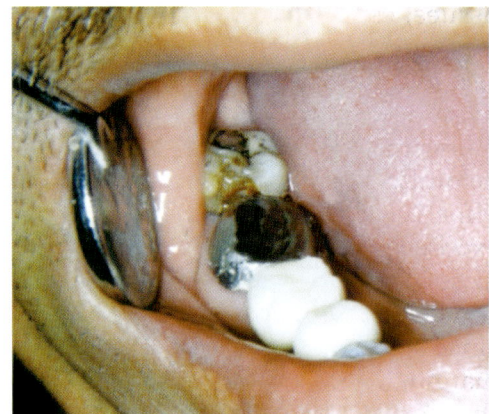
Fig. 13.2: Poorly positioned food table

exercised, as regard choice of the restoration over the tooth/teeth with compromised bone support.

b. *Oversized occlusal table:* The oversized or poorly positioned occlusal table usually leads to stagnation of food and may lead to abnormal pressure under the tissues. An attempt is made to narrow the bucco-lingual configuration of the occlusal table by reducing the lingual cusps and/or opening the lingual embrasure. Creating auxiliary escape grooves through marginal ridges to buccal and lingual areas of the restorations can also be helpful. Such modifications are preferred in case of full crowns and bridges where full crowns are given as abutments (Fig. 13.2).

c. *Inadequate/improper contact area:* The inadequate contact area may force the restoration towards or away from the approximating teeth (Fig. 13.3). The configuration of contact area in a restoration should be examined at the time of try-in seating. The contact area is modified as per need; alternatively, the restoration can be re-fabricated.

d. *Overprotected or underprotected gingiva:* The overprotected and underprotected gingival tissues lead to swelling and bleeding from the gums. In case of overprotection, the embrasures and contours can be reshaped; whereas in case of under protection, the

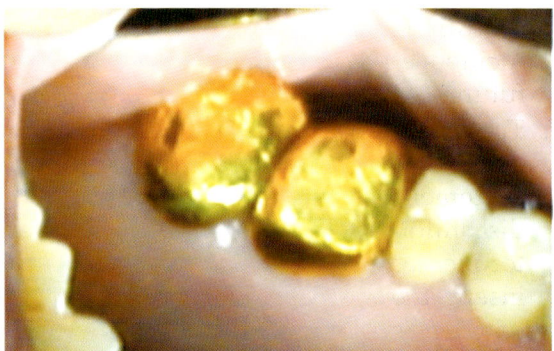
Fig. 13.3: Inadequate contact area

restoration is preferably re-fabricated (Fig. 13.4).

e. *Sensitive cervical areas:* The sensitivity at the cervical areas is the most common complaint of the patients. The cervical areas may get exposed due to displacement of the gingival

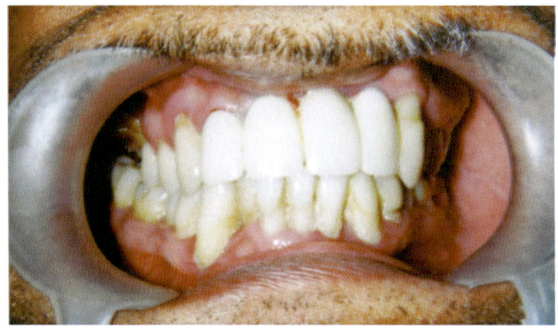
Fig. 13.4: Under protected gingival tissues

tissues, especially placing overextending temporary crowns for a longer period and also ill fitting, under extended restorations (Fig. 13.5). The desensitizing agents such as potassium nitrate, zinc chloride, etc. can be helpful in initial stages. Iontophoresis is also effective. In case of metal crowns, the exposed cervical area can be restored with glass-ionomer cement/composite; however, composite is avoided under ceramic crowns since it may lead to discoloration at the margins. A few authors are of the view that the sensitivity should not be treated immediately. One should wait for a week or two so as to enable the natural phenomenon to occur. The newer bonding agents and modified techniques may minimize the incidence of postoperative sensitivity in future.

f. *Torque generated during placement of restoration:* The torque generated during placement of indirect restoration leads to discomfort to the patient. The intensity of torque depends upon the changed path of insertion or misfitting castings. The torque can be minimized by modifying the preparation so as to have single path of insertion. The inner surface of the casting should be thoroughly checked for any irregularity, during try-in procedures and corrected.

2. Loose Restoration

Loose restoration (crowns, bridges, inlays and onlays) is a common finding (Figs 13.6a and b).

The restoration is cemented again and again only to escape operator's failure in providing appropriate form to the cavity preparation. The looseness of the restoration is due to the following reasons:

a. Deformation of the metal castings: The deformation can be because of:
   • Insufficient tooth reduction (Fig. 13.7).
   • Shallow preparations
   • Excessive/abnormal occlusal forces leading to wear.
   • The sharp cusp of the opposing tooth putting abnormal stresses.
   • When the opposing restoration is of harder metal or unglazed porcelain.
   • When the yield point of the alloy is low.
   In case of deformity, cause may be any; the restoration is to be re-fabricated.

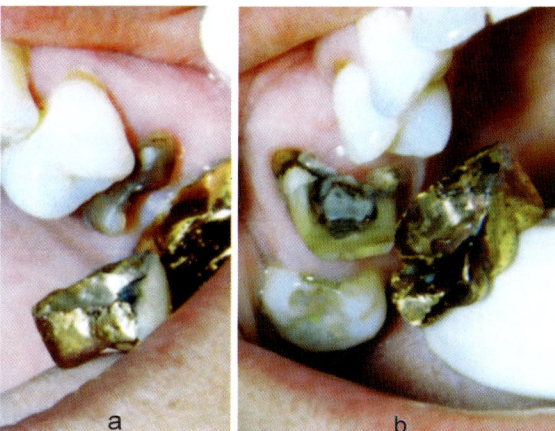

Fig. 13.6a and b: (a) Loose restoration (improper surface area); (b) Loose restoration (lacks mechanical features)

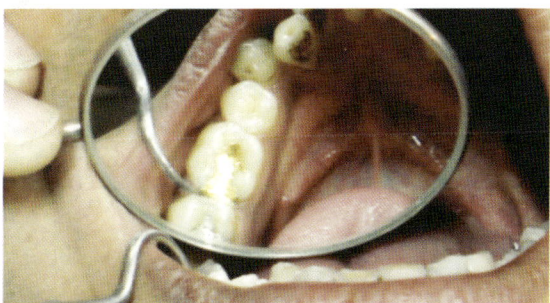

Fig. 13.5: Under extended restoration

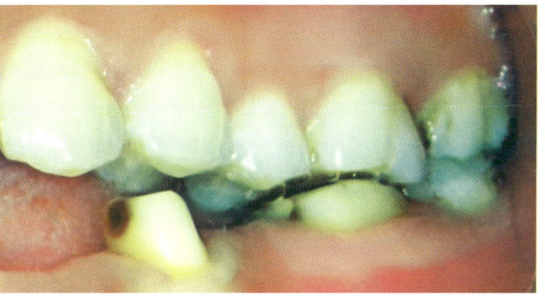

Fig. 13.7: Insufficient tooth reduction

b. *Torque movement:* The abnormal torque movements lead to loosening of the cement at the tooth-restoration interface. Such torque movements are mainly due to premature contacts in lateral excursion. Different types of restoration in a bridge (for example, full crown at one end and inlay at another), lead to such torque movements. The torque is minimized or even eliminated by equilibration of the occlusion and by re-contouring the occlusal table.

c. *Luting cements:* The technique of cementation and the solubility of luting cement in oral fluids is also a reason for loosening of the restoration. In case, the cements are not mixed properly or the tooth surfaces are not cleaned, the cementation remains ineffective. Dissolution of the cement is mainly because of gap at the margins; however, sometimes a small hole is created in casting during occlusal equilibration, also leads to cement dissolution. Wear of luting cement at these surfaces may lead to sub-margination of the restoration.

d. *Recurrent caries:* Recurrent caries can lead to loosening of the indirect restorations. Caries can develop because of gaps, gingival recession and/or exposed tooth surfaces. Basically, caries and loosening are interrelated; caries may lead to loosening of the restoration and loose restorations can lead to caries. In case, caries has undermined the restoration, the restoration is to be removed, caries treated and the tooth is to be prepared again for fresh fabrication of the restoration.

e. *Bridge with one retainer as inlay:* Such restorations cause abnormal stresses onto the tooth, subsequently loosening of the restoration. In case of single inlay restoration, such problems do not arise (Fig. 13.8).

3. Recurrence of Caries

One of the major causes of failure of indirect restorations is recurrence of caries, mostly at

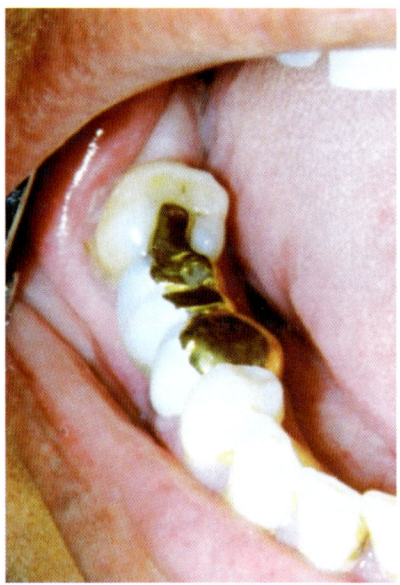

Fig.13.8: Inlay as retainer causes problem

the cervical margins (Fig. 13.9). The initiation of recurrent caries is due to:
- Short castings/open margins
- Loose restoration (multiple paths of insertion)
- Overcontoured restorations filling the embrasures (Figs 13.10a and b)
- Wear of the restoration occlusally
- Prolonged temporary restorations leading to gingival recession
- Metals which cannot be burnished, especially at the margins
- Poor oral hygiene
- Cement dissolving especially at cervical margins

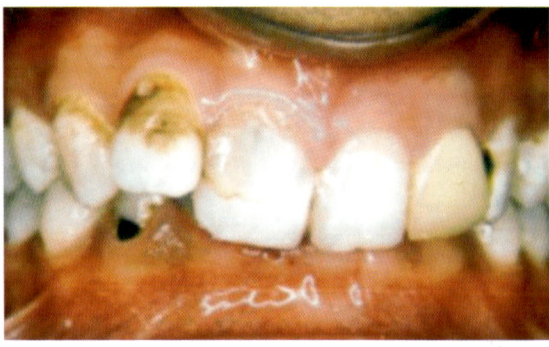

Fig. 13.9: Secondary caries

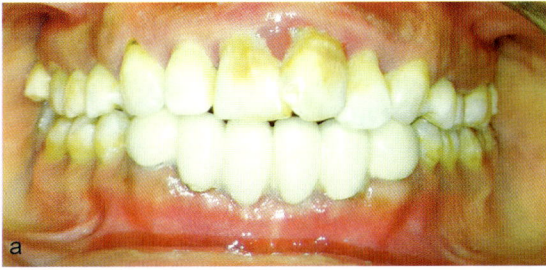
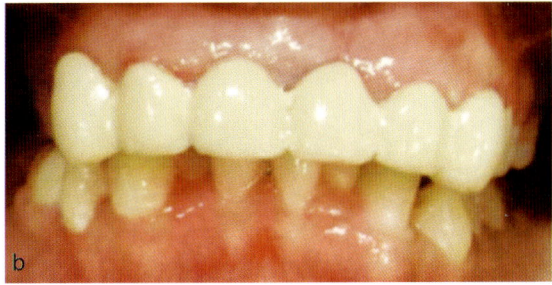

Fig. 13.10a and b: Overcontoured restoration

4. Loss of Supporting Structures

The supporting periodontal tissues aid in better prognosis of the indirect restorations. The features which lead to loss of supporting structures are:

- Overextension of the margins
- Size of the food table
- Proximal contours and embrasures
- Length of the span of bridge
- Inability to clean the area
- Patient prone to periodontal problems

The overextended margins and the contours can be corrected during try-in of the restoration. In case, the contours cannot be modified, re-fabrication is indicated. Long span bridges should only be planned if the abutment teeth are suitable both in numbers and in periodontal health. The food table or the occlusal table should be shortened in order to decrease the load during mastication. The periodontal problems should be periodically treated and evaluated so as to minimize loss of support to these restorations.

5. Degeneration of the Pulp

The preparation of the tooth should be carried out slowly along with using coolants so as to avoid any damage to the pulp. Pulp is affected because of the heat generated due to rapid tooth cutting and especially when coolants are not used. An utmost care is exercised during tooth preparation, more so in metal-ceramic crowns, where excessive labial/occlusal reduction is required. In case, pulp is near to exposure, the cutting/finishing is stopped immediately and the pink spot is covered with calcium hydroxide. In case of full veneers, the temporary crown is fabricated or pre-fabricated polycarbonate crown is selected and fitted using zinc oxide eugenol as sealer. The temporary seal with zinc oxide eugenol cement is indicated since the time gap between the preparation and the final restoration is deleterious to the pulpal health. Premature contacts and the minor occlusal interferences, if not corrected, leads to pulpal involvement. The root canal treatment becomes mandatory if the irreversible pulpitis is confirmed in the prepared tooth/teeth.

6. Fracture of Restoration and/or Tooth

Fracture of restoration, especially separation of porcelain from the metals in metal ceramic restorations is quite common. The possible reasons for fracture of porcelain attachments can be:

a. The difference in modulus of elasticity between metal and ceramic material is the main cause of fracture of porcelain attachment. When feldspathic porcelain is cooled, the leucite crystals contract more than the surrounding glass matrix; subsequently the tangential stresses around the leucite particles may lead to microcracks within the ceramic crystals.

b. The silicate bonds in the glassy ceramic matrix are susceptible to hydrolysis by moisture in the environment (oral cavity) coupled with mechanical stresses. The oral environment does affect longevity of the restoration.

c. Cracks within the ceramics are also a major reason of failure of ceramic restorations.

The minute scratches present on the ceramic surface may behave as sharp notches whose tips are susceptible to fracture. The crack tip is extended through the body of the material.

d. The microporosities developed during sintering can predispose to crack initiation and propagation; subsequently leading to fracture of the restoration. The laboratory procedures, if not followed meticulously, may lead to failure of ceramic restoration.

e. Inadequate occlusal cutting during tooth preparation leading to too little interocclusal space for the porcelain is also a major cause of porcelain fracture from the metal surface.

The acrylic facings can also be separated from the underlying metals. The major cause of the fracture of the acrylic attachments is the abnormal trauma from occlusal interferences. The occlusal interferences should be corrected prior to planning the tooth preparation as well as during temporary restorations. Resin restorations can also fracture under heavy loads (Fig. 13.11)

7. Loss of Functions

The restoration, by all means, should restore the functions. In case, the patient feels difficulty in chewing, may be immediately after placing the restoration or after lapse of some time, the cause should be looked into. Patients unable to chew, immediately after placing the restoration may be due to abnormal occlusal contacts or underlying periodontal problems. The occlusion should be thoroughly checked and corrected in all movements. The delayed functional loss can be due to extraction of the opposing tooth. The loss of occlusal contact may lead to tilting of teeth or even rotation of the restored teeth.

The over-carving and under-carving of the occlusal surfaces also disturbs the functioning of the indirect restorations.

8. Loss of Esthetics

The main aim of restorative dentist is to achieve pleasing esthetics; more importantly in anterior teeth. Unable to restore esthetics or placing conspicuous restorations amount to failures. The maintenance of color, shape, texture, etc. should be evaluated with passage of time leads to failure (Fig. 13.12). The cause of such change is to be looked into and repaired. In case, repair is not feasible, then the re-fabrication is planned.

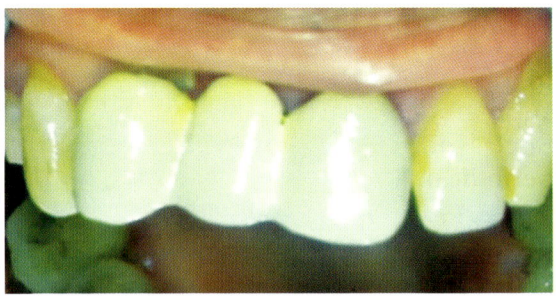

Fig. 13.12: Unaesthetic restoration

Risk Factors associated with Failures of Indirect Restorations

Various factors affect the longevity of indirect restorations. The failure of such restorations is multifactorial. Certain factors enhance the risk of failure of these restorations. Such factors may not have direct influence for failure, but certainly increase the probability of failures.

The various risk factors associated with failure of indirect restorations are as follows:

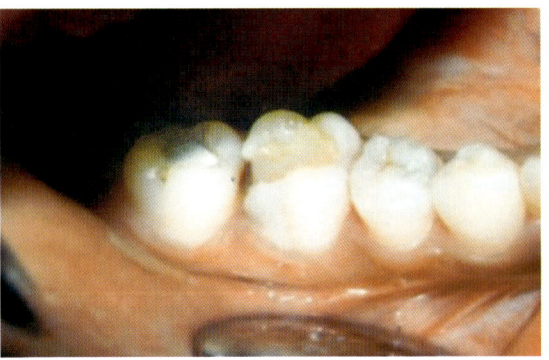

Fig. 13.11: Fractured restoration

1. Factors Related to Patients

a. History: A thorough history is always essential along with observing para-functional habits prior to suggesting type of indirect restoration.

Patients wearing partial denture, may like facial flanges; the patient's psychological requirement should be considered.

Patient should be made aware of minor and major complications associated with the tooth preparation (hot and cold sensation or even pulp involvement). A fully informed patient copes better with the 'pre-warned' complications.

b. Oral hygiene: The patient's ability to clean and maintain his/her dentition affects the performance of indirect restorations. The plaque control around fixed restorations is more difficult as compared to natural teeth. Poor oral hygiene subsequently leads to periodontal problems, especially around abutments, which is one of the main causes of failure of indirect restorations.

In case, the patient is susceptible to caries, his/her cleaning regime should be supplemented with fluoride supplements. Such patients should be evaluated periodically.

c. Smoking: Although smoking is not directly related to failure of indirect restoration, however, continuous smoking does stain the ceramic surface giving it the unesthetic appearance. The smokers, especially the chain smokers should be advised to minimize smoking and follow preventive measures.

2. Factors Related to Restorations

a. Single unit restorations survive better than bridges. Gold crowns have better survival than porcelain fused to base metal crowns. All ceramic crowns should be preferred, especially when the bridge span is less. In case of inlay, the increase in thickness considerably reduces stresses at the base; subsequently less chances of failure.

b. Long span bridge designs lead to high risk of failure. The choice of abutments in such cases is important.

c. All metal crowns/bridges have better survival than porcelain fused to metal restorations. A common cause for failure of PFM restoration is fracture of the veneering ceramic.

d. Bitewing radiographs should routinely be used to diagnose recurrent caries, early bone loss and also for assessing the amount of sound tooth tissues above the crestal bone. All these features, if not managed, lead to failures.

REPAIR OF VENEERS

Small pieces of separated acrylic/porcelain especially in posterior teeth can be repaired with composites; however, large pieces of separated covering need re-fabrication of the restoration.

The preparation designs should allow for sufficient bulk of the ceramics, which improve upon the longevity of the restoration. The luting cements with etching-bonding protocol aid in long-term success of the restorations.

Repair of Porcelain Veneers

The esthetic veneers may break, discolor or wear in due course of time. Chipping of the porcelain in porcelain fused to metal (PFM) restorations can occur because of the various bond failures:

Type I: Metal Porcelain

When the metal surface is totally depleted of oxide layer prior to firing procedure, the metal porcelain bond fails; e.g. gold alloys. This type of failure also occurs on contaminated porous surface.

Type II: Metal Oxide Porcelain

This type of failure occurs in base metal alloys. The porcelain fractures at the metal oxide surface leaving the oxide firmly attached to the metal.

Type III: Cohesive within Porcelain

This type of failure occurs because of the mechanical properties of the porcelain.

Various material aspects of the porcelain (all ceramic) may create residual stresses in the restoration that promote chipping, such as:

i. *Coefficient of thermal expansion:* Chipping during function signals the presence of tensile stresses, likely associated with the zirconia-porcleain surface. Some researchers have suggested that a mismatch in thermal expansion coefficient of the two materials is responsible for failure.

ii. *Thermal conductivity:* During cooling, residual stresses arise in the veneering porcelain because of a temperature gradient between the cool outer surface and the warm inner surface adjoining the coping. As a result, tensile stresses develop in the depth of the veneering material and accelerate crack propagation. The faster the cooling and the lower the thermal conductivity of the core material, the higher the residual stresses inside the veneering porcelain.

iii. *Phase transition:* The property of phase transition serves as toughening mechanism to inhibit crack propagation and is responsible for the extraordinary high flexural strength of zirconia. However, at porcelain zirconia interface, phase transition leads to tensile stresses on the bottom of the veneering porcelain, probably resulting in starting points for cracks.

Aging

Low temperature degradation on aging process is also responsible for a number of severe fractures of artificial hips made of zirconia. Other factors that influence chipping are:
- The design of the framework
- Ratio of the framework thickness to the veneering porcelain thickness

Consideration should be given to conservative repair of veneers if the remaining tooth and restoration are sound. The material most commonly used for repairs is light-cured composite.

Re-contouring and polishing can often correct small chipped areas on veneers; whereas if a sizeable area is broken, it should be replaced.

The direct composite veneers, should be repaired with the same material that was used originally. After cleaning the area and selecting the shade, the damaged surface is roughened with a coarse, round-end diamond instrument to form a chamfered margin at the edges.

Roughening with micro-etching is also effective. Mechanical locks may be placed in the remaining composite restoration for additional retention. The exposed area is etched. A bonding agent is applied to the etched area and polymerized. The defective area is restored with composites. Indirect composite veneers are repaired in a similar manner.

The defective/chipped porcelain cannot be repaired with porcelain; however, the defect can be repaired with composite or glass-ionomer cement depending upon the area of defect. Clinical cases showing repair of chipped porcelain are shown in Figs 13.13a–f and 13.14a–c.

To repair porcelain veneers, mild hydrofluoric acid is used to etch the defective porcelain. Hydrofluoric acid gels are available in approximately 10% buffered concentrations that are intended for intraoral porcelain repairs. Sand blasting and micro-abrasion has also been used to create micro-mechanical retention areas (intraoral sand blasting kits are available). Full strength hydrofluoric acid should never be used intraorally for etching porcelain. The porcelain veneer to be repaired should be isolated with a rubber dam to protect the gingival tissues from the irritating effects of hydrofluoric acid. The roughened

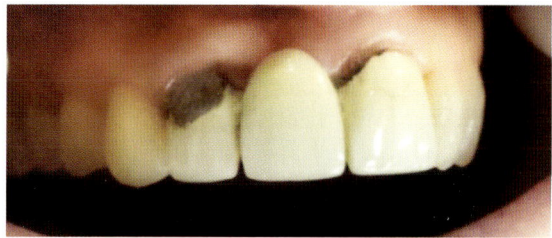

Fig. 13.13a: Preoperative (showing chipped off porcelain at the cervical area)

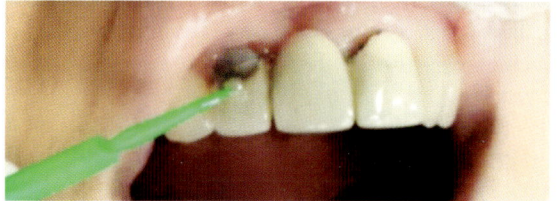

Fig. 13.13b: Acid etching

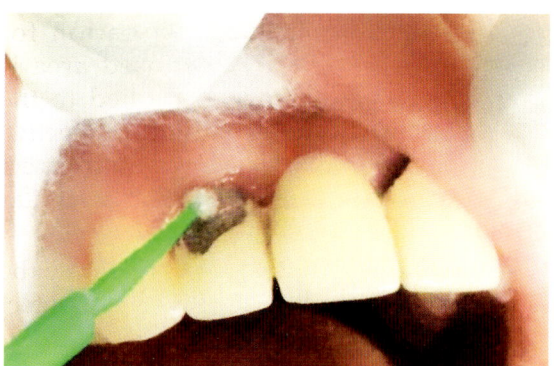

Fig. 13.13c: Application of primer

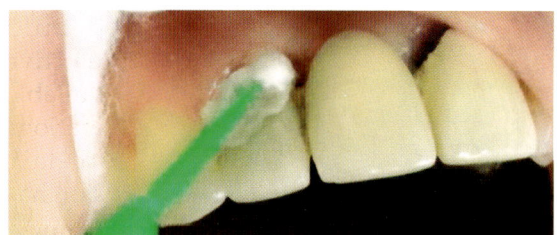

Fig. 13.13d: Application of composite

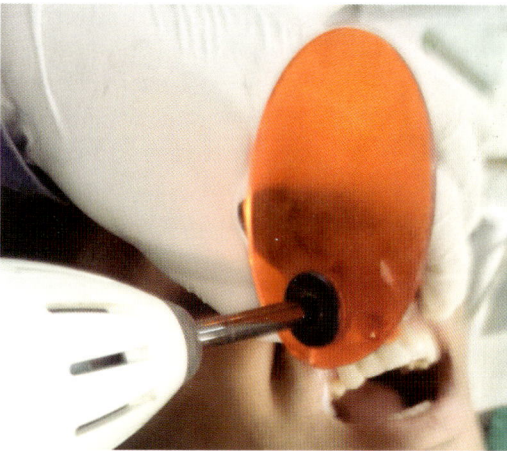

Fig. 13.13e: Light curing

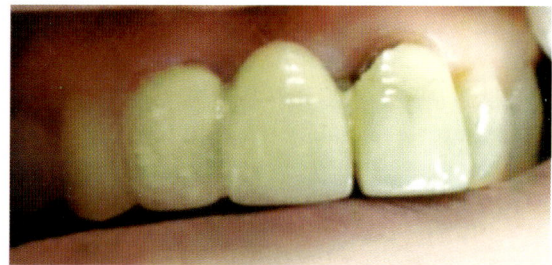

Fig. 13.13f: Postoperative

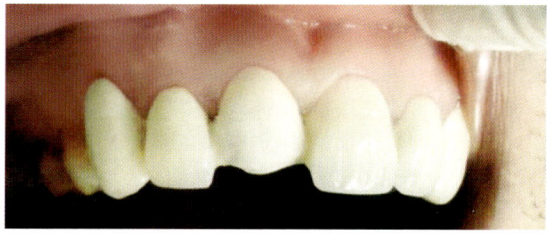

Fig. 13.14a: Preoperative (showing fractured crown on incisal edge)

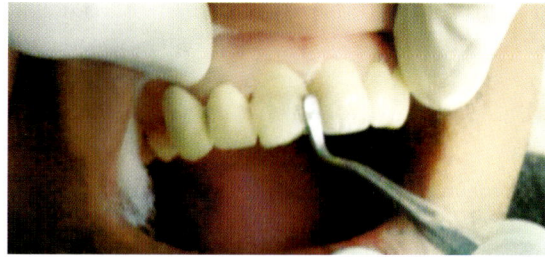

Fig. 13.14b: Application of composite

surface can be primed with appropriate adhesive and the matching shade of the composite is placed and cured. The area, so filled, is finished and polished in routine.

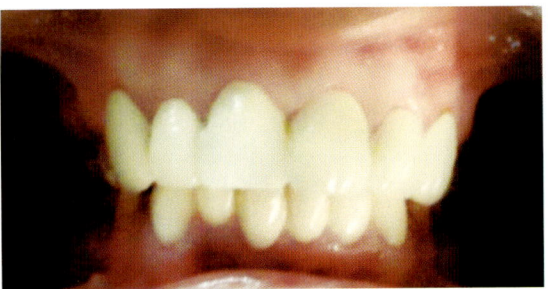

Fig. 13.14c: Postoperative

Bibliography

1. Al-Omiri MK, Mahmoud AA, Rayyan MR and Abu-Hammad O. Fracture resistance of teeth restored with post-retained restorations: an overview. J. Endod.: 2010;36:1439–49.

2. Aquilino SA and Caplan DJ. Relationship between crown placement and the survival of endodontically treated teeth. J. Prosthet. Dent.: 2002;87:256–63.

3. Beier US, Kapferer I and Dumfahrt H. Clinical long-term evaluation and failure characteristics of I,335 all-ceramic restorations. Int. J. Prosthodont.: 2012;25:70–8.

4. Blatz MB. Long term clinical success of all ceramic posterior restorations. Quint. Int.: 2002;33:415–26.

5. Brochu JF and Mowafy O El. Longevity and clinical performance of IPS—Empress ceramic restorations: A literature review. J. Can. Dent. Assoc.: 2002;68:233–7.

6. Bru E, Forner L, Llena C and Almenar A. Fibre post behavior prediction factors: A review of literature. J Clin. Exp. Dent.: 2013;5:e150–3.

7. Chaudhuri AR and Shah K. Avoiding and managing the failure of conventional crowns and bridges. Dent. Update: 2012;39:78–84.

8. Cheung GS. A preliminary investigation into the longevity and causes of failure of single unit extracoronal restorations. J. Dent.: 1991;19:160–3.

9. Chrepa V, Konstantinidis I, Kotsakis GA and Mitsias ME. The survival of indirect composite resin onlays for the restoration of root filled teeth: a retrospective medium-term study. Int. Endod. J.: 2014;47:967–73.

10. Conigleo I, Magni E, Cantoro A, Goracci C and Ferrari M. Push-out bond strength of circular and oval-shaped fiber posts. Clin. Oral Invest.: 2011; 15:667–72.

11. Cubas GB, Habekost L, Camacho GB and Pereira-Cenci T. Fracture resistance of premolars restored with inlay and onlay ceramic restorations and luted with two different agents. J. Prosthodont. Res.: 2011;55:53–9.

12. Etemadi S and Smales R. Survival of resin-bonded porcelain veneer crowns placed with and without metal reinforcement. J.Dent.: 2006;34:139–45.

13. Frankenberger R, Petscheldt A and Kramer N. Leucite reinforced glass ceramic inlays and onlays after six years: clinical behaviour. Oper. Dent.: 2000;25:459–65.

14. Frankenberger R, Taschner M, Garcia-Godoy F, Petschelt A and Kramer N. Leucite-reinforced glass ceramic inlays and onlays after 12 years. J. Adhes. Dent.: 2008;10:393–8.

15. Friedel W and Kern M. Fracture strength of teeth restored with all-ceramic posts and cores. Quint. Int.: 2006;37:289–95.

16. FronChabious H, Smail Faugeron V and Attal JP. Clinical efficacy of composite versus ceramic inlays and onlays: a systematic review. Dent. Mater.: 2013;29:1209–18.

17. Gallasatos AA and Bergou D. Six-year clinical evaluation of ceramic inlays and onlays. Quint. Int.: 2008;34:407–12.

18. Goodacre CJ and Spolnik KJ. The prosthodontic management of endodontically treated teeth: a literature review. Part I. Success and failure data, treatment concepts. J. Prosthodont.: 1994;3:243–50.

19. Goodacre CJ, Bernal G, Rungcharassaeng K and Kay YN. Clinical complications in fixed prosthodontics. J. Prosh. Dent.: 2003;90:31–41.

20. Hamdy A. Effect of full coverage, endocrowns, inlays restorations on fracture resistance of endodontically treated molars. J. Dent. Oral Health: 2015;1:1–5.

21. Haselton DR, Diaz-Arnold AM and Hilli SL. Clinical assessment of high strength all ceramic crowns. JPD: 2000;83:396–401.

22. Hayashi M, Takahashi Y, Imazato S and Ebisu S. Fracture resistance of pulpless teeth restored with post-core and crowns. Dent. Mater.: 2006;22:477–85.

23. Jiang W, Bo H, Yongchun G and Long XN. Stress distribution in molars restored with inlays or onlays with or without endodontic treatment: a three-dimensional finite element analysis. J. Prosthet. Dent.: 2010;103:6–12.

24. Lange RT and Pfeiffer P. Clinical evaluation of ceramic inlays compared to composite restorations. Oper. Dent.: 2009;34:263–72.

25. Magne P and Belser UC. Porcelain versus composite inlays/onlays: effects of mechanical loads on stress distribution, adhesion, and crown flexure. Int. J. Periodontics Restorative Dent.: 2003;23:543–55.

26. Martin N and Jedynakiewicz NM. Clinical performance of Cerec ceramic inlays: a systemic review. Dent. Mater.: 1999;15:54–61.

27. Mehl A, Kunzelmann KH, Folwaczny M and Hickel Q. Stabilization effects of CAD/CAM ceramic restorations in extended MOD cavities. J. Adhes. Dent. Autumn: 2004;6:239–45.

28. Molin MK and Karlsson SL. A randomized 5 years evaluation of 3 ceramic inlay system. Int. J. Prosthodont.: 2000;13:194–200.

29. Morimoto S, Vieira GF, Agra CM, Sesma N and Gil C. Fracture strength of teeth restored with ceramic inlays and overlays. Braz. Dent. J.: 2009; 20:143–8.

30. Naumann M, Blankenstein F, Keissling S and Dietrich T. Risk factors for a failure of glass fiber reinforced composite post restorations: a prospective observational clinical study. Eur. J. Oral Sci.: 2005;113:519–24.

31. Nikolopoulou F and Loukidis M. Critical review and evaluation of composite/ceramic onlays versus crowns. Dentistry: 2014;4, s261.

32. Nissan J, Parson A, Barnea E, Shifman A and Assif D. Resistance to fracture of crowned endodontically treated premolars restored with ceramic and metal post systems. Quint. Int.: 2007; 38:120–3.

33. Oden A, Andersson M, Krystekm-Ondracek I and Magnusson D. Five year clinical evaluation of Procera All Ceramic Crowns. J.Prost.Dent.: 1998; 80:450–6.

34. Ona M., Watanabe C., Igarashi Y and Wakabyashi N: Influence of preparation design on failure risks of ceramic inlays: A finite element analysis. J Adhes Dent 2011;13:367–73.

35. Otto T and De Nisco S. Computer aided direct ceramic restorations: a 10-years prospective clinical study of Cerec CAD/CAM inlays and onlays. Int. J. Prosthodont.: 2002;15:122–8.

36. Patras M., Naka O., Doukadakis S and Pissiotis A: Management of provisional restorations' deficiencies: A literature review. J Esthet Restor Dent 2012;24:26–9.

37. Reitemeier B, Hansel K, Kastner C and Walter MH. Metal ceramic failure in noble metal crowns: 7-year results of a prospective clinical trial in private practices. Int. J. Prosthodont: 2006;19: 397–9.

38. Sahafi A, Peutzfeldt A, Asmussen E and Gotfredsen K. Retention and failure morphology of prefabricated posts. Int. J. Prosthodont.: 2004; 17:307–12.

39. Sailer I, Pietursson BE, Zwahlen M and Hammerle CHF. A systematic review of the survival and complication rates of all-ceramic and metal-ceramic reconstructions after an observed period of at least 3 years. Part II : fixed dental prostheses. Clin. Oral Impl. Res.: 2007;18:86–96.

40. Schmitter M, Rammelsberg P, Gabbert O and Ohlmenn B. Influence of clinical baseline findings on survival of 2 post systems: a randomized clinical trial. Int. J. Prosthodont.: 2007;20:173–8.

41. Schulte AG, Vockler A and Reinhardt R. Longevity of ceramic inlays and onlays luted with a solely light-curing composite resin. J.Dent.: 2005;33, 433–42.

42. Scotti R, Catapano S and D'Elia A. A clinical evaluation of in-ceram crowns. Int. J. Prosthodont. 1995;8:320–3.

43. Silva RHBT, Ribeiro APD, Catirze ABCE, Pinelli LAP and Fais LMG. Clinical performance of indirect esthetic inlays and onlays for posterior teeth after 40 months. Braz J Oral Sci.: 2009;8:154–8.

44. Smales RJ and Etemadis S. Survival of ceramic onlays placed with and without metal reinforcement. J. Prosth. Dent.: 2004;91:548–53.

45. Strub JR, Stiffler S and Scharer P. Causes of failure following oral rehabilitation : Biological versus technical factors. Quint. Int.: 1988;19:215–22.

46. Suzuki S, Nagi E, Taira Y and Minesaki Y. In vitro wear of indirect composite restoratives. J. Prosthet. Dent.: 2002;88:431–6.

47. Tagtekin DA, Ozyoney G and Yanikoglu F. Two-year clinical evaluation of IPS Empress II ceramic onlays/inlays. Oper. Dent.: 2009;34:379.

48. Turner CH. Post retained crown failure: a survey. Dent. Update: 1982;9:221, 224–6, 228–9.

49. Vira DE. Failure of endodontically treated teeth: Classification and evaluation. J. Endod.: 1991;17: 338–42.

50. Wilson NA, Whitehead SA, Mjor IA and Wilson NHF. Reasons for the placement and replacement of crowns in general dental practice. Primary Dent. Care: 2003;10:53–9.

51. Yang A and Lamichanne A: Remaining coronal dentin and risk of fibre-reinforced composite post-core restoration failure: A meta analysis. Int J Prosthodont. 2015;28:258–64.

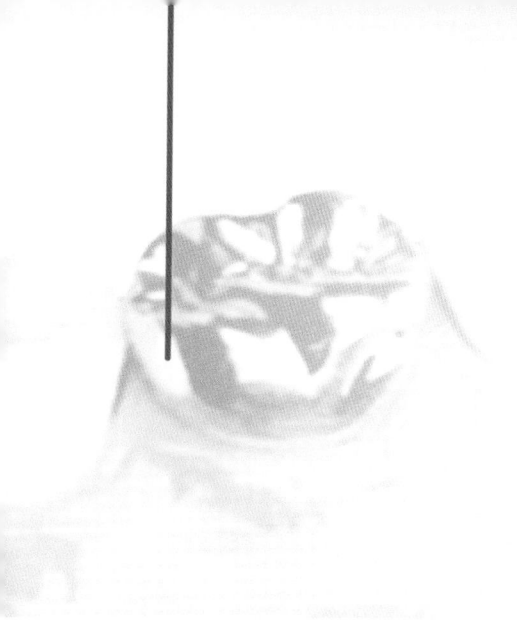

Glossary

A

Abrasion: The wearing away of teeth by mechanical means.

Abrasive: A substance used for abrading, smoothing or polishing.

Abutment: That part of a structure that directly receives thrust or pressure, an anchorage or a tooth implant that serves to support and retain prosthesis.

Acquired eccentric relation: The relationship of mandible relative to maxilla (whether conditioned or habitual), which will bring teeth in contact.

Adhesion: The property of remaining in close proximity, as that resulting from the physical attraction of molecules to a substance or molecular attraction existing between the surface of bodies in contact.

Adhesive failure: Failure at the interface between the adhesive and the adhered, or the material to be bonded.

Adhesive: Any substance that creates close adherence to or on adjoining surfaces.

Agar: It is used as a gelation agent in dental impression materials.

Ala-tragus line: An imaginary line running from inferior border of the tragus of ear to the ala of the nose (usually considered to be parallel to occlusal plane).

Alloy: A mixture of two or more metals that are mutually soluble in molten state; distinguished as binary, ternary, or quaternary, etc. depending on number of metals within the mixture.

Alloying element: Metallic/non-metallic elements added to pure metal for achieving required properties in that metal.

Aluminium oxide: A constituent of dental porcelain that increases hardness and viscosity or a high strength ceramic crystal dispersed throughout a glossy phase to increase its strength as in aluminous dental porcelain.

Aluminous porcelain: A ceramic material composed of glass matrix phase with 35% or more of aluminium oxide, by volume.

Anatomic crown: The portion of natural tooth that extends coronal from cemento-enamel junction.

Anatomic landmarks: A recognizable anatomical structure used as a point of reference.

Anatomic occlusion: An occlusal arrangement wherein posterior artificial teeth have masticatory surfaces that closely resemble those of natural healthy dentition and articulate with similar natural or artificial surfaces.

Anatomic teeth: Artificial teeth that duplicate the anatomic forms of natural teeth.

Angle's classification: The classification is based on the relationship between mesiobuccal cusp of the maxillary first permanent molar and buccal groove of the mandibular first permanent molar.

Class I: The mesiobuccal cusp of the maxillary first molar occluding in line with the buccal groove of the mandibular first molar, i.e. the maxillary first molar is slightly posteriorly positioned relative to the mandibular first molar.

Class II: The mesiobuccal cusp of the maxillary first molar occluding anterior to the buccal groove of the mandibular first molar, i.e. the maxillary first molar is incline with or anteriorly positioned relative to the mandibular first molar.

Class II is further divided in to Div.1 and Div. 2.

Class II Division 1: Class II molars with normally inclined or proclined maxillary central incisors.

Class II Division 2: Class II molars with retroclined maxillary central incisors.

Class III: The mesiobuccal cusp of the maxillary first molar occluding posterior to the buccal groove of the mandibular first molar, i.e. the maxillary first molar is severely posteriorly positioned relative to the mandibular first molar.

Anneal: To heat a material such as metal/glass followed by controlled cooling to remove internal stresses and create desired degree of toughness, temper or softness of a material and/or to homogenize the amalgam alloy by heating.

Antagonist: A tooth in one jaw, which articulates with tooth in other jaw.

Ante's Law: The law states that the combined pericemental surface area of all abutment teeth supporting a fixed dental prosthesis should be equal to or greater in pericemental surface area to the tooth or teeth to be replaced.

Anterior guidance: The influence of the contacting surfaces of anterior teeth on tooth limiting mandibular movements.

Anterior tooth form: The outline as viewed in any selected plane and related contours of an anterior tooth.

Anterior: In the front or in the frontal portion.

Antero-posterior curve (Curve of Spee): The anatomic curve established by the occlusal alignment of teeth as projected onto median plane, beginning with the cusp tip of mandibular canine and following buccal cusp tips of premolar and molar teeth, continuing through the anterior borders of mandibular ramus, ending with anteriormost portion of mandibular condyle.

Antiflux: The chemicals, which limit the flow of metals.

Anxiety: A response to an anticipated experience that the person perceives as threatening.

Arcon articulator: Articulator, which follows arcon design.

Arcon: Synonym for *articulator* and *condyle*, used to describe the articulator containing condylar path elements within its upper member and condylar elements within lower elements.

Articulating paper: Ink coated paper strips used to locate and mark occlusal points; available in different thickness and colors.

Articulation: The static and dynamic contact relationship between occlusal surfaces of the teeth during function.

Artificial crown: An ornamental covering of metal, plastic or ceramic that covers three or more axial surfaces and occlusal/incisal edge of tooth.

Attrition: The wearing of occlusal or incisal surfaces of teeth as a result of functional or parafunctional occlusal contacts.

Auto-polymerizing resin: A resin whose polymerization is initiated by a chemical activator.

Axial contour: The shape of a body that is in its long axis.

Axial inclination: The relationship of long axis of the body to a designated plane.

Axial wall: Any wall parallel to the long axis of tooth and facing the pulp.

Axis of preparation: The planned path of placement and removal of dental restoration.

Axis: A line around which body may rotate or about which a structure should turn if it could revolve.

B

Back pressure porosity: Porosity produced due to the inability of gases to escape from the mold during the casting procedure.

Backing: A metal support that attaches a facing (composite, ceramic) to the prosthesis.

Balanced articulation: A bilateral, simultaneous, anterior and posterior occlusal contact of teeth in centric and eccentric positions on an articulator.

Balanced occlusion: It is bilateral, simultaneous, uniform anterior as well as posterior contacts of maxillary and mandibular teeth during centric and eccentric movements in the oral cavity.

Balancing occlusal surfaces: The occlusal surfaces of teeth on the balancing side (antero-posteriorly or laterally) that are developed for purpose of stabilizing occlusion.

Base metal: Any metallic element reactive to air/oxygen.

Base: Any material placed under the restoration, which acts as a substitute for lost dentin. It controls the thickness of the restoration and acts as thermal and chemical barrier to the pulp.

Beilby layer: The molecular disorganized outer surface layer of polished metals.

Bevel: Any abrupt incline between the two surfaces of prepared tooth or between the cavity wall and the cavosurface margins in the prepared cavity.

Bi-maxillary protrusion: A simultaneous dental/skeletal protrusion of both maxillary/mandibular jaws/teeth.

Biocompatibility: Ability of a material to elicit an appropriate biological response in living tissues.

Biologic width: The combined width of connective tissue and junctional epithelium.

Block out: Elimination of undesirable undercuts on a cast.

Body porcelain: A porcelain material used for the bulk of a ceramic restoration.

Bonding Agent: A material used to promote adhesion between two different substances; or between a material and the natural tooth.

Bonding: Joining together with an adhesive substance.

Bonwill triangle: A four inch equilateral triangle bounded by lines connecting the contact points of the mandibular central incisors, incisal edge (or the midline of mandibular residual ridge) to each condyle (usually its mid-point) and from one condyle to the other.

Brittle: Easily broken or shattered; fragile or crisp.

Bruxism: The parafunctional grinding of teeth. A habit consisting of involuntary rhythmic or spasmodic non-functional gnashing, grinding or clenching of teeth other than in chewing movements of mandible, which may lead to occlusal trauma or a condition in which patients grinds his/her teeth.

Bruxomania: Grinding of teeth, occurring as neurotic habit during waking state.

Burnish: To create shine or luster by rubbing; to facilitate marginal adaptation of restoration by rubbing the margin with an instrument.

Burnishability: The ease with which a material can be burnished.

Burnout: See wax elimination.

Butt joint: To bring any two flat-ended surfaces into close contact without overlapping.

C

CAD-CAM: Computer Aided Designing-Computer Aided Manufacturing

Calcium hydroxide: An odourless white powder, soluble in water and insoluble in alcohol. Aqueous and non-aqueous suspension of calcium hydroxide is often used as cavity liners to protect the pulp.

Camper's line/plane: A plane formed by inferior border of right or left ala of the nose and the superior border of tragus of both ears—ala-tragus line.

Canine eminence: A labial prominence on the maxillary alveolar process corresponding to the position of root of maxillary canine.

Canine protected articulation: The form of mutually protected articulation in which vertical and/or horizontal overlap of canine teeth disengage the posterior teeth in the excursive movements of the mandible.

Cantilever: Prosthesis supported only at one end.

Cast post and core: A one-piece casting that comprises a post within the root canal and a core replacing missing coronal structure to form the tooth preparation.

Cast: To produce a shape by thrusting a molten liquid or plastic material into a mold possessing the desired shape. In dentistry it is formed by pouring gypsum into the impression.

Castable ceramic: A glass-ceramic material which can be cast using lost wax process.

Castable: Any refractory material that has a bonding agent added and can be mixed with water or other liquid agents and poured in a mould to set.

Casting ring: The metal tube or ring that provides refractory material into which metal is cast.

Casting wax: A combination of various waxes with desired properties for making wax patterns to be formed in metal castings.

Casting: An object formed by the solidification of liquid or molten metal that has been poured or injected into a mold.

Catalyst: A substance that accelerates a chemical reaction without affecting the properties of the materials involved.

Cement: Binding element or agents used to make objects adhere to each other or substance that hardens to act as base or filling material.

Cementation: The process of attaching indirect restoration to natural teeth by means of cement.

Cemento-dentinal junction: The area of union of dentin and cementum.

Cemento-enamel junction: The area of union of cementum and enamel.

Cementoid: The uncalcified layers of cementum including incorporated connective tissue fibers.

Cementum: A thin calcified tissue of mesodermal origin that covers the root of teeth.

Centric jaw relation: The maxillo-mandibular relationship in which condyles articulate with the thinnest avascular portion of their respective disks with complex in antero-superior position against shapes of the articular eminences.

Centric stop: Opposing cuspal/fossae contacts that maintain the occlusal vertical dimension between opposing arches.

Centric: Located in or at a center.

Ceramic crown: A ceramic restoration that restores a clinical crown without supporting metal substructure.

Ceramic flux: A glass modifier; metallic ions such as calcium, potassium or sodium; usually as carbonates, which interrupt the oxygen/silica bond, thus enhancing fluidity.

Ceramic: Any non-metallic mineral, which can withstand high heat.

Cervical: In dentistry, pertaining to the region at or near the cement-enamel junction.

Chamfer angle: The angle between a chamfered surface and one of the original surfaces from which the chamfer is cut.

Chamfer: A finish line design usually for lingual part of tooth preparation having obtuse angle and width less than 0.5 mm.

Chroma: Relative saturation of color.

CIE LAB System: It relates the tristimulus values to a color space. This space accounts for the illuminant and the observer. By establishing a uniform color scale, color measurements can be compared and movements in color space defined.

CIE: Acronym for Commission International d'Eclairage.

Clinical crown: That portion of tooth that extends from the occlusal table or incisal edge up to the free gingival margin.

Cohesion: Force of attraction between two or more particles of similar nature.

Cohesive failure: Bond failure within dental material due to a tensile or shearing force (a failure in the bulk layer of the adhesive).

Collarless metal ceramic restoration: A metal ceramic restoration whose cervical metal collar has been eliminated.

Color blindness: Abnormal color vision or the inability to discriminate certain colors, most commonly along the red–green axis.

Color constancy: The perceived color of object remains relatively constant under varying illumination conditions.

Color deficiency: A general term for all forms of color vision that yield chromaticity discrimination below normal limits such as monochromatism, dichromatism and anomalous trichromatism.

Color difference: Magnitude and character of the difference between two colors under specified conditions; referred to as delta E.

Color scale: An orderly arrangement of colors showing graduated change in some attribute or attributes of color as a value scale.

Color: The quantity of an object or substance with respect to light reflected or transmitted by it. Color is usually determined visually by measurement of hue, saturation and luminous reflectance of the reflected light.

Complementary colors: Two colors that, when mixed together in proper proportions, result in a neutral color.

Complete crown: A restoration that covers all the axial and occlusal tooth surfaces.

Components of occlusion: The various elements that are involved in occlusion, such as temporomandibular joints, the associated musculature, the teeth and the associated supporting structures.

Condylar guidance: Mandibular guidance generated by the condyle and articular disc traversing the contour of the glenoid fossae.

Connector: The portion of fixed partial denture, which unites the retainer and pontic. It can be rigid or non-rigid type.

Contra Bevel: An external bevel arising from the occlusal surface or edge of a preparation and placed at an angle that opposes or contrasts the angle of surface it arises from.

Coping impression: An impression, usually encompassing an entire dental arch, that uses metal or resin copings placed on prepared teeth. The copings are repositioned before pouring of working cast.

Coping: A thin covering.

Copper band: A copper cylinder employed as a matrix for making an impression.

Core: A restoration that serves as a substitute for tooth structure providing resistance and retention form to the final restoration (portion outside the root in the coronal portion)

Coronoplasty: An alteration or change in morphology of the coronal portion of natural teeth by use of abrasive instruments.

Corrosion: The action, process or effect of corroding; a product of corroding; the loss of elemental constituents to the adjacent environment.

Counter-die: The reverse image of a die; usually made of a softer and lower fusing metal than the die.

Covalent bond: A chemical bond between two atoms or radicals formed by sharing of a pair, two pairs, or three pairs of electrons.

Craze: Production of minute cracks on any surface.

Creep: The slow change in dimensions of an object due to prolonged exposure to high temperature or stress.

Crossbite: An occlusal relationship in which the maxillary facial surfaces of one or several teeth are positioned lingual to the facial surface of the opposing mandibular tooth.

Crown fracture: Micro or macroscopic cleavage in coronal portion of a tooth.

Crown slitter: A mechanical device used to slit the axial surface of an artificial crown to facilitate its removal.

Crown: An artificial replacement that restores missing tooth structure by surrounding part or all of the remaining structure with a material such as cast metal, porcelain, or a combination of materials such as metal and porcelain.

Crown–root ratio: The physical relationship (radiographically) between the portion of tooth within the alveolar bone compared with the portion not within the alveolar bone.

Crucible former: The base to which a sprue former is attached while the wax pattern is being invested in refractory investment.

Crucible: A vessel or container made of any refractory material (as porcelain) used for melting or calcining any substance that requires high degree of heat.

Curve of Monson: For proposed ideal curve of occlusion in which each cusp and incisal edge touches or conforms to a segment of the surface of a sphere of 8 inches in diameter with its center in region of glabella.

Curve of occlusion: The average curve established by the incisal edges and occlusal surfaces of anterior and posterior teeth in either arch.

Curve of Spee: The anatomic curve established by the occlusal alignment of the teeth, as projected onto the median plane, beginning with cusp tip of the mandibular canine and following the buccal cusp tips of the premolar and molar teeth, continuing through the anterior border of the mandibular ramus, ending with the anteriormost portion of the mandibular condyle.

Curve of Wilson: The curvature of the cusps as projected on the frontal plane; the curve in the lower arch being concave and the one in the upper arch being convex.

Cusp angle: The angle made by average slope of a cusp with the cusp plane measured mesiodistally or buccolingually.

D

Davis crown: A dental restoration supported by a dowel in the root canal over which a porcelain tooth is given in direct contact with root face of the tooth.

Decision pathways: Protocols which identify the range of treatment options, indicating key points leading to appropriate treatment decision.

Decision trees: Protocols specifying treatment options—include research based success rates for each of these options.

Defective color vision: The condition in which color discrimination is significantly reduced.

Definitive diagnosis: A pattern of findings that point clearly to a specific disease entity or problem.

Dental implant: A prosthesis device made of alloplastic material implanted into the oral tissues beneath the mucosal or periosteal layer, and on/or within bone to provide retention and support from a fixed or removable dental prosthesis.

Dental impression wax: Any thermoplastic wax used to make impressions of oral and dental tissues.

Dental impression: A negative replica of oral and dental tissues used to produce a positive replica or cast.

Dental plaster: The β-form of calcium sulfate hemihydrate. It is a fibrous aggregate of fine crystals with capillary pores that are irregular in shape and porous in character.

Dental prosthesis: An artificial replacement of one or more teeth and associated alveolar structures.

Dental stone: The α-form of calcium sulfate hemihydrate with physical properties superior to β-form.

Devest: The retrieval of casting or prosthesis from an investing material.

Devitrification: To eliminate vitreous characteristics (recrystallization).

Dew point: Temperature at which moisture in air begins to condense.

Diagnosis: Utilization of scientific knowledge in identifying a disease process and to differentiate the same from other disease processes.

Diagnostic cast: Reproduction of a part or parts of the oral cavity and/or facial structures for the purpose of study and treatment planning.

Diastema: A space between two adjacent teeth in the same dental arch.

Die spacer: An agent applied to a die to provide space for the luting agent in finished casting.

Die: The positive reproduction of the form of a prepared tooth in any suitable substance.

Differential diagnosis: The process of identifying a condition by comparing the signs and symptoms of all pathologic processes that may produce similar signs and symptoms.

Dilaceration: Sharply angular or deformed roots.

Dimensions of color: Terms used to describe the three-dimensional nature of color. In the Munsell color system, the dimensions are named Hue, Value and Chroma.

Direct lift technique: A means of fabricating porcelain labial margins whereby porcelain is condensed directly onto the die.

Dis-occlusion: Separation of opposing teeth during eccentric movements of the mandible.

Divergence angle: The sum of angles of taper of opposing walls of a tooth preparation that diverge away from each other.

Dovetail: A widened portion of a prepared cavity (shape varies) used to increase retention and/or resistance.

Dowel pin: A metal pin used in stone casts to remove die sections and replace them accurately in original position.

Dowel: A post, may be of metal or any other material, that is fitted into the root canal of natural tooth.

Draw: The taper or convergence of walls of a preparation for a restoration.

Ductility: The ability of a material to withstand permanent deformation under a tensile load without rupture.

Dysplasia: Abnormal tissue development or pathological alteration in size, shape and organization of cells.

E

Eccentric jaw relation: Any relationship between jaws other than the centric relation.

Edge to edge articulation: Articulation in which the opposing anterior teeth meet along their incisal edges, when the teeth are in maximum intercuspation.

Elastic modulus: The stiffness or flexibility of a material within the elastic range.

Elasticity: The quality that allows a structure or material to return to its original form on removal of an external force.

Elastomer: A natural or synthetic polymer having elastic preparations [a polymer with viscoelasticity (both viscosity and elasticity) and weak intermolecular forces].

Elastomeric impression material: A group of polymers, which are either chemically or physically cross-linked.

Embedment: The relation of using ceramic powder mixed with water to surround glass ceramic casting.

Erosion: Chemical dissolution of the tooth structure (enamel/dentin).

Esthetic: Pertaining to the study of beauty and the sense of beautiful.

Etch: To produce a retentive surface, especially on glass or metal, by corrosive action of an acid.

Exostosis: Bony overgrowths, usually non-malignant.

External resorption: Resorption of external root surface initiated primarily in periodontium.

Extracoronal retainer: That part of fixed partial denture uniting the abutment to the other elements of fixed partial denture that surrounds all or part of prepared crown.

Extracoronal: Outside or external to the crown.

Extrinsic coloring: Applying color to the external surface of a prosthesis.

F

Facial form: The outline form of the face from an anterior view.

Facial profile: The outline form of the face from a lateral view.

Facial: The surface of a tooth or other oral structure approximating the face.

Feldspathic porcelain: Porcelain fabricated from feldspar (natural mineral group).

Ferrule: A metal band over the coronal aspect of the remaining crown to enhance the resistance form.

Film thickness: A property of luting cements, this dimension is measured after pressure is applied between two flat surfaces.

Final impression: The impression that represents the completion of the registration of the surface or object.

Finish line: The peripheral extension of a tooth preparation or the terminal portion of the prepared tooth.

Fissure: Any superficial or deep groove, normally present or otherwise; a ditch in the outer surface of a tooth, usually due to imperfect fusion of adjoining enamel lobes.

Fixed partial denture: The partial denture that is luted or otherwise securely retained to the natural teeth, roots and/or dental implant abutments.

Fluorescence: A process by which a material absorbs radiant energy and emits it in the form of energy in a different wavelength band, all or most of whose wavelengths exceed that of the absorbed energy.

Fluorescent: Having or relating to fluorescence.

Flux: These are the agents, which improve the flow of metal during soldering.

Force: Any pressure or influence that, when exerted on a body, tends to set the body into motion or to alter its present state of motion.

Forces of mastication: The motive force created by the dynamic action of the muscles during the physiological act of mastication.

Fracture strength: Strength at fracture based on the original dimensions of the specimen.

Free gingiva: The part of the gingiva that surrounds the tooth and is not directly attached to the tooth surface.

Free gingival groove: The line demarcating the junction between free and attached gingival tissue.

Free gingival margin: The unattached gingiva surrounding the teeth in a collar-like fashion and demarcated from the attached gingiva by a shallow linear depression termed the free gingival groove.

Frit: The calcined or partly fused matter of which glass is made.

Frontal plane: Imaginary plane parallel with the long axis of the body and at right angle to the median plane, dividing the body into front and back parts.

Fulcrum line: A theoretical line passing through the point around which a lever functions and at right angles to its path of movement.

Functional malocclusion: Abnormal relations of teeth in dentition may prevent stable closure of mandible in occlusion or interfere with eccentric gliding movements, thereby creating disharmony in teeth and joint.

Functional/physiological occlusion: Occlusion which can function efficiently without pain and remains in state of health regardless of maxillary and mandibular teeth relations.

G

Galvanism: Accelerated corrosion of a metal due to electrical contact with a more noble metal in a corrosive electrolyte.

Gelation: The transformation from a hydrocolloid solution to a gel.

Gingival retraction: The process of retracting the soft tissue or gingiva to provide the maximum exposure of the operating site.

It can be achieved by either mechanical means (copper band, retraction cord, rubber dam) or chemical (racemic chloride, aluminium chloride, alum, aluminium sulfate) or surgical (rotary curettage, electrosurgical retraction)

Glass ceramic: A solid material, partly crystalline and partly glassy, formed by controlled crystallization of a glass.

Glass ionomer: A cement, luting or restorative agent, composed of glasses, polyacrylic acid and water.

Glaze: The attainment of smooth and reflective surface or to cover with smooth coatings.

Groove: A long narrow channel or depression, such as the indentation between tooth cusps or the retentive features placed on tooth surfaces to augment the retentive characteristics of crown preparations.

Group function occlusion: Group function occlusion implies simultaneous gliding contact of teeth on lateral and protrusive side during lateral and protrusive movement.

Guidance: Providing regulation or direction to movement.

H

High fusing ceramic: A ceramic with a maturation or fusion range of 1290° to 1370°C.

High fusing solder: Any soldering alloy formulated to melt at approximately 1100°C used to form connectors before ceramic application.

Horizontal plane: Any plane passing through the body at right angles to both the median and frontal planes, thus dividing the body into upper and lower parts.

Hue: The dominant color of an agent, e.g. red, green or blue.

Hydrocolloid: A colloid system in which water is the dispersion medium; those materials described as a colloid sol with water that are used in dentistry as esthetic impression material.

Hydrophilic: Tendency of strong affinity for water.

Hydrophobic: Lack of affinity to water.

Hydroxyapatite ceramic: A composition of calcium and phosphate in physiologic ratios to provide a dense, non-resorbable, biocompatible ceramic used for dental implants and residual ridge augmentation.

Hygienic pontic: A pontic that is easier to clean because it has a domed or bullet-shaped cervical form and does not overlap edentulous ridge.

Hygroscopic expansion: Expansion due to the absorption of moisture.

Hypercementosis: An excessive deposition of cementum.

Hyperplasia: The abnormal multiplication or increase in the number of normal cells in normal arrangement in a tissue.

Hypertrophy: An enlargement or overgrowth of an organ or tissue beyond that considered normal as a result of an increase in the size of its constituent cells without tumor formation.

I

Iatrogenic complication: An adverse condition in a patient of unknown aetiology.

Illuminance: Density of luminous flux on a surface.

Imbibition: Process of water sorption.

Implant: To graft or insert a material such as an alloplastic substance, an encapsulated drug, or tissue into the body of a recipient.

Impression material: Any substance or combination of substances used for making an impression or negative reproduction of any object.

Impression technique: A method and manner used in making a negative replica.

Impression tray: A container into which suitable impression material is placed to make a negative replica.

Impression: The negative replica of any object; an imprint of teeth and adjacent structures for use in dentistry.

Incipient: Beginning, commencing.

Incisal guidance: The contact of maxillary and mandibular anterior teeth and their influence on mandibular movement.

Inclined plane: The inclined surfaces of a tooth from cusp tips.

Indirect restoration: A restoration that is fabricated outside the patient's oral cavity, preferably in laboratory.

Induction: Activation of free radicals, which in turn initiate growing polymer chains.

Infra-occlusion: The occluding surfaces of teeth are below the normal plane of occlusion.

Inlay: Anything laid inside the tooth. In dentistry, it is primarily an intracoronal restoration that is designed to restore occlusal and/or proximal surfaces of posterior teeth without covering the cusps.

Interarch distance: The vertical distance between the maxillary and mandibular arch with or without teeth.

Interdental papilla: A projection of the gingiva filling the space between the proximal surfaces of two adjacent teeth.

Interim prosthesis: A dental prosthesis, designed to enhance esthetics, stabilization and/or function for a limited period of time, after which it is to be replaced by a definitive prosthesis.

Intermediate abutment: A natural tooth located between terminal abutments that serve to support a fixed or removable prosthesis.

Interocclusal distance: The distance between the occluding surfaces of maxillary and mandibular teeth when the mandible is in a specified position.

Interrupted bridge: A fixed dental prosthesis with one or more non-rigid connectors.

Intraeruption: Failure to erupt in the established plane of occlusion.

Intrinsic coloring: Coloring from within; the incorporation of a colorant within the material of a prosthesis or restoration.

Intrusion: Movement of a tooth in an apical direction.

Investment: Refractory material used to form a mold cavity for cast metals or hot pressed ceramics.

J

Junctional epithelium: Layers of non-keratinizing cells adhering to the tooth surface at the base of the gingival crevice.

K

Key teeth: Important teeth that serve as abutments for fixed restoration. Loss of key tooth may adversely affect the treatment options.

Keyway: An interlock between the two units. Used in post and core and fixed partial dentures.

L

Labial: Towards the lip.

Laminates: The restorations, which restore only the facial surface of the tooth mostly fabricated with composite resins or ceramics and bonded to the etched surfaces.

Lengthening of the clinical crown: A surgical procedure designed to increase the extent of the clinical crown by apically positioning gingival margin.

Lesion: Abnormality in any tissue.

Light-cure impression material: Impression material contains methacrylate resin activated by light.

Lightness: Achromatic dimension necessary to describe the three-dimensional nature of color, the others being hue and saturation.

Line angle: The point of convergence of two planes in a cavity preparation.

Linear coefficient of thermal expansion: The fractional change in length of a given material per degree change in temperature.

Lingual: Towards the tongue.

Lingualized occlusion: This form of denture occlusion articulates the maxillary lingual cusps with the mandibular occlusal surfaces in centric working and non-working mandibular positions.

Liquidus temperature: Temperature at which an alloy begins to freeze on cooling or at which the metal is completely molten on heating.

Lost-wax casting technique: The casting of a metal into a mold produced by surrounding the wax pattern with a refractory slurry that sets at room temperature, after which the pattern is removed by the use of heat.

Luting agent: See cement/cementing agent.

M

Maintenance phase: The portion of a comprehensive treatment plan that is intended to promote the long-term oral health of the patient and manage any persistent and chronic oral problems.

Malocclusion: Any deviation from a physiologically acceptable occlusion.

Margin: The outer edge of crown, inlay, onlay or other restorations, or the boundary surface of tooth preparation.

Master impression: The negative likeness made for the purpose of fabricating a prosthesis.

Masticatory cycle: A three-dimensional representation of mandibular movement produced during the chewing of food.

Masticatory efficiency: The efficiency by which the masticatory cycle is completed.

Mesial drift: Movement of teeth towards the midline.

Mesial: Near or towards the centre line of dental arch; towards medial sagittal plane of the face following the curvature of dental arch.

Metal ceramic restoration: A fixed restoration that uses a metal sub-structure on which ceramic veneer is fused.

Metal: An element whose atomic structure readily loses electrons to form positively charged ions.

Metamerism: Pairs of objects that have different spectral curves but appear to match when viewed in a given hue exhibit metamerism.

Model: A positive full arch replica of teeth and soft tissues used as a diagnostic aid.

Modified ridge lap pontic: A ridge lap surface of pontic that is adapted to only facial or buccal aspect of pontic.

Modifier: A substance that changes the color or properties of a substance.

Monochromatic vision: Vision in which there is no color discrimination.

Mucositis: An inflammation of the mucous membrane.

N

Natural glaze: The production of glazed surface by the vitrification of material itself and without addition of other fluxes or glasses.

Noble metal: Those metal elements that resist oxidation, tarnish and corrosion during heating, casting or soldering.

O

Occlusal balance: A condition in which there are simultaneous contacts of opposing teeth or tooth analogues on both sides of opposing dental arches during eccentric movements within the functional range.

Occlusal force: The result of muscular force applied on opposing teeth; the force created by the dynamic action of the muscles during the physiologic act of mastication.

Occlusal form: The form of occlusal surface of a tooth or a row of teeth.

Occlusal pattern: The form or design of masticatory surfaces of tooth or teeth based on natural or modified anatomic or non-anatomic teeth.

Occlusal plane: The average plane established by the incisal and occlusal surfaces of teeth.

Occlusal position: The relationship of the mandible and maxilla when the jaw is closed and the teeth are in contact; this position may or may not coincide the centric occlusion.

Occlusal table: The occlusal surfaces of posterior teeth that lies within the perimeter of the cusp tips and marginal ridges (the functional portion of the occlusal surfaces of posterior teeth).

Occlusion: The act or process of closure or of being closed.

One-half crown: It restores one-half of the clinical crown. Such restorations are preferred in tilted molars or in mandibular second molar where third molar is erupting or abnormally erupted.

Onlay: It is a combination of intracoronal and extracoronal cast restoration when one or more cusps are covered; but not all the cusps of teeth or an indirect restoration that covers one or more cusps, but not all the cusps.

Opaque porcelain: The first porcelain layer applied in the metal-ceramic technique to the underlying metal framework to establish the bond between the porcelain and metal while simultaneously masking the dark color of the metallic oxide layer.

Opaque: Property of a material that can absorb all light and prevent transmission of light.

Operculum: Soft tissue flap covering the crown of an erupting tooth.

Over-glaze: The production of a glazed surface by the addition of a fluxed glass that usually vitrifies at a lower temperature.

Overhang: An overcontoured portion of a restoration on a proximal surface.

P

Partial veneer crown: A restoration that does not restore all the coronal and axial surfaces of the tooth (restores only portion of the clinical crown).

Path of insertion: The specific direction in which a prostheses is placed and removed on the abutment teeth.

Percussion: A diagnostic procedure, which involves tapping of a tooth and recording discomfort to the patient.

Phases: Segments of the treatment plan.

Phosphorescence: A form of photo-luminescence based on the properties of certain molecules to absorb energy, and emit it in the form of visible radiation at a higher wavelength.

Photoactive: Reacting chemically to visible light or ultraviolet radiation.

Physiologic occlusion: Occlusion in harmony with the functions of the masticatory system.

Pier: An intermediate abutment of fixed partial denture.

Pigment: Finely ground, natural or synthetic, inorganic or organic, insoluble dispersed particles, which, when dispersed in a liquid vehicle, may provide in addition to colour, many other essential properties such as opacity, hardness, durability and corrosion resistance.

Pinlay/pin ledge: A modified form of inlay/onlay where retention is gained through pins attached with the restoration.

Pin-retained cast metal core/crown: A casting wherein pins are integral part of core/crown.

Pleasure curve: A curve of occlusion which when viewed in the frontal plane, conforms to a curve that is convex from the superior view, except for the last molars, which reverse the pattern.

Plunger cusp: A cusp abnormally located, usually tends to force the food interproximally or abrade the opposing tooth surface.

Polish: To make smooth and glossy surface, usually by friction.

Polyether: An elastomeric impression material of ethylene oxide and tetrahydrofluoro copolymers that polymerizes under the influence of an aromatic ester.

Polymer: Chemical compound consisting of larger organic molecule formed by the union of smaller units, the monomer.

Polymerization: The forming of a compound by joining together of molecules of small molecular weights into a compound of large molecular weight.

Polysulfide: An elastomeric impression material that cross-links under the influence of oxidizing agents such as lead peroxide.

Polyvinyl siloxane: An elastomeric impression material of silicone polymers having terminal vinyl groups that cross-link with silanes on activation by salts of platinum/palladium which acts as catalyst.

Pontic: An artificial tooth on a fixed partial denture that replaces a missing natural tooth, restores its function; or the suspended member of a fixed partial denture.

Porcelain: A ceramic material formed of infusible elements. Dental porcelains are usually glasses and are used in the fabrication of teeth for dentures, pontics and facings, metal ceramic restorations, crowns, inlays, onlays and other restorations.

Postcore crown: A restoration in which the crown and cast post is in one unit.

Posttreatment assessment: A comprehensive evaluation of the patient's oral condition after the treatment. This is accomplished at the conclusion of definitive phase.

Precious metal alloy: An alloy predominantly composed of elements such as, gold, platinum, palladium, etc.

Precious metal: A metal containing primarily elements of the platinum, palladium and gold.

Precision attachment: A retainer consisting of metal receptacle and closely fitting unit.

Precision rest: A prefabricated, rigid metallic extension in fixed partial denture that fits immediately into a box or keyway portion of precision attachment of cast restoration.

Primary colors: Three basic colors used to make most other colors by mixture, either additive mixture of lights or substractive mixture of colorants.

Primary flare: The extension of proximal box walls into the embrasure areas. The proximal box walls are extended at an angle of 110–120° from the axial-proximal line angle, depending upon the contact areas. In case of wider contacts, the angle is increased so as to fall in embrasures.

Prognosis: An estimation of the probable outcome for a disease after treatment or the prediction of duration, course and termination of the disease process.

Proportional limit: That unit of stresses beyond which deformation is no longer proportional to the applied load.

Protrusion: Position of mandible forward from centric relation (condition of being forward or projecting).

Proximal groove: One of the extra-retentive feature; the groove given on proximal surface(s).

Pumice: A polishing agent to finish and polish restoration and teeth.

R

Radiolucent: Permitting the passage of radiant energy (X-rays) without any absorption (dark areas on radiographs).

Radiopaque: A structure that strongly inhibits the passage of radiant energy (X-rays); appear as white areas on radiographs.

Recurrent caries (secondary caries): Caries occurring at restoration-tooth interface or under an existing restoration.

Refractory cast: A cast made of material that will withstand high temperatures without disintegrating.

Refractory investment: An investment material that can withstand high temperatures (used in soldering or casting).

Refractory mold: A refractory cavity in which an object is shaped or cast.

Re-mineralization: Process of restoring mineral content in demineralized tooth structure.

Resilient: Characterized or noted by resilience as: (a) capable of withstanding shock without permanent deformation or rupture; (b) tending to recover from or easily adjust to change.

Resin bonded prosthesis: A prosthesis that is luted to tooth structures, primarily enamel, which has been etched to provide mechanical retention for the resin cement.

Resin crown: A resin restoration that restores a clinical crown without a metal substructure.

Resin-veneered restoration: A fixed restoration that uses a metal framework on which an esthetic resin veneer is applied.

Retention form: The feature of tooth preparation that resists dislodgement of a restoration in vertical direction or along the path of placement.

Reverse three quarter crown: Similar to three quarter crown except that the lingual surfaces are excluded (preferred in lower molars).

Rheology: Study of deformation and flow characteristics of matter.

Richmond crown: A dowel retained crown made for an endodontically treated tooth using a porcelain facing.

Ridge lap pontic: The pontic whose tissue surface is concave and envelops both buccal and lingual surfaces of the residual ridge.

Rochette bridge: A resin bonded prosthesis incorporating holes within the metal framework and lutes to the lingual aspect of teeth adjacent to edentulous space that replaces one or more teeth.

Rouge: A compound composed of ferric oxide used to impart high luster to a polished surface.

S

Saddle pontic: A pontic with a broad concave facio-lingual area of contact with the residual ridge.

Sagittal plane: Any vertical plane parallel to the median plane of the body that divides a body into right and left portions.

Sanitary pontic: Usually given in posterior region, having free space underneath; esthetically not pleasing.

Saturation: The attribute of color perception that expresses the degree of departure from gray of the same lightness. All grays have zero saturation.

Secondary flare: The secondary flare is like a cavosurface bevel given on the proximal walls in case of gold inlays.

Sectional impression: A negative replica that is made in sections.

Semi-precious metal alloy: An alloy composed of precious and base metals in different ratios.

Separating medium: A coating applied on the surface and serving to prevent adherence of one surface to other.

Seven-eighth crown: A modification of three-quarter crown whereby seven surfaces out of eight of the clinical crowns are restored. The mesio-buccal areas of the maxillary first molars are excluded for esthetic reasons.

Shade: A term used to describe a particular hue, or variation for a primary hue, such as a greenish shade of yellow.

Shell crown: An artificial crown that is adapted like a shell or cap over the remaining clinical crown of a tooth.

Shoulder: A finish line design for tooth preparation in which the gingival floor meets the external axial surfaces at approximately right angle. The width should be more than 0.5 mm.

Shrink spot porosity: An area of porosity in cast metal that is caused by shrinkage of a portion of the metal as it solidifies from the molten state without flow of additional molten metal from surrounding areas.

Signs: Findings discovered by clinician during examination.

Sinter: To become coherent mass by heating without melting.

SOAP note: The documentation of patient's visit. The components are (S) subjective findings, (O) objective findings, (A) assessment and (P) plan for treatment. Usually used for acute conditions.

Solder: A fusible metal alloy used to unite the edges or surfaces of two pieces of metal.

Soldering antiflux: A material such as oxide (rouge) when dissolved in a suitable solvent (turpentine) to confine the flow of molten solder on a metal surface.

Soldering flux: A material such as borax, glass ($Na_2B_4O_7$) applied to a metal surface to remove oxides or prevent their formation in order to facilitate the flow of solder.

Spatula: A flat bladed instrument used for mixing or spreading materials.

Speaking space: A space that occurs between the incisal and/or occlusal surfaces of maxillary and mandibular teeth during speech.

Split dowel crown: An artificial crown supported and retained by a dowel that was split longitudinally in an attempt to use spring retention in an undersized dowel space.

Sprue button: The material remaining in reservoir of the mold after dental casting.

Sprue former: A wax, plastic or metal pattern used to form the channel allowing molten metal to flow into a mold to make a casting.

Sprue: The channel or hole through which plastic or metal is poured or cast into the mold.

Stability: The quality of maintaining a constant position in the presence of forces that threaten to disturb it.

Stain: A soiled or discoloured spot; a spot of color in contrast to the surrounding area.

Strain: Change in length per unit length when stress is applied; the change in length/original length.

Stress: Force per unit area; a force exerted on one body that presses on, pulls on, pushes against, or tends to invest or compress another body, the deformation caused in a body by such a force; an internal force that resists on externally applied load or force.

Subgingival margin: The restoration margin or tooth preparation's finish line, that is located apical to the free gingival tissues.

Sublingual: Pertaining to the regions or structures located beneath the tongue.

Suck back porosity: A shrinkage void in a solidified casting opposite the location of the sprue attachment. The hot spot is created by lingering of molten metal after the casting has solidified.

Supporting cusps: Those cusps or incisal edges of teeth that contact and support centric occlusion. Usually, buccal cusps of mandibular posterior teeth and the palatal cusps of maxillary posterior teeth are designated as supporting cusps.

Suprabulge: That portion of tooth crown that converge towards the occlusal surfaces, i.e. above the height of contour.

Supraeruption: Movement of a tooth or teeth above the normal occlusal plane.

Surface tension: A property of liquid in which the exposed surface tends to contact the smallest possible area, as in the spherical formation of drops; this is a phenomenon attributed to the attractive forces or cohesion, between the molecules of liquid.

Surveyor: A paralleling instrument used in construction of prosthesis to locate and delineate the contours and relative positions of abutment teeth and associated structures.

Symptoms: Findings revealed by the patient. Usually the one causing problems.

Syneresis: Expression of fluid over the surface of gel structure.

T

Taper: The convergence of two opposing external walls of a tooth preparation as viewed in a given plane. The extension of those lines within that plane form an angle, described as angle of convergence.

Technique (direct): The temporary is altered, adapted and cemented over the prepared tooth surface in patient's oral cavity.

Technique (direct–indirect): The temporary crown is checked for fit and finish in patient's oral cavity. Later, the tissue surface of preformed crown is customized in laboratory.

Technique (indirect): The temporary crown is fabricated in the laboratory.

Telescopic crown: An artificial crown constructed to fit over the coping.

Temporization or provisional restoration: A temporary, protective and functional restoration which is fabricated over the prepared tooth to be used until fabrication of final prosthesis (also known as transitional or prototype restorations).

Thixotropic: Property of certain material to become liquefied (less viscous) when stirred or shaken.

Three-quarter crown: Crown covering occlusal and three out of four axial surfaces (excluding facial surfaces).

Tissue displacement: The change in the form or position of tissue as a result of mechanical or chemical means.

Tooth color selection: The determination of the color and other attributes of appearance of an artificial tooth or set of teeth for given individual.

Tooth preparation: Mechanical alteration of a tooth (defective, diseased, injured or normal) in such a way so as to receive a restorative material that will re-establish the healthy state for the tooth, including the functions of mastication, phonetics and esthetics as well.

Tooth selection: The selection of a tooth or teeth of a shape, size and color to harmonize with the individual characteristics of a patient.

Torque: A twisting or rotary force; the movement of system of forces producing rotation.

Toughness: The ability of a material to withstand stresses and strains without breaking.

Translucent: In between complete opaque and complete transparent.

Traumatic occlusion: The occlusion of teeth, which is capable of producing injury to oral structures.

Treatment objective: Certain goals that represent the intents or rationale for a treatment plant.

Treatment planning: The diagnostic findings, systemic or local, which influence the clinical procedures. It also depends on patient's mental attitude, systemic status, past dental history as well as local oral conditions.

U

Ultraviolet: Radiant energy of wavelengths shorter than extreme violet and lying beyond the ordinarily visible spectrum.

Undercut: That portion of the surface of an object that is below the height of contour in relation to the path of placement.

Uniform color space: Color space in which equal distances are intended to represent threshold or above threshold perceived color differences of equal size.

V

Vacuum casting: The casting of metal or plastic in presence of partial vacuum.

Vacuum investing: The process of investing pattern within a partial vacuum.

Vacuum mixing: A method of mixing a material such as plaster of Paris or casting investment below atmospheric pressure.

Value: Relative darkness or lightness of a color.

Varnish: A solution of natural gum and resins dissolved in a volatile solvent such as acetone, ether or chloroform.

Veneer: A layer of tooth color material usually porcelain or composite, placed on facial surface of the tooth.

Vent: A vertical indentation in the post to minimize stresses during cementation.

Vertical dimension: The distance between two points when occluding arches are in contact.

Viscoelastic: Ability of a polymer to have properties of both elastic and viscous.

Viscosity: Resistance of fluid to flow.

Vision: An image or idea of what the patient's dentition will look like when the treatment is complete.

W

Wax addition technique: The process used to develop a wax pattern through organized sequential addition of wax to shape the individual components of desired anatomic form.

Wax elimination: Removal of wax from the mold, usually by heat.

Wax expansion: A method of expanding a wax pattern to compensate for shrinkage of gold during casting process.

Wax pattern: The wax forms that is positive likeness of an object to be fabricated.

Wax: One of the several esters of fatty acids with higher alcohols; usually monohydric alcohols.

Wear facet: Any wear surface on a tooth caused by attrition.

Weld: To unite or fuse two pieces by rendering them soft by heat and adding fusible material in between.

Working occlusion: The occlusal contacts of teeth on the side to which the mandible moves.

Wrought metal: Cold worked metal that has been plastically deformed to alter the shape of the structure and certain mechanical properties.

Wrought: Worked into shape.

Zirconia ceramic post: A ceramic post, manufactured from Zirconia, used in the restoration of endodontically treated teeth.

Index